relish

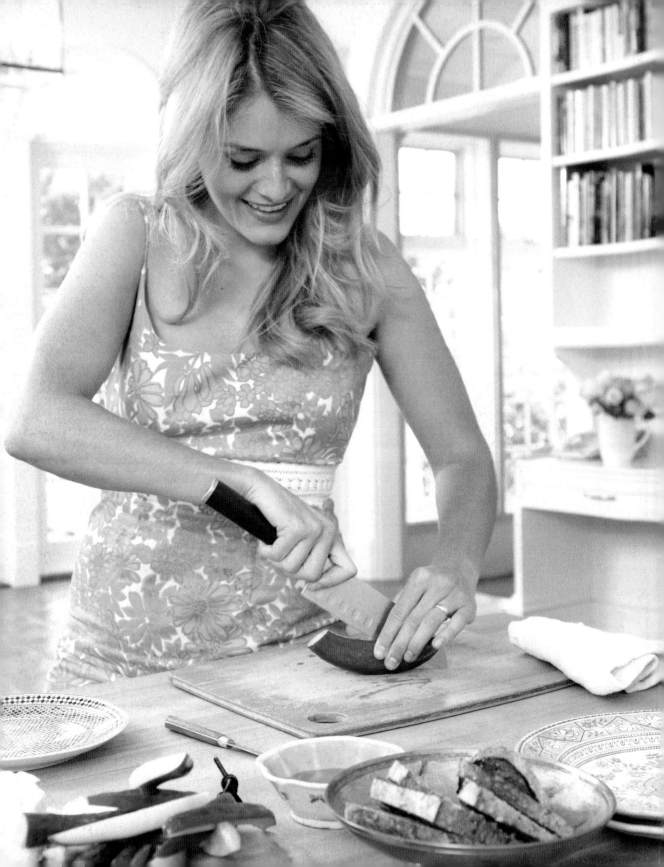

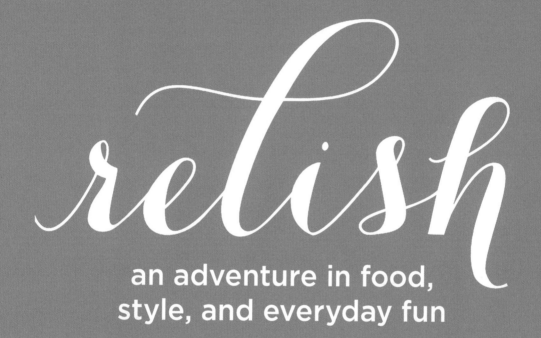

relish

an adventure in food, style, and everyday fun

daphne oz

PHOTOGRAPHS BY ELLEN SILVERMAN

WM
WILLIAM MORROW
An Imprint of HarperCollinsPublishers

ALSO BY DAPHNE OZ
The Dorm Room Diet

Photographs by Ellen Silverman except for the following: family photographs and candids courtesy of Daphne Oz; pages 218 and 219 by SPREADhouse; pages 270, 271, and 272 © by Lou Rocco/American Broadcasting Companies, Inc.; pages 290, 296, and 301 by Brian Adams Photographics.

HarperCollins books may be purchased for educational, business, or sales promotional use. For information please write: Special Markets Department, HarperCollins Publishers, 10 East 53rd Street, New York, NY 10022.

FIRST EDITION

Designed by Kris Tobiassen

Library of Congress Cataloging-in-Publication Data has been applied for.

ISBN 978-0-06-219686-6

13 14 15 16 17 ID5/QGT 10 9 8 7 6 5 4 3 2 1

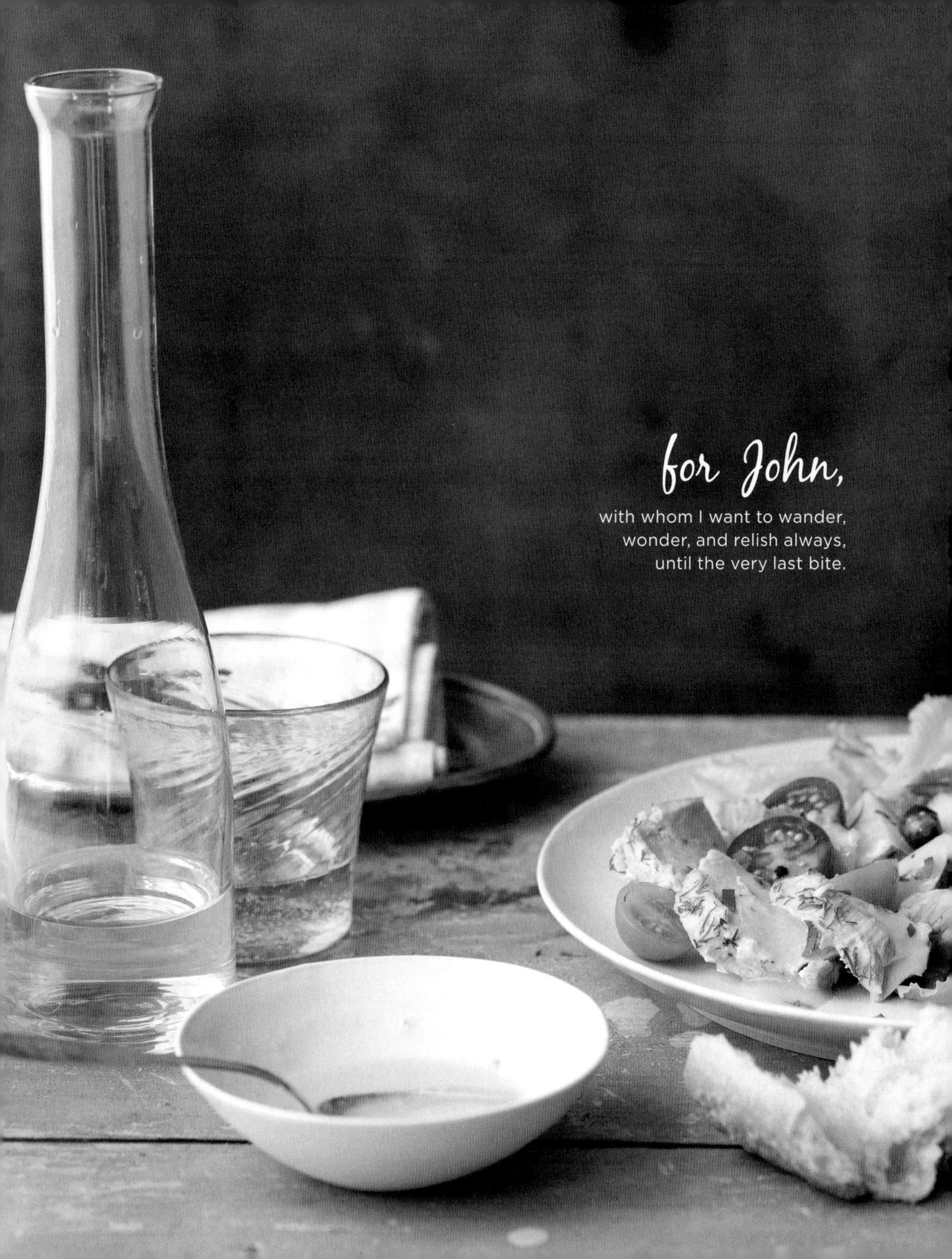

for John,

with whom I want to wander,
wonder, and relish always,
until the very last bite.

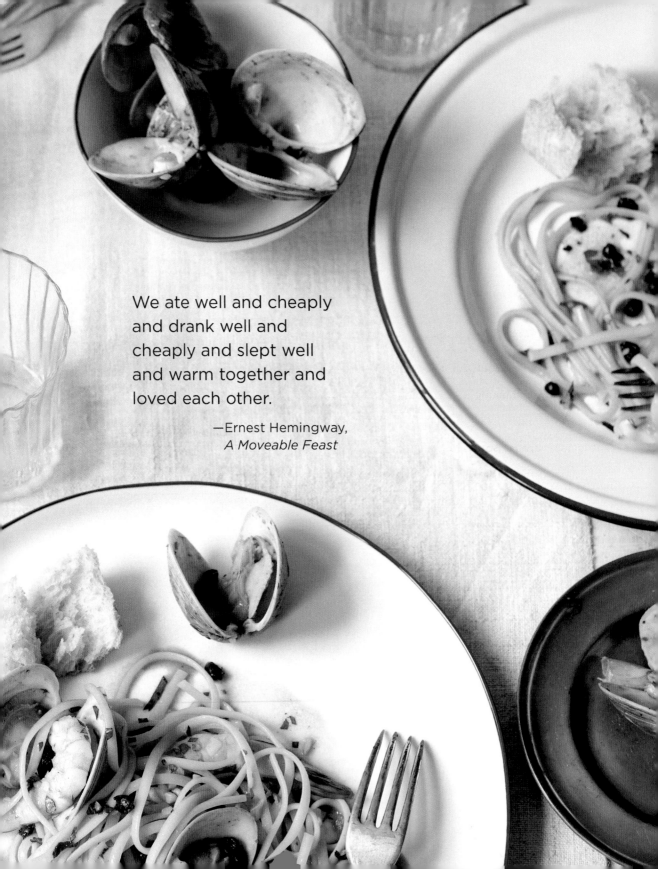

We ate well and cheaply and drank well and cheaply and slept well and warm together and loved each other.

—Ernest Hemingway,
A Moveable Feast

CONTENTS

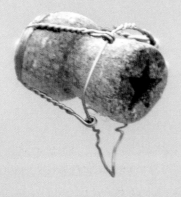

One cannot think well, love well,
sleep well, if one has not dined well.

—Virginia Woolf,
A Room of One's Own

INTRODUCTION

I love food. I love to eat it, I love to prepare it, I love to explore through it.

Food is the basis of a joyful, happy life—a life worth relishing—and eating well is a framework through which I see all the other things that make life rewarding, exciting, and fun. Sharing food with people turns strangers into friends and friends into family, and it gives me an excuse to sit down with my nearest and dearest and dish about the day. It's how we bond, how we get close, how we nourish ourselves and take care of each other.

For me, life builds around and from the kitchen. A homemade meal brings family to the table and grounds a happy home. A happy home begets a confident lady. A confident lady presents herself well: She has purpose, drive, and zest for life. Zest for life leads to longing for adventure. Adventure means travel and experience that bring friends and more-than-friends back to the home table. A well-rounded life begins with a well-balanced meal. And a well-rounded life is what I want—and what this book is all about.

I wrote this book for a reader who is a lot like I was—and in some ways still am. Someone who relishes life and wants to live the biggest and best that she can but often lets life get in the way. Who cares about her health and wants to keep fit but doesn't always have time for the gym and, frankly, would often rather spend her cash on a killer blazer than a session with a trainer. Who adores going out to eat on the weekends but could do with fewer mediocre, rushed meals out of a box or a bag on Monday through Thursday.

Does that sound like you? If I'm right, your home is your castle, but you wouldn't say no to a personal organizer. Custom curtains are a few pay bumps away, but you know what you like and you fill your current digs with a mix of retail-store gems, flea-markets finds, and family heirlooms—aka hand-me-downs—that you've made your own. You clean up nice, but your closet is full of things you never wear (and never will unless you drop two sizes and crushed velvet comes back in style). You like to entertain and mean to have people over more. Just like you mean to go to the farmers' market more often. Just like you mean to remember birthdays. Just like you mean to go to Tulum. . . .

Am I getting warm? How about the rest of your life? Are you happy, fulfilled, excited? Are you an emotional giver or taker? What do your family and friends like best about you? Do you like these things about yourself? Would *you* want to marry you?

Speaking of which, are you married? Or seeing anybody? If no, do you want to be? If yes, are you being the best partner possible or just coasting? How about your job—are you in love or simply paying bills? When was the last time you took a vacation? What do you do for fun; what gets you giddy? What do you nerd out over? And how do you give back? What's your purpose for getting out of bed every day? Where do you see yourself in twenty years? What makes you tick?

I'm sure you ask yourself these questions all the time. How am I so sure? Because I ask *myself* the same ones. I wonder if I'm doing it right, if I'm making mistakes, if I could be creating bigger and better opportunities for myself. And so do all of my friends! Sure, life is good, and we've got so much to be grateful for. But in our minds, we know life could be even better if we could figure out what we wanted and how to put a plan in action to get us there.

Most of us have at least an inkling of what we might like our better lives to resemble. What holds us back from going for that goal, I've found, is a combination of not being sure how to get started and worrying/expecting/hoping that the moment to embark down that path isn't right now. For some reason or another, we convince ourselves that we'd better just sit tight and hold off on going for gold because we're not supposed to have it until we're pushing retirement. Even though we have absolutely no idea what the future holds, we're putting all our betting money on it to make our wildest dreams come true while we go plugging along doing what we think is good enough for now.

What confuses me is why we think we have to wait for this better life. Who taught us that the life we've been waiting for kicks in when we're older, wiser, wrinklier? Why does it have to be the life we've been waiting for instead of the life we've been living all along or at least practicing to live? In fact, if we don't get a jump-start now, how can we be guaranteed that better life will find us down the road? When do we start making choices and taking action?

This is what I ask myself: Am I paving the way to make my dream life not only possible but probable? Or am I sitting on my heels, waiting for that life to land in my lap?

FINDING THE SWEET SPOT

I spent my early twenties trying hard instead of trying smart. Focused on the wrong goals, relying on ineffective techniques, I found myself treading water instead of forging ahead full-steam. I knew that I was doing some things right and that I wanted to be doing lots of things better, but I wasn't sure how to make those changes without becoming an insane, workaholic maniac! I wanted to be able to enjoy life and enjoying living it, too.

In many ways, I was waiting for my twenties to end because I assumed real life, and all the things I thought (and think) I want as part of that life, would hit in my thirties and forties. The part of the equation I was forgetting is that to have that life down the line, you need to start living like you want it—laying the foundation, acting the part, doing the searching and finding—now.

In the meantime, I had my placeholder life: I lived in a white box apartment that looked like an insane asylum because I refused to invest in decorating a rental—even though I spent two years there. I ate bland meals because I didn't want to "waste time" preparing delicious courses if I was the only one who was going to be eating them. I allowed clutter to collect, metaphorically and physically, and let it cloud my ability to see clearly. I worked a job that I knew wasn't the be-all and end-all. I was very lucky to have met my boyfriend (now husband!) in college, but I wasn't taking full advantage of all the wonderful things he and I could have been exploring together when we moved to New York City after graduation.

Bottom line: I kept making choices that put my maximized life—the life I want for myself—on hold.

And you know what? My placeholder life came really easily: It was comfortable and gave me a kind of free pass to go about my business rather than approach every day like the shiny, new opportunity it represented. I was happy, but I also recognized that this life wasn't totally filling me up. I looked around and saw so many people, places, and things I wanted to meet and visit and try. But busy days kept turning into busy weeks, and busy months became busy years, and I felt like I was missing out.

About the time I started feeling like life was passing by way too quickly, I realized that days where I'm busy and engaged fly by but feel substantial—like an incredible meal with great company that passes in a blink but leaves you full of sustenance on every level—whereas lazy, disconnected days speed away without a trace. I wanted to make my mark, and I wanted to do it in a way that would give me many volumes of memories to leaf through when I'm old and gray.

So I started trying new things and doing research and asking questions. I experienced failures and successes, read dozens of books and magazine articles about living in the moment, posed thousands of questions to everyone I met—from world experts, to friends and family, to average Joes and Janes—about what makes them blissfully, exuberantly happy.

Here's a pared-down version of what I learned: *Happiness is an attitude, but it's easier to have that happy outlook when you're living a life that is just right for you.*

Relish is about adding a little something special that changes everything, about not only *living* in the moment but *loving* that moment, too. It's about savoring highs and lows, gives and takes, and seeing that maximizing joy, potential, and growth while minimizing fear, worry, or (gasp!) boredom begins when you find that balance between effort and laissez-faire. Where you're working toward something better but loving where you are and making the most of every day. Half the fun of getting to your destination is the journey itself!

A desire to *relish* our lives comes naturally; it's no secret we all want to enjoy the best there is, to be happy, fulfilled, nourished on the inside and out. The trick is not to work harder, longer, more to have this abundance; you just need to work smarter and remind yourself of what to pay attention to, what to forget, and what to savor. *Relish* is an exciting, active approach to life that embraces the adventure of every moment without letting you lose sight of the big picture.

As my grandmother loves to say, "Only boring people get bored." In other words, you're responsible for creating a life worth *relishing*.

RELISH IS A VERB

Verbs mean action—as in *Get up and do this now.* I'm challenging you to dig out that laundry list of things you always mean to do and *do* them. Don't let self-sabotage get in the way. Don't let doubt or fear masquerade as logic in your life. A perfect example of this is when we put our dreams on hold, "just until we get settled."

Perhaps you're not totally, fully, 100 percent maximizing this time in your life because you, like I once did, think that real life starts later. What you're telling yourself is that you're not ready now. Or maybe you're working so hard to try to get to that "later" faster that you're not enjoying this precious moment the way you should. Maybe money is a barrier, location is a barrier, partners or kids (or lack thereof) are barriers, your job is a barrier, not having a job is a barrier, time is a barrier . . . you get the idea. These aren't barriers; they're all merely excuses you can list off when you think about why you're putting life on pause or rushing by in a hurry.

If your plan is to get through the next few years—decades, even—waiting for the moment when a timer will go off and you can finally start investing in yourself the way you want to, then here's some cold, hard truth: Life won't wait around until you're ready. If you don't live in the moment, you cannot adequately plan or prepare for the future you want; if you don't set yourself up for the shot—heck, if you're not even on the court—you're never going to sink a basket and win the game.

Whether you've been postponing the home design redo, the fitness plan, or that trip of a lifetime overseas, taking that cooking class or asking for the raise you deserve, I'm here to tell you that waiting until an undefined "later" is probably the biggest mistake you're making.

This is your real life, and no matter how much you have to be grateful for, you can make it even better.

HOW TO START RELISHING THE MOMENT

Relish is about seeing your potential and reaching for it. It's about waking up to the reality of those areas of your life—physical, mental, emotional—you're doing right and those you could be improving.

I've broken the book into chapters that focus on eating well, living well, and loving well, offering the essential tools you need to find that centered place of happiness and balance that will let you achieve your perfect-fit, full-plate life right now.

We'll get the party started in the kitchen, continue through the rest of your home, send you out into the world ready for anything, make time for the places you want to go and people you want to see, and then bring you home to roost full of memories and inspiration and no regrets.

All great achievements take hard work—and I would consider creating a life you'll love nothing short of a great achievement—but the masters make it look effortless because they love the process! And that's the trick: Having more fun in the kitchen, at home, and in life is just about jumping in headfirst, learning how to do little things a little bit better, and enjoying the ride!

LET FOOD LEAD THE WAY

I'll say it again: I love food, and I believe it promotes joy in every part of our lives. For this reason, I've let food thread this text much the way delicious meals punctuate our days. You'll find recipe chapters for breakfast and brunch, lunch, cocktails, dinner, and dessert laced in between all the other good stuff we'll be talking about—from home, to style, to beaus and

BFFs. After all, growing gals need good eats! And we'll be doing lots of growing (and eating) together in the coming pages.

Eating well is a wonderful way to see firsthand the difference it makes when you invest effort in homemade goodness instead of simply accepting what's on the hot line at the cafeteria. Good food nourishes us, and the disparity between processed, packaged junk and fresh, delicious meals is analogous to the difference between falling out of bed with a one-night stand and falling in love with Mr. Right, between accepting a job that pays the bills and discovering a path that is your passion.

Of course, this book isn't just about food. Food is simply the starting point that can open the door for conversations about everything else going on in your life—your style, your home, your work, your playtime, your hobbies, your heart.

My journey toward a relished existence began in the kitchen. It's where I learned firsthand how small changes can yield big results right away, and that's why we're starting our adventure together with food first.

READY, SET, COOK!

There are two basic things you need to become the master of your kitchen:

1. You need to love to eat. (I think we've got this covered.)
2. You need a reliable arsenal of easy, delicious recipes that will have you comfortable in the kitchen in no time.

To help you get started, I chose a selection of my favorite everyday recipes to include in this book—ideas for grab-'n'-go breakfasts that power me up, scrumptious brunches, and lazy lunches; weeknight dinners and weekend feasts; cocktail-hour favorites; and decadent desserts. They're all based in wholesome ingredients you'll easily find at your local grocery store (or even more easily order online for delivery straight to your front door). Best of all, you'll be shocked by how simply all these recipes come together.

I'm no Iron Chef, but a good home cook knows how to play to her strengths, and these are the dishes that make me look damn good. I turn to these over and over again, whether I want to eat well for one, impress for two, or throw an epic dinner party for twelve, because they deliver maximum results for minimum effort every time.

You'll notice that I use butter, full-fat dairy, white flour, and forms of sugar in some of my recipes. Don't be alarmed! I want to give you a sampling of how I like to eat in my everyday

When it comes to getting a recipe down pat, it helps to have some tricks up your sleeve. For those dishes where a bit of expert knowledge will make your life easier, or a little something extra will make your results ten times tastier, I've included some pointers under the heading DASH, which stands for Delicious Additions and Smart Help. You'll see these quick DASH tips as you work your way through the book, and they'll make the journey even more delicious!

life, the recipes that keep me happy *and* healthy, along with a balance of foods that are super-healthful, supereasy, or superdelicious—preferably all three!

Eating food that helps you look and feel the way you want is crucial to creating a relish-worthy life. That means having plenty of easy, healthful recipes up your sleeve. But part of letting food add all its possible richness to our lives is making sure we leave *plenty* of room for worthy indulgences!

I'll begin with recipes for breakfast and brunch and then dish about the basics of smart, nutritious eating, giving you all the tools you need to navigate the supermarket and your kitchen like a pro.

After a nice lunch, I'll invite you to think about how you feel inside and how you look on the outside. From meditation and mindfulness techniques to help you reach center, to cultivating a personal appearance that has style and verve without relying too heavily on trends so you can show your best self to the world, it's all about creating a personal ethos and aesthetic that supports who you are.

Then it's on to cocktails to get your creative juices flowing as you turn into a domestic goddess! I'll help make you the mistress of your domain and the hostess with the mostess with simple tips for decorating, organizing, and cleaning your home and how to show it off when you throw some killer, stress-free parties.

Dinner, as always, invites deeper conversations about work, playtime, and your many relationships—families, friends, and sweethearts. Even the most independent women need a support team . . . and a vacation. Speaking of which, I'll also give you all my favorite tips for strategic packing and trip planning to make your time away from home as relaxing as it should be.

And then, naturally, we have dessert—because life is a celebration, and sometimes the best way to have your cake is to eat it, preferably with a glass of bubbly!

But first, breakfast.

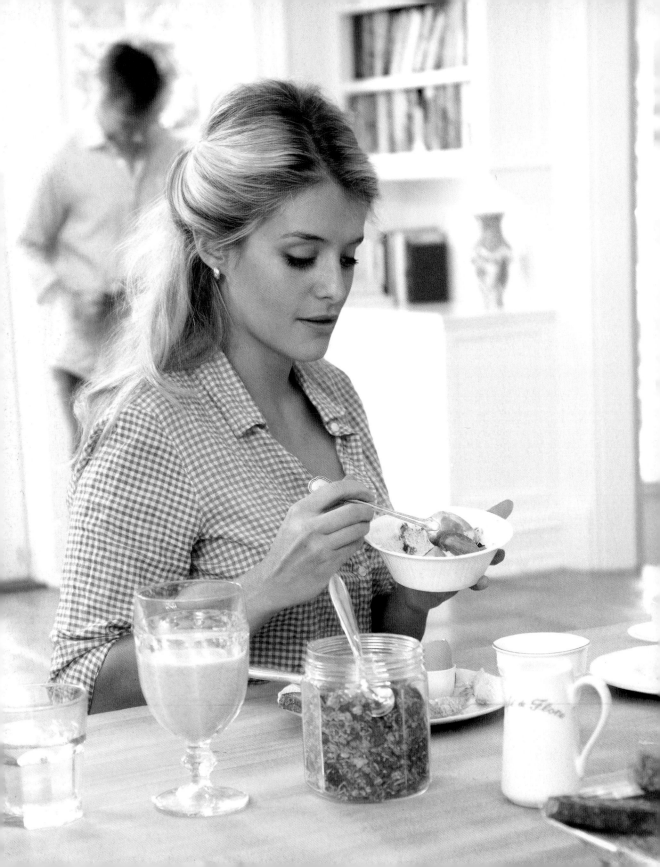

ONE

START SMART

breakfast and brunch

First we eat, then we do everything else.
—M. F. K. FISHER

WAKE UP YOUR PALATE, YOUR PLATE, AND YOUR PLAYMATES with these fast-to-fix, easy-to-enjoy treats. For luxurious mornings of leisure, Whole-Wheat Blueberry Sticky Buns are a pleasure to share along with the weekend paper. Caught in the fast pace of the daily grind? You'll never have to skip breakfast on a busy morning—with recipes like Fudgy Chocolate Banana Flax Muffins or Hot Grains with Coconut Cream, you'll be fabulously fueled in no time flat. Savories and sweets, forkfuls and hand-to-mouth treats—from Banana-Pecan Buttermilk Pancakes to a Black Bean and Onion Frittata to Avocado Toast with Harissa, this chapter is full of morning nourishment, perfect for boys who breakfast and ladies who brunch.

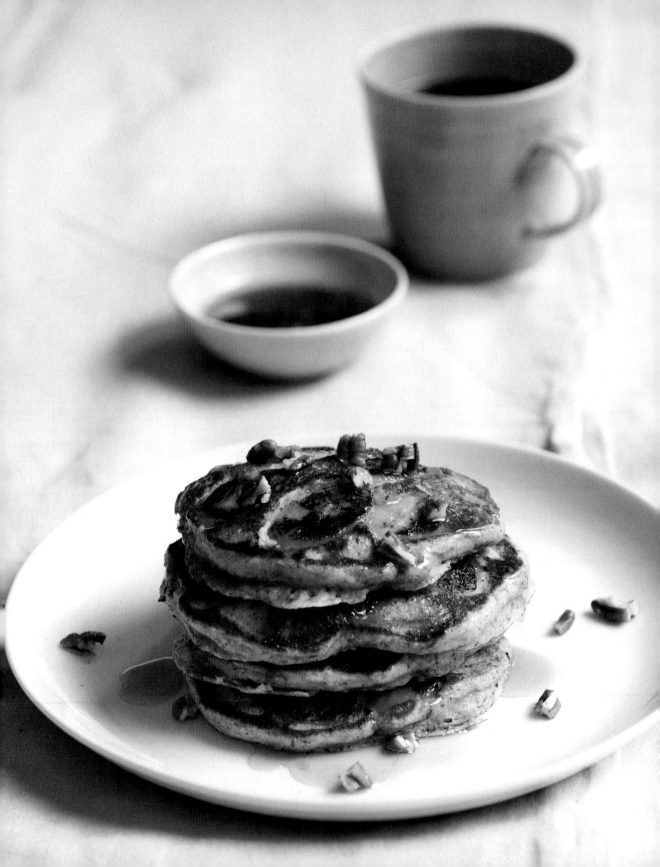

BANANA-PECAN BUTTERMILK PANCAKES

makes eighteen 4-inch pancakes

EVERY SUNDAY DURING our family summers up in Maine, we would spend the morning feasting on pancakes. Sometimes we made them with heaping handfuls of wild Maine blueberries, but the sweet caramel of bananas and buttery pecans has always been my favorite. My mom would get up early to get the batter started, and by the time my siblings and I came down, there would be perfect cakes lining the griddle. We piled them high, poured on the maple syrup, and then went back for seconds . . .

3/4 cup pecans, toasted, plus more for garnish

1 3/4 cups whole-wheat flour

1/2 cup all-purpose flour

2 tablespoons sugar

2 tablespoons baking powder

1/4 teaspoon iodized salt

4 tablespoons ground flaxseed (optional)

3 large eggs

4 tablespoons (1/2 stick) unsalted butter, melted, plus more for the pan

1 cup milk, whole or 2%

1 1/2 cups buttermilk (see Note)

1 teaspoon pure vanilla extract

3 large ripe bananas, sliced into 1/4-inch-thick rounds (reserve some for garnish)

Buttered Maple Syrup (recipe follows)

1. Preheat the oven to 200°F and place a cooling rack on a baking sheet.

2. Finely grind 1/2 cup of the pecans in a food processor, or chop them to a fine powder. Coarsely chop the remaining 1/4 cup pecans and reserve. Transfer the ground pecans to a large bowl. Add the flours, sugar, baking powder, salt, and flaxseed (if using) and whisk until combined.

3. In a medium bowl, whisk the eggs, butter, milk, buttermilk, and vanilla until frothy. Pour the wet ingredients into the dry ingredients and stir until just combined (don't overmix or your pancakes won't rise properly). Fold the reserved 1/4 cup of chopped pecans into the batter.

4. Heat a griddle or large skillet over medium heat. Brush the griddle with butter; keep the surface buttered well throughout cooking to prevent the bananas from sticking. Pour 1/4 cup of the batter onto griddle for each pancake. Lay about 5 banana slices onto each

Note: If you don't have buttermilk, simply add 1 tablespoon white distilled vinegar or lemon juice to 1-cup measure and complete the cup with whole or 2% milk to yield 1 cup "buttermilk"! Let stand for 5 minutes and then use as needed.

pancake and cook until small bubbles form and pop on the surface and the bottom is golden brown. Flip the pancakes and cook until golden brown, 6 to 8 minutes.

5. Place the pancakes on the cooling rack on top of the baking sheet and keep them warm in oven until ready to serve. Drizzle with Buttered Maple Syrup and garnish with bananas and pecans. Serve warm.

= DASH =

- Start in one spot and lift your spoon or ladle up as you pour over the same spot to form well-shaped circles.
- Flip the pancakes only once so that they stay light and fluffy.
- Store your pancakes in the oven on a cooling rack over a baking sheet to keep the pancakes from steaming.

BUTTERED MAPLE SYRUP

1½ cups pure maple syrup

4 tablespoons (½ stick) butter

2 ounces bourbon whiskey (optional)

In a small saucepan, warm the syrup and butter over medium-low heat; whisk to combine. If desired, stir in bourbon to give these pancakes an adult zing!

BROILED GRAPEFRUIT WITH CANDIED GINGER AND BASIL

serves 2

DIET FOOD for people who don't diet. You'll thank me later.

1. Place the sugar in a small bowl. Use a Microplane or ginger grater to grate the ginger into the sugar, being sure to catch all the juice and pulp; stir to combine. Set it aside for at least 20 minutes in an airtight container until ready to use.

2. Sprinkle each grapefruit half with 1 teaspoon of the ginger sugar. Place under the broiler until the sugar has just begun to melt and caramelize and the grapefruit is slightly warm—but don't let it burn! Top with shredded basil and enjoy on the spot.

¼ cup sugar

One 1-inch piece peeled fresh ginger

1 grapefruit, cut in half horizontally

3 large basil leaves, cut into thin ribbons

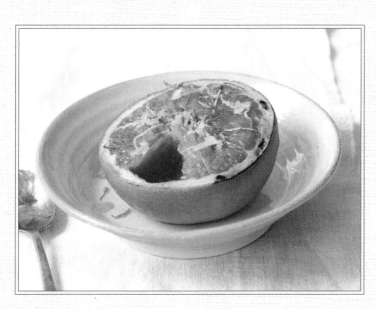

HOT GRAINS WITH COCONUT CREAM

makes about 3 cups

⅓ cup amaranth

⅓ cup quinoa

⅓ cup millet

3 ½ cups water

2 tablespoons flaxseeds, ground (see DASH below)

3 tablespoons coconut milk, "lite" if preferred

1 tablespoon pure maple syrup

Dash of ground cinnamon

OATMEAL GETS OLD, fast, but it's the breakfast of choice for people looking to eat smart on the run, especially if you're interested in managing that waistline, so I came up with something triple delicious and easy to put together when you're craving a warm bowl of hot cereal to rev up your morning. I make a big batch on Mondays and reheat portions over the rest of the week.

Amaranth, quinoa, and millet are all good choices for anyone sensitive to gluten—a protein found in wheat and other grains—and they pack both a powerful protein-fiber double whammy to keep you full, and plenty of healthful complex carbohydrates to energize. I keep a can of coconut milk in the pantry for an indulgent addition to this morning meal. Shake the can to combine the separated coconut cream and water, spoon some over your cereal, and save the rest for a smoothie or curry later in the week.

1. Rinse the soaked (see DASH on next page) or dry grains under running water for 1 minute. Place them in a medium saucepan and toast over a medium-low flame, stirring frequently to evaporate the excess water and develop a nutty flavor for the cereal. The grains are done toasting after 2 or 3 minutes, or when you start to smell a warm, nutty aroma.

=== DASH ===

You can either grind whole flaxseeds in a coffee or spice grinder or buy the seeds already ground, but remember that it's a good idea to keep all nuts and seeds—especially ground—in the fridge to keep the oils from going rancid.

2. Add the water, stir, and bring to a boil over medium heat. Lower the heat to a gentle simmer and cook, partially covered, until the water has evaporated, 20 to 25 minutes, stirring occasionally. Remove the pot from heat and stir in the flaxseed. Allow to sit, covered, for 5 minutes.

3. You will end up with about 3 cups of cooked grains, enough to last you a few days. Serve yourself ½ to ¾ cup of the cereal, spoon the coconut milk on top, drizzle with syrup, and top with the cinnamon. Next stop: mouth party!

=== DASH ===

Soaking is a big part of this recipe because it's how you break down enzyme inhibitors—naturally occurring compounds that stop your body from efficiently absorbing nutrients found in all kinds of grains, seeds, and nuts. If you remember, put the amaranth, quinoa, and millet in a medium bowl and cover with twice the amount of water in an airtight container and place in the fridge overnight; in the morning, rinse and drain well before cooking. If you forget, don't worry about it; you can just skip to the rinsing process.

CRISPY BAKED BREAKFAST POTATOES

serves 4

3 medium russet potatoes, peeled and cut into ½-inch cubes

1 red bell pepper, cored, seeded, and chopped

1 large yellow onion, diced

½ cup olive oil

1 tablespoon garlic powder

1 tablespoon onion powder

¼ to ½ teaspoon cayenne

½ teaspoon sea salt

¼ teaspoon fresh-cracked black pepper

THESE MAY BE MY favorite way to start a lazy Saturday morning—or close a Friday night out. Extra crispy without ever being fried, with soft, tender potato inside, these are what hash browns should be. Guard your plate with your fork.

1. Place the potatoes in a large bowl and cover them with cold water. Allow to soak for 15 to 20 minutes. If you're really patient, drain and rinse the potatoes, then cover with water and soak for another 20 minutes; this will make them even crispier. (Alternatively, you can place the potatoes in a bowl with water and leave in your fridge overnight for the next morning.) Drain the potatoes and pat dry in a dish towel.

2. Preheat the oven to 450°F.

3. In a large bowl, combine the potatoes, bell pepper, and onion. Add the oil and toss well to coat. In a small bowl, combine the garlic powder, onion powder, cayenne, salt, and pepper and toss with the potatoes.

4. Spread the potato mixture in a thin layer on a rimmed baking sheet (a rim will allow you to move the potatoes around while baking; thinner/uncoated sheets tend to give a better crisp, too). If you want to pop the sheet in the oven while it preheats, the heat of the tray will help get the browning action going. Bake 30 to 40 minutes, shaking the pan or using a rubber spatula every 8 to 10 minutes to ensure all sides of the potatoes are a deep, golden brown.

5. Serve them hot out of the oven. I like mine with ketchup and plenty of hot sauce.

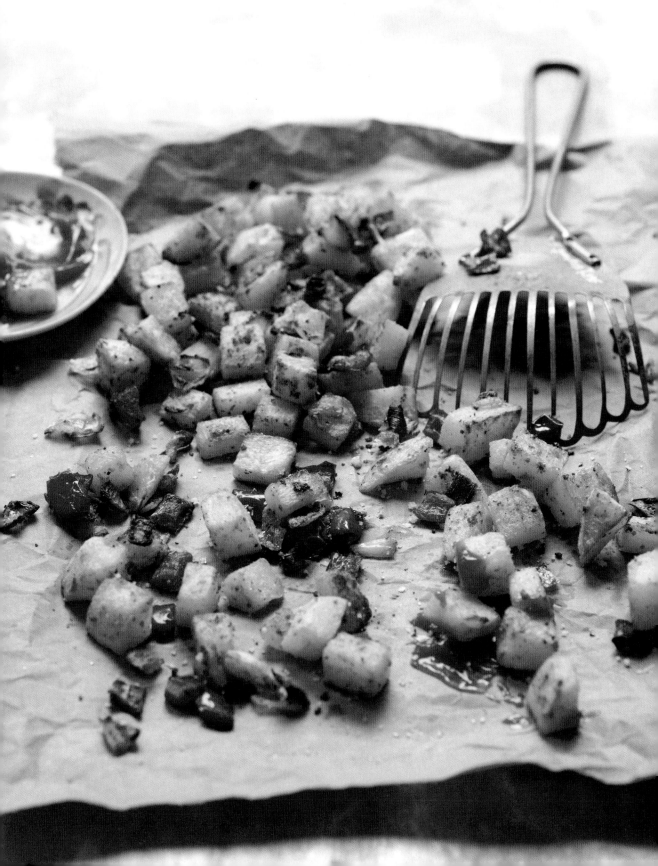

FUDGY CHOCOLATE BANANA FLAX MUFFINS

makes 12 to 14 muffins

½ cup organic coconut oil, softened to room temperature or melted

¼ cup packed light brown sugar

4 medium overripe bananas, mashed

2 tablespoons unsweetened applesauce

1 teaspoon pure vanilla extract

¼ cup water

2 large eggs

1½ cups whole-wheat flour

¼ cup good-quality cocoa powder

½ cup wheat germ

2 tablespoons ground flaxseed

1½ teaspoons baking soda

½ teaspoon salt

⅓ cup semisweet chocolate chips, pulsed in food processor or chopped

THIS IS NOT YOUR AVERAGE breakfast muffin. Imagine a fudgy brownie—chocolatey, rich, ringing every bell—and then picture yourself dancing around your kitchen, exuberant with the knowledge that these babies are truly guilt-free, since (almost) all the sinfully sweet goodness is derived from bananas, applesauce, and cocoa powder. That's something to get up for in the morning! And I'll say what I want to say without saying it: Fiber never tasted so good.

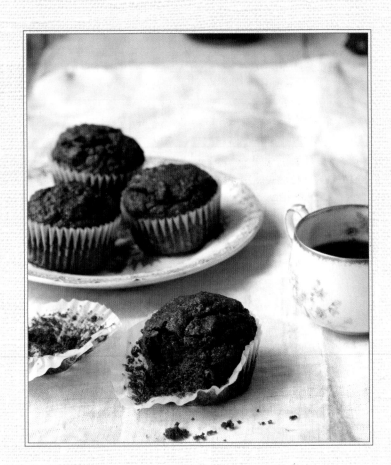

1. Preheat the oven to 350°F. Line a large muffin pan with paper liners.

2. Using the paddle attachment on a stand mixer, a hand mixer, or two forks, cream the oil and sugar. Add the bananas, applesauce, vanilla, and water and beat until smooth. Beat in the eggs.

3. In a separate large bowl, whisk together the flour, cocoa powder, wheat germ, flaxseed, baking soda, and salt. Add the wet ingredients to the dry ingredients and mix just until combined. Fold in the chocolate chips.

4. Spoon the batter into the muffin liners until they are almost full. Bake for 12 to 15 minutes, or until a toothpick inserted into the center of a muffin comes out just damp with small crumbs attached. Place the muffins on a cooling rack and let them cool for at least 5 minutes before digging in!

DASH

- To store the muffins, place them in a zip-top bag with 1 paper towel and remove as much air as possible; store in cool, dry place.

- To freeze leftover batter, pour into a zip-top bag, remove the air, and seal, or spoon into a lined muffin pan, wrap tightly with plastic wrap, and place in freezer for about 24 hours until the batter is solid. Once frozen, remove the cups from the pan and put them into a zip-top bag, removing as much air as possible. Double-wrap them in a second zip-top bag to prevent freezer burn.

- To bake, you have two options. You can thaw the batter in the bags and pour it into lined muffin tins (cut the bottom corner off the bag to make this easy!) and bake as usual, or you can place the frozen muffins in a muffin pan and place the pan in a cold oven. Set the oven to 350°F and add 20 to 30 minutes to baking time to allow the oven to preheat and the muffin batter to thaw.

POACHED EGGS AND ROASTED ASPARAGUS ON HONEY WHOLE-WHEAT TOAST

serves 1

6 asparagus spears

½ tablespoon olive oil, plus extra for drizzling

Sea salt and fresh-cracked black pepper

1 teaspoon white wine vinegar

2 eggs

Honey Whole-Wheat Bread (page 14) or other crusty bread

Fresh basil leaves, finely sliced

Tabasco (optional)

Ketchup (optional)

BREAKFAST FOR ONE or breakfast for a few: The technique is the same. The only skill you'll need is the ability to poach an egg. Here's the CliffsNotes version: Add a bit of vinegar to boiling water, gently crack the egg in, and swirl with a wooden spoon. The result is tender cooked whites enveloping molten yolk gold that will drench your toast with just the right amount of rich, buttery goodness.

1. Preheat the oven to 400°F.

2. Place the asparagus spears on a rimmed baking sheet, drizzle with oil, and sprinkle on salt and pepper. Bake for 10 minutes. Shake the pan to rotate the asparagus spears and bake for 5 minutes more. The spears should be tender and slightly shrunken, with a golden brown char. If you want them a bit darker, pop them under the broiler for 1 or 2 minutes, but watch them closely or you'll end up with charcoal! Chop the spears in half.

3. Fill a medium saucepan halfway with water and bring to a low simmer over medium-low heat (tiny bubbles just barely breaking the surface). Add the vinegar and whisk vigorously. One at a time, crack the eggs into a small bowl and gently drop them into the water while stirring the water gently with a slotted spoon. Keep swirling the water gently to help the eggs form into little balls. Skim away any foam on the surface so that you can keep an eye on the eggs. You will have perfectly poached eggs with runny yolks in about 3 minutes. Cook longer if you prefer a firmer yolk. Remove the eggs with a slotted spoon and place them on a dish towel or paper towel to drain.

4. Slice yourself a nice hunky piece of bread and toast it if you like. Top with the asparagus spears and poached eggs. Sprinkle with salt, pepper, basil, and a drizzle of olive oil. If desired, add a dash of Tabasco and some ketchup as well. Swoon!

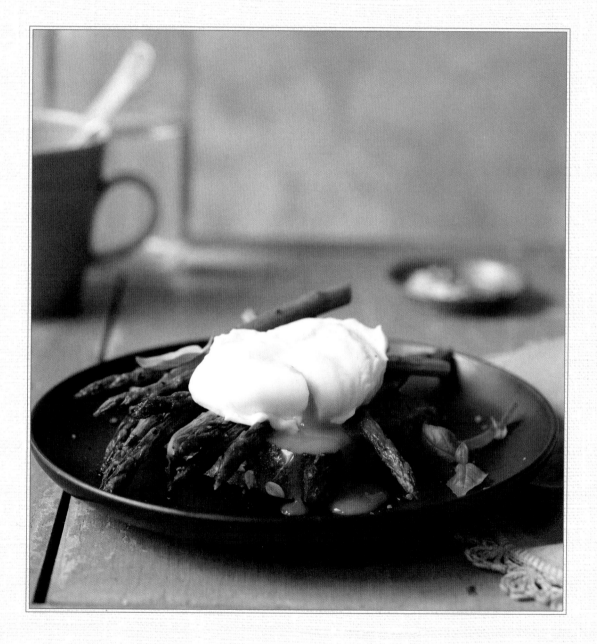

HONEY WHOLE-WHEAT BREAD

makes 1 loaf

2 tablespoons coconut oil, plus more for the pan

2 cups warm (130°F) water

1 packet active dry yeast (about 2 ¼ teaspoons)

3 cups whole-wheat flour

1 cup rolled oats (not instant or quick-cooking)

2 tablespoons wheat germ

2 tablespoons ground flaxseed

½ cup coarsely chopped walnuts

3 tablespoons raw sunflower seeds

1 teaspoon sea salt

¼ cup honey

2 tablespoons unsweetened applesauce

HEY, HONEY. Like a good relationship, this recipe is worth putting your heart and soul into. Inspired by a loaf in Sophie Dahl's Voluptuous Delights *(a delicious book cover to cover!), this is one of my all-time favorite easy bread recipes, perfect for even the non-bread-baking wizards among us. It's equally delicious for a sandwich, under eggs (see page 12), or with Strawberry Honey Butter (page 16) and jam.*

1. Preheat the oven to 375°F and oil a standard loaf pan with coconut oil.

2. Pour the water in a large bowl and sprinkle the yeast over the top. Let stand until the yeast is foamy, about 5 minutes.

3. In another large bowl, whisk together the flour, oats, wheat germ, flaxseed, walnuts, sunflower seeds, and salt.

4. Stir the coconut oil and honey into the water-yeast mixture until combined.

DASH

Any whole-wheat flour or whole grain should be kept in a cool, dark place and stored in dark containers that keep out the light. Because whole grains still contain the fat originally found in seeds and grains, they must be protected from sunlight and heat that could turn the fat rancid. If you have room, keep them in the fridge!

Trim your rising time! Heat the oven to 175°F for 5 minutes, then shut it off. Place the dough in an oiled heat-safe bowl, covered with plastic wrap, and put it in the oven to rise. Creating this "rising box" cuts the rising time by more than half.

5. Using a wooden spoon, stir the dry ingredients into the wet ingredients and mix well. The dough will be dense and very sticky. Cover the bowl with plastic wrap and set in a warm place for 20 minutes.

6. Use a large wooden spoon to fold the dough from the perimeter into the center of the bowl onto itself, rotating the bowl as you fold, for 2 minutes. This will knead the dough and help develop the gluten for a nice, chewy bread.

7. Pour the dough into the prepared loaf pan. Lightly dampen your fingers with water and spread out the dough to fill the pan. Cover with plastic wrap and return the pan to a warm spot for another 20 minutes.

8. Remove the plastic and place the pan in the middle of the oven. Bake for about 50 minutes, or until the crust is a deep golden brown. Or, turn the bread out of the pan and thump it on the bottom—it should sound hollow.

9. Turn the bread out onto a cooling rack and cool completely before serving.

STRAWBERRY HONEY BUTTER

makes about 1 cup

1 pint fresh strawberries, hulled

8 tablespoons (1 stick) unsalted butter, softened

2 tablespoons raw honey

¼ teaspoon kosher salt plus extra for serving

COMPOUND BUTTERS—basically, just softened butter mixed with add-ins—are a really simple way to add tons of flavor to your food. Traditionally, compound butters are made with herbs, such as fresh chives and parsley, but sweet compound butters are equally delicious.

This particular combination draws straight from my childhood. I grew up loving strawberry butter on popovers, which my mom would make for us on special weekend mornings, and you'll usually find a roll sitting in my freezer for emergencies. After an audience member at The Chew *suggested this trick, I started adding it to my baked goods for an extra blissful pop of flavor. Give it a try in my Strawberry Cake with Caramel Fleur de Sel Whipped Cream Frosting (page 327)—you won't be sorry.*

1. Puree the strawberries in a food processor and pour into a small saucepan. Place over medium heat, stirring frequently to prevent burning, until the mixture is reduced by half, about 10 minutes. Transfer the strawberry puree to the freezer until completely cool, about 15 minutes.

2. In a food processor, combine the strawberry puree, butter, honey, and salt and process until well combined and fluffy. If using right away, spoon it into serving ramekins or small dishes, sprinkle with a pinch of extra salt, and chill in the refrigerator until ready to serve. If storing, scrape the mixture onto wax paper and roll into a log; store it in the refrigerator or freezer until ready to use.

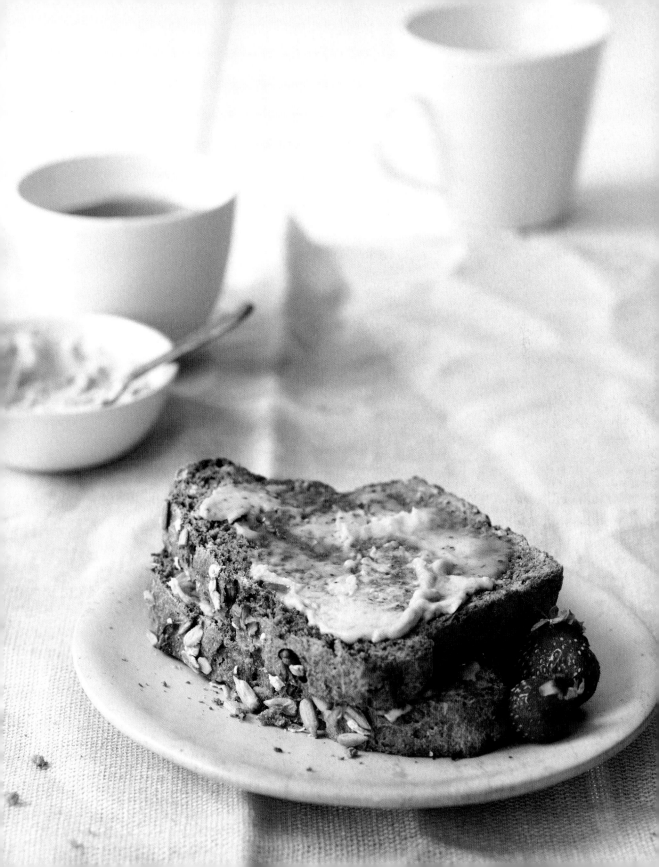

AVOCADO TOAST WITH HARISSA

serves 1

1 slice Honey Whole-Wheat Bread (page 14) or your favorite whole-grain bread

½ tablespoon Harissa Paste (optional; recipe follows)

½ ripe avocado

1 teaspoon olive oil

1 teaspoon honey

Sea salt

Dried chile flakes

HARISSA IS A DELICIOUS chile paste traditionally used to spice up Moroccan dishes. It adds exotic flair and a mild-to-killer heat (depending on the chiles you get!) that pair beautifully with creamy avocado in this sweet-and-savory easy breakfast toast.

Toast the bread. Spread it with the harissa, if desired, and mash the avocado on top. Drizzle with the oil and honey and top with a pinch of sea salt and chile flakes.

HARISSA PASTE

makes 1 heaping cup

9 dried red chile peppers, seeded and stemmed (ancho for a mild heat; chile de arbol for fire-breathers)

3 garlic cloves, peeled

1 teaspoon ground coriander

1 teaspoon ground cumin

1 teaspoon iodized salt

¼ cup olive oil plus extra for storing

1. Soak the dried chiles in hot water for 45 minutes. Drain and remove the stems and seeds; squeeze out the extra water. Use a food processor or blender (or mortar and pestle if you're feeling brawny) to combine the peppers, garlic, coriander, cumin, and salt. Add in the oil and blend to a smooth paste.

2. Store in an airtight container and top with a thin layer of olive oil to form a hermetic seal. The harissa will keep in the refrigerator for up to 1 month.

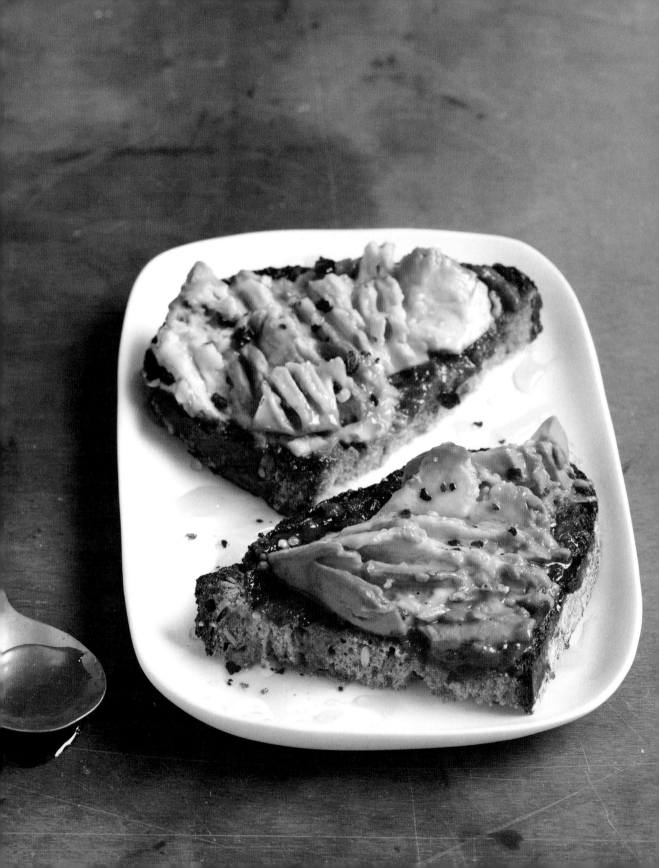

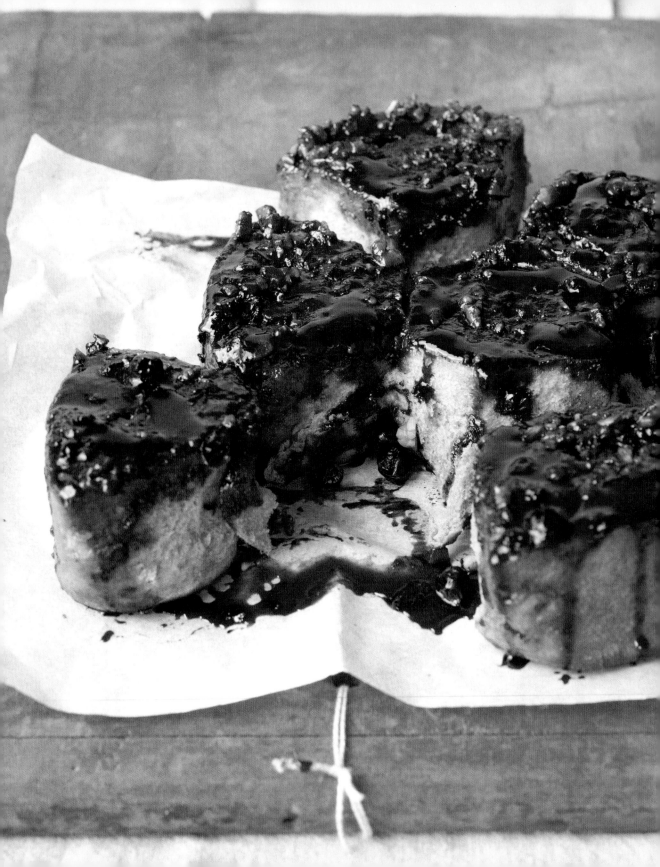

WHOLE-WHEAT BLUEBERRY STICKY BUNS

makes 6 to 8 buns

WHOLE-WHEAT BLUEBERRY sticky buns. Say it slowly. Let it sink in. These breakfast gems, dripping with maple syrup and bursting with juicy blueberries, are just healthful enough to justify their decadence—and so much more satisfying than their white bread counterparts. Pull them sweet and fragrant out of the oven. Then stand back and let the hordes devour.

¼ cup warm (about 100°F) water

1 packet active dry yeast, about 2¼ teaspoons

1 cup whole or 2% milk, at room temperature

1 large egg, lightly beaten, at room temperature

¼ cup honey

3½ tablespoons organic coconut oil, melted

4 cups whole-wheat flour plus more if needed

2 teaspoons ground cinnamon

1¼ teaspoons iodized salt

½ cup packed light brown sugar

1½ cups blueberries

⅓ cup pure maple syrup

½ cup walnuts or pecans, chopped

2 tablespoons (¼ stick) unsalted butter, cut into ¼-inch pats

1. Pour the warm water into a medium bowl, sprinkle with the yeast, and let stand in a warm spot until foamy, about 5 minutes. Whisk in the milk, egg, honey, and 1½ tablespoons of the oil.

2. In large bowl, whisk together the flour, 1 teaspoon of the cinnamon, and the salt. Add the wet ingredients into the dry and mix with a wooden spoon until the mixture comes together.

3. Turn out the dough onto a floured surface and knead for 10 minutes, adding flour as needed to form a sticky but not wet dough. Transfer the dough to a large, lightly oiled bowl and cover with plastic wrap; let stand in a warm place for 45 minutes (the dough may not rise much, but you are giving the yeast time to activate).

4. On a lightly floured surface, roll the dough into a 14 x 12-inch rectangle that's about ¼ inch thick. Brush the dough with the remaining 2 tablespoons of oil. Sprinkle with the remaining tea-spoon of cinnamon, ¼ cup of the sugar, and the blueberries. With the longest side facing you, roll the dough into a tight log and cut the last ½ inch off the ends (this helps to make sure each of your buns contains enough filling). Cut the remaining log in half and

- Depending on the weather, you may need to add more flour. Damp or humid days will make your dough wetter.
- As a time-saver, you can use store-bought whole-wheat pizza dough in place of homemade dough. Thaw it overnight in the fridge, then let it come to room temperature on the counter (1 to 2 hours), and proceed with step 4.

---

cut each half into 3 buns, to make six roughly 2-inch-wide rounds. If you want to cut smaller rounds, you can get up to 8 buns.

5. Preheat the oven to 350°F.

6. Pour the syrup into a 9-inch-round cake pan, sprinkle it with the remaining ¼ cup sugar and the chopped walnuts or pecans, and dot it with pats of butter. Place the dough rounds in the cake pan cut side down on top of the sticky mixture, leaving about 1 inch in between each roll to allow for rising. Cover with plastic wrap and let stand in a warm place until slightly risen, about 15 minutes.

7. Remove the plastic wrap and bake until the buns are deep golden brown, about 40 minutes. Cool the sticky buns in the pan. Turn them out onto a rack set on a parchment-lined baking sheet or straight onto a serving dish to save any excess glaze.

BLACK BEAN AND ONION FRITTATA WITH SALSA FRESCA

serves 4 to 6

THE BEST TIME TO MAKE a frittata is when you're about to have a table full of brunch guests and you'd rather be hobnobbing than staking out the stove. And don't worry about late arrivals! This baby is as good hot out of the oven as room temp in the afternoon.

1. Preheat the oven to 350°F.

2. If using dried beans, measure the beans into a bowl or container, cover with fresh water, and soak overnight in the refrigerator. In the morning, rinse with clean water and place in a medium soup pot with 4 cups water. Bring the water to a boil, then reduce to a simmer and cook the beans, partially covered, for 40 to 45 minutes, or until tender (easily crushed between thumb and forefinger but not falling apart). Drain well and set aside.

If using canned beans, drain the beans and rinse them until the water runs clear. Set them aside to drain thoroughly over a bowl or paper towel.

3. Peel the potato and shred it using a grater or a food processor. Place the shredded potato in a clean dish towel and wring out any extra liquid. (Work those muscles! The less liquid, the crispier it'll get.)

4. In a 10-inch cast-iron or stainless-steel skillet, melt the butter over medium heat. Add the potato and onion and sweat them for about 3 minutes, stirring often so nothing burns. Add a pinch of

½ cup dried black beans, or one 15-ounce can black beans

1 medium russet potato

2 tablespoons (¼ stick) butter or organic coconut oil

1 medium yellow onion, thinly sliced

Sea salt and fresh-cracked black pepper

1 medium jalapeño, minced (discard the seeds and ribs if you want less heat)

1 bunch of scallions (white and light green parts), sliced thin (about ⅔ cup)

8 eggs

2 egg whites

1 teaspoon ground cumin

1 teaspoon dried chile flakes

Leaves from 1 bunch of cilantro or parsley, half chopped, half left whole for garnish

4 ounces Monterey Jack cheese, shredded

2 cups Salsa Fresca (recipe follows)

Sour cream for serving

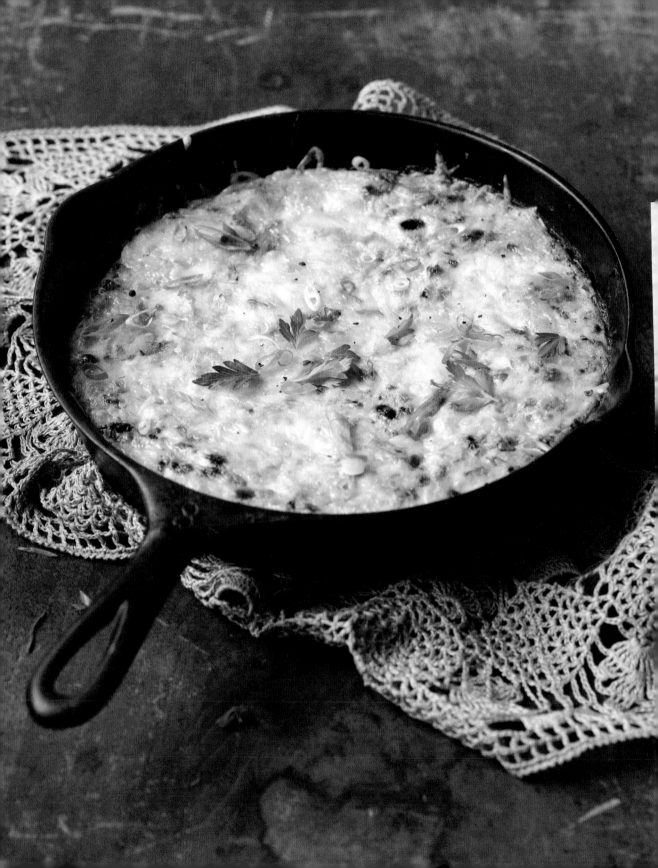

salt and some pepper and continue stirring for another 3 minutes. Both the potato and onion should be softened and the onion should be translucent. Add the black beans and minced jalapeño and stir to combine. Allow beans to heat for 2 minutes. Arrange in an even layer on the bottom of the pan and sprinkle with the scallions (holding back 2 tablespoons for garnish).

5. Crack the eggs and egg whites into a clean bowl and whisk until frothy. Season with the cumin, chile flakes, and more salt and pepper and add the chopped cilantro; whisk to combine. Pour the egg mixture over the sautéed veggies. Lower the heat to medium-low and use a spatula to bring the mixture from the outer corners into the middle (the eggs should look like very loose curds, and new eggs should run to fill the empty space). Gather the mixture to the center 6 times and allow the eggs to re-form into a circle shape. Top the frittata with shredded cheese and bake for 20 minutes, or until the eggs are entirely cooked through and the frittata is firm but springy.

6. Serve slices straight from the skillet, topped with Salsa Fresca (see recipe below) and sour cream and a sprinkling of the reserved cilantro and scallions.

SALSA FRESCA
makes 3½ cups

1. Combine all the ingredients in a bowl and allow to sit for 15 minutes. Taste and adjust the seasonings.

2. The salsa will keep for 3 days in the fridge, covered.

3 ripe red tomatoes, cored and chopped

½ small red onion, minced

½ jalapeño, minced (discard the seeds and ribs if you want less heat)

2 scallions (white and light green parts), finely chopped

1 or 2 garlic cloves, peeled and minced

2 tablespoons fresh lime juice

½ teaspoon salt

VANILLA, DATE, AND PISTACHIO GRANOLA

makes 7 cups

6 tablespoons raw honey, room temperature

3 tablespoons pure maple syrup, room temperature

2 tablespoons organic coconut oil, melted, plus extra for the baking sheets

2 tablespoons unsweetened applesauce, at room temperature

1 tablespoon pure vanilla extract (or scrapings from 1 vanilla pod if you're feeling fancy!)

3 cups rolled oats (not quick-cooking)

1 cup raw pistachios

½ cup raw walnuts, chopped

½ cup raw sunflower seeds

½ cup raw sesame seeds

1 cup unsweetened shredded coconut

3 tablespoons ground flaxseed

1 teaspoon ground cardamom

1 teaspoon ground cinnamon

1 teaspoon sea salt

10 Medjool dates, seeded and chopped

10 dried apricots, chopped

STAND ASIDE, HIPPIES—we're not in Vermont anymore (I love hippies and Vermont, PS!). This breakfast staple is loaded up with spices straight out of the bazaar. Dates, coconut, and pistachios lend sweetness and exotic appeal, while flaxseed packs in the omega-3 fatty acids, meant to give you quick wits and beauty inside and out! Enjoy like cereal, over yogurt (or ice cream! Not for breakfast, silly), or as an eminently portable snack on-the-go.

1. Preheat the oven to 325°F.

2. In a medium bowl, add the honey, syrup, oil, applesauce, and vanilla and whisk well to combine.

3. In a large bowl, combine the oats, nuts, seeds, coconut, flaxseed, cardamom, cinnamon, and salt and stir well. Pour the wet mixture into the dry and stir well to coat all the oats, nuts, and seeds.

4. Grease 2 rimmed baking pans well with melted oil (or line them with parchment paper). Spread the granola mixture across the pans in an even ½-inch layer. Bake for 40 to 45 minutes, using a plastic spatula or wooden spoon to stir periodically so all the ingredients cook evenly, until the granola is golden brown and fragrant. (The finished granola will be slightly moister and less clumpy than most granolas you've known.)

5. Set the granola aside to cool for 20 minutes. It will crisp up as it cools, and you will be able to invert the pan onto a clean dish towel and break the granola apart into bite-size crumbles. Toss the granola with the chopped dates and apricots—or any dried fruit you like! Cherries are a tart addition—and give it bright flavor!

6. Store the granola in an airtight container or zip-top bag in the fridge for up to a month.

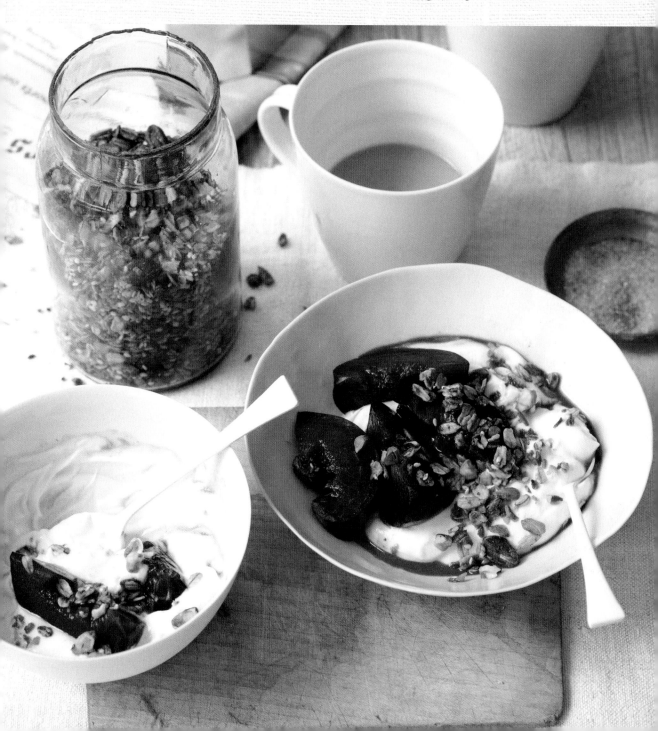

CHAI-RASPBERRY CHIA SEED PUDDING

serves 5

2 ½ cups unsweetened coconut or almond milk, "lite" if preferred

2 chai tea bags (I like Zhena's Gypsy Fair Trade Organic Coconut Chai)

4 tablespoons pure maple syrup plus more for serving

½ cup chia seeds

½ teaspoon ground cardamom

½ teaspoon ground cinnamon

1 teaspoon pure vanilla extract

½ cup unsweetened shredded coconut

1 cup fresh raspberries

PUDDING FOR BREAKFAST?? Better believe it!! Chia is a tiny but powerful seed that's loaded with antioxidants, fiber, and healthful fats. Aztec warriors used to eat it before a battle—so surely it's a good choice to arm yourself for a Monday morning meeting. This recipe is best made the night before, which will give you an extra few minutes of shut-eye. Enjoy a little caffeine kick from the chai tea—or swap in your favorite noncaffeinated option!

1. In a small saucepan over medium-low heat, heat the coconut milk to scalding, being careful not to boil; there will be a thin skin on the sides of the pan when you swirl it. Remove from the heat, add the tea bags, and steep, covered, for 5 minutes to infuse their flavor. Set the pan aside and cool milk to room temperature. When cool, remove tea bags and add the infused milk, syrup, chia, cardamom, cinnamon, and vanilla to an airtight glass container or jar. Shake vigorously for 30 seconds. Refrigerate the mixture for 4 hours or overnight, swirling, stirring, or shaking every 30 minutes for the first few hours, until the chia starts to form a gel.

2. Place the coconut in a small skillet and toast it over low heat, gently shaking the pan until the coconut is golden brown and crispy, about 6 minutes.

3. Puree ½ cup of the raspberries in a blender to form a liquid. Stir it into the chia pudding just before serving. Top each portion with a few whole raspberries, a sprinkle of toasted shredded coconut, and a drizzle of extra syrup.

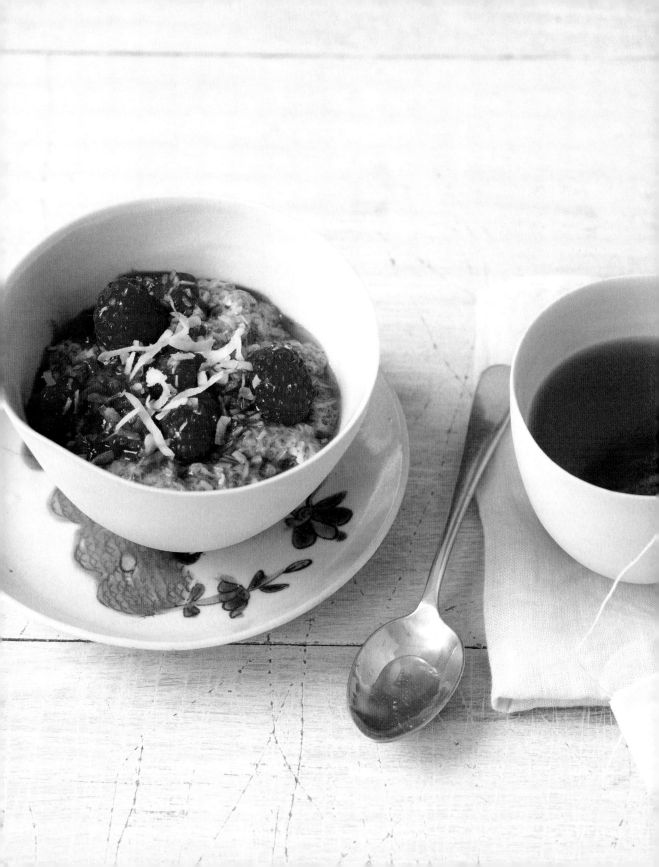

MUSHROOM, LEEK, AND GOAT CHEESE QUICHE

serves 6

WHENEVER I MISS PARIS, I make this simple quiche—and John never complains. We love to re-create the meal we had after a long walk around the city on our honeymoon: a piping-hot slice of quiche next to a lightly dressed mixed green salad with chives, and pistachio macarons with fresh berries and cream for dessert. Bliss all over again!

So, yes, real men eat quiche. And so do their wives.

2 tablespoons olive oil

2 leeks (white and light green parts), cleaned and sliced into thin half-moons (see DASH)

2 cups thinly sliced assorted mushrooms (shiitake, button, cremini)

Leaves from 2 fresh thyme sprigs

½ teaspoon salt plus more for seasoning

Fresh-cracked black pepper

6 large eggs

½ teaspoon ground nutmeg

1 cup whole or 2% milk

1 frozen deep-dish 9-inch piecrust, thawed (you can also make your own using my recipe on page 32)

6 ounces goat cheese

1. Preheat the oven to 400°F.

2. Heat the oil over medium heat in a saucepan large enough to fit all the vegetables. Add the leeks and cook for 2 minutes, stirring to sweat until softened, taking care to avoid burning. Add the mushrooms and thyme and stir to incorporate. The mushrooms will release a good amount of water. Cook, stirring often, until all the liquid is evaporated and the mushrooms are turning a deep golden brown, 10 to 12 minutes. Season to taste with salt and pepper. Remove from the heat and set aside.

3. In a large bowl, whisk the eggs and nutmeg. While you whisk, slowly incorporate the milk to make a nice froth.

4. Score the piecrust by giving the bottom 4 or 5 pokes with a fork. If using a frozen crust, bake for 5 to 8 minutes, until the bottom is slightly puffy and golden brown. Arrange the sautéed vegetables in the shell and crumble the goat cheese on top. Whisk ½ teaspoon salt into the egg and milk mixture and pour it into the pie shell, filling to just below the rim, about 2 cups. Save any extra wet mix for tonight or tomorrow's omelets.

To clean leeks, cut off the dark green tops and discard. Cut off the bottom bulb and discard. Slice the leeks in half vertically and then into your desired shape (thin half-moons for this recipe). Soak the leeks in a bowl of cold water, swirling with your hands to loosen any silt trapped between the layers. Rinse and repeat. Lift leeks from the water and onto a dry dish towel to remove some of the extra water before using.

5. Reduce the oven temperature to 375°F and bake for 35 to 40 minutes, or until the top is golden brown and the egg and milk custard is cooked through.

6. This quiche also holds up nicely covered with wax paper or plastic wrap if you want to sample some in the morning and then leave it on the kitchen counter for an afternoon snack.

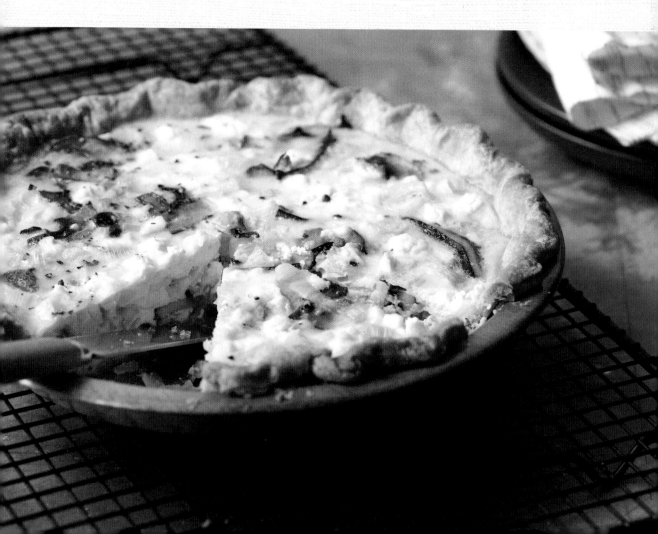

SUPER-EASY ALL-BUTTER PASTRY CRUST

makes one 9-inch piecrust

1 cup plus 2 tablespoons
all-purpose flour

½ teaspoon salt

⅓ cup butter, chilled and cut
into ½-inch pieces

3 to 4 tablespoons milk

IF YOU'RE FEELING UP TO doing everything from scratch, you can make this easy pastry crust. It goes really well with all sorts of savory fillings, or you can add 1 or 2 tablespoons sugar to the dry ingredients to give the dough a slightly more cookielike taste for sweet tarts.

1. In a large mixing bowl, sift together the flour and salt. Use a pastry cutter or two knives to cut in the butter, dispersing it into the flour and salt until only pea-size or smaller butter pieces remain. The mixture should have a sandy consistency. You want to touch the dough with your hands as little as possible to keep the butter chilled throughout.

2. Using a spatula or wooden spoon, mix in the milk, 1 tablespoon at a time, just until you can pinch a piece of dough between your fingers and it sticks together. Gently use your hands to gather the dough into a ball, wrap it tightly in plastic wrap, and gently press into a disc, then refrigerate for 20 minutes.

3. On a well-floured surface, roll the dough to about ¼ inch thick. Use the rolling pin to lift the dough off the counter (you can use a spatula to help get it off the counter surface) and place it over a greased 9-inch tart or pie pan, taking care to sink the dough into the deepest part of the dish so you don't get holes or stretching. Leave about 2 inches of dough hanging over the edge of the pan. Tuck 1 inch under the outside rim of the dish so that you get a lifted ridge, and use your fingertips to form any fun decorative fluting pattern you like.

4. To prevent the bottom of your crust from becoming soggy, blind-bake at this point by stabbing the crust bottom with a fork a few times, then lining the crust with parchment paper, weighting it down with about 3 cups of dried beans, and baking it in a 400°F oven for 20 minutes. Remove the beans and parchment and bake another 5 to 10 minutes, until the bottom begins to brown, taking care not to burn the edge. Cool the crust slightly on a rack.

5. Now it's ready to be filled with any quiche or savory tart filling you like and baked again! Once you add the filling, you need to bake it another 15 to 30 minutes, depending on the filling—just until the filling is cooked through and set (a toothpick inserted at the center should come out clean, but you don't want to see any liquid separating out on the surface; this means the eggs are overcooked)—just be careful not to burn the edges of the crust.

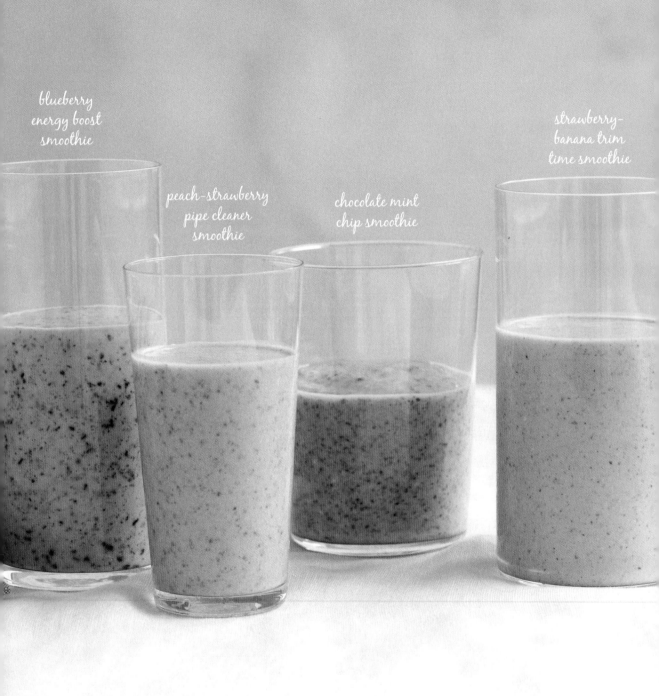

blueberry
energy boost
smoothie

peach-strawberry
pipe cleaner
smoothie

chocolate mint
chip smoothie

strawberry–
banana trim
time smoothie

BLUEBERRY ENERGY BOOST SMOOTHIE

serves 1

SOME MORNINGS NEED *a little more help than others, and this smoothie is a riff on the old standby of delicious blueberries and banana with green tea thrown in for a nice little jolt of caffeine and plenty of age-defying antioxidants. You'll be off and running in no time.*

Place all the ingredients in a blender and blend on high until smooth.

½ cup fresh or frozen blueberries

½ ripe banana

½ cup whole or 2% plain yogurt

¾ cup ice

½ cup brewed and chilled green tea

1 to 3 teaspoons psyllium husk powder or chia seeds (see DASH on page 36)

1 tablespoon flaxseed oil or Total EFA oil

1 teaspoon honey or maple syrup (optional)

¾ cup ice (reduce to ½ cup if using frozen blueberries)

DASH

All the smoothies shown in this book can easily be poured into ice pop molds and frozen for a deliciously healthy breakfast or snack on the go! See the photo on page 37 for inspiration.

PEACH-STRAWBERRY PIPE CLEANER SMOOTHIE

serves 1

½ cup fresh, frozen, or canned peaches, diced or cut into small pieces (avoid fruit stored in syrup and discard any liquid)

½ cup fresh or frozen strawberries, cleaned

¼ cup whole or 2% plain yogurt

1 to 3 teaspoons psyllium husk powder or chia seeds (see DASH)

1 tablespoon flaxseed oil or Total EFA oil

1 scoop greens powder (optional; I like Barlean's organic greens powder)

½ cup water or water plus fruit juice, to help blend

1 teaspoon raw honey or pure maple syrup (optional)

¾ cup ice (reduce to ½ cup if using frozen fruit)

PREPARE TO BE CLEANED. This smoothie is a superfast, supereasy way to start the day with plenty of powerful phytonutrients (plant-based nutrition!) and healthy probiotics to boost your immune system. Plus, you're getting a good bit of fiber to fill you up and keep those pipes running smoothly, if you catch my drift. And good elimination means your body can detox and keep you looking and feeling fresh, shiny, and new! Bottoms up!

Place all the ingredients in a blender and blend on high until smooth. More ice or liquid may be added to reach your desired consistency.

=== DASH ===

A NOTE ON SMOOTHIES THAT CONTAIN PSYLLIUM: Start with 1 teaspoon psyllium and wait to try more the next time you make the smoothie, to give your body time to adjust. Make sure to drink 8 to 16 ounces of additional water along with the smoothie to help your body digest this fiber properly.

STRAWBERRY-BANANA TRIM TIME SMOOTHIE

serves 1

FIBER, HEALTHFUL FAT, *good, complex carbs and a bit of protein make this breakfast smoothie a powerhouse for those looking to take charge over midmorning snacking and get back into those skinny jeans.*

Place all the ingredients in a blender and blend on high until smooth.

½ ripe banana

½ cup strawberries, fresh or frozen

¼ cup whole or 2% plain yogurt

1 teaspoon almond butter

¼ cup rolled oats (quick cooking)

1 tablespoon flaxseed oil or Total EFA oil

½ cup water or juice

1 teaspoon honey or pure maple syrup (optional)

¾ cup ice (reduce to ½ cup if using frozen strawberries)

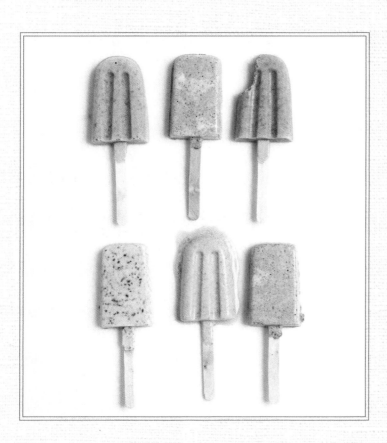

CHOCOLATE MINT CHIP SMOOTHIE

serves 1

½ ripe banana

¼ cup frozen spinach (trust me, you won't know it's there)

¼ ripe avocado

1 to 2 tablespoons unsweetened shredded coconut (optional)

1 to 2 teaspoons psyllium husk powder or chia seeds (see DASH on page 36)

1 tablespoon flaxseed oil or Total EFA oil

½ teaspoon peppermint extract

½ cup coconut milk

1 teaspoon honey or pure maple syrup (optional)

¾ cup ice

2 tablespoons semisweet chocolate chips or carob chips

LIKE ICE CREAM—but good for you! This gets its luscious creaminess from coconut milk and avocado, and its sweetness from honey—which just happens to be antibacterial to boot. This is one smoothie that I particularly love as a breakfast or snack-time frozen pop. No, you don't have to share.

Place the banana, spinach, avocado, coconut (if using), psyllium, oil, peppermint, coconut milk, honey (if using), and ice in a blender and blend on high until smooth. Add the chocolate chips and blend to break them up and distribute throughout the smoothie.

GLOW JUICE

makes two 8-ounce servings

ALKALINE EATING is all the rage, and for good reason. It's supposed to help you lose weight, brighten eyes, clarify skin, and prevent cancer—and this alkalizing vegetable juice is an easy way to give it a try. It tastes great while loading you full of vitamins and minerals to help your body run optimally from the inside out.

I dropped a pretty penny on my Breville Ikon juicer, but it's been with me for years and shows no signs of slowing. The best juicers on the market are quite a bit more expensive because they use technology that doesn't heat (and kill) the enzymes in fresh juice. But the Breville works fast, doesn't heat up too much, is easy to clean, and gives me good-quality juice anytime I want it.

Since this recipe makes about 16 ounces of juice, I like to have 8 ounces for breakfast and 8 ounces for an afternoon snack, but any time is a good time to reach for this healthful hydration!

3 celery stalks, scrubbed

1 large handful of kale or spinach, stems removed

1 cucumber, scrubbed

1 bunch of parsley

1 bunch of mint

1 Granny Smith apple, cored, or ½ cup chopped fresh pineapple

1 lemon, peeled

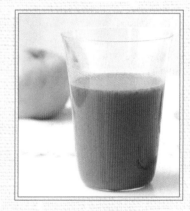

1. Process all the ingredients through a juicer and enjoy.

2. You can store the juice in an airtight container in the fridge for up to 3 days, but it's best to make it fresh daily to maximize nutrient availability.

DASH

Make sure you eat a little bit of fat with or shortly after your juice—whether it's a shot of flaxseed oil or cod liver oil, some coconut milk, or even some yogurt—to help your body maximally absorb all the nutrients.

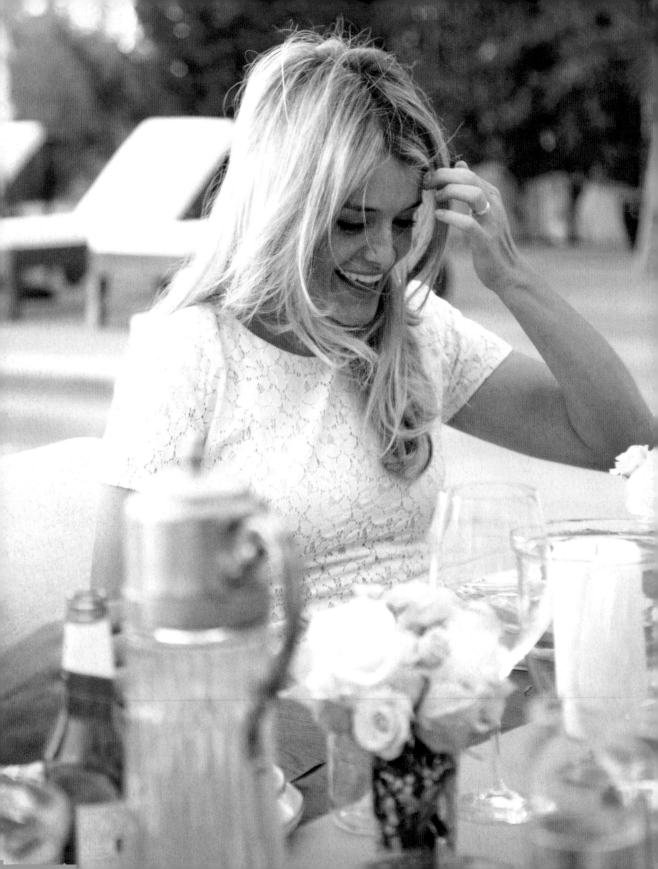

TWO

EAT HAPPY

making friends with your kitchen

A good cook is like a sorceress who dispenses happiness.
—ELSA SCHIAPARELLI

MOST GIRLS WHO GREW UP IN NEW JERSEY LOVE THE MALL. Me? I love grocery stores. I love the sight of ripe produce, the smell of baking bread and pastries, the taste of local dairy and fresh eggs. In our family, cooking was all about experimenting, remaking, and reimagining with total freedom to achieve maximum taste from wholesome ingredients. I rarely saw my mother and grandmother consult a recipe. With them, there was a dash of this and a splash of that. If you weren't present in the kitchen, peering over their shoulders into the pot, you'd miss the magic. So the kitchen was where I came to play. I made myself a fixture at the stove and never left.

Today any kitchen at all, really, is my happy place—especially if somebody else is doing the dishes. When I visit someone's house for the first time, the first thing I ask to see (okay, fine, the first place I *snoop*) is the kitchen. You can learn everything you need to know about a person by peering into their fridge and pantry and understanding how he or she likes to eat. Is their kitchen a temple or is it a closet? Do they have food in their fridge or just a few beer bottles? I'm not judging, I'm just saying that, for me, the kitchen is the most basic source of creativity in a home. If you're treating it as a large shoe box, you're missing out. And it's one of the only places where it's okay for us to make messes as adults! Don't squander that opportunity.

My adventure with eating has taught me many things, but chief among them is that food can always surprise and excite you. Just when I think I've mastered a recipe, someone teaches me an easier, healthier, or tastier way to do it. We develop family favorites, cherish secret ingredients, crave our version of comfort food, discover somebody else's—but somehow the unknown is always just one bite away.

Man, woman, or child: If you rely on a box to feed you, you'll never know the full taste of life. (I'm here all night, folks!) The fanciest restaurant meal cannot compare with the satisfaction that comes from enjoying a homemade supper. Once you learn a few basic techniques, every cookbook, food blog, and meal becomes a source of inspiration to take you to new heights. Refuse to settle into recipe ruts and you'll never be bored—how could you, with all the dishes left to try! And know this: If you know how to cook, you will never be lonely.

People flock to good cooks. Preparing good-quality food creates warmth in a home, and sharing a meal creates an immediate bond. Unless you're a sadist, you should break bread only with people you like and want to get to know better—and yes, cooking will make you friends! The intimacy of offering someone a plate that you spent time creating, or receiving one from them, is about as primal as it gets. You can't help but feel all warm and rosy.

If you want to be truly happy, knowing how to cook for yourself and others is absolutely essential. And understanding how to eat healthfully and well is the basis of the best cooking—the kind that nourishes while it delights and brings us back to the table for more.

TOO MUCH OF A GOOD THING

I grew up in a huge Irish, Italian, Swedish, and Turkish clan in which food has always been at the locus of family communing. Family dinners brought us together around long farm tables laid high with generous helpings of homemade deliciousness. We had whole spice bazaars in our cupboards, racks of unusual teas, and random condiments cluttering our shelves. Anytime

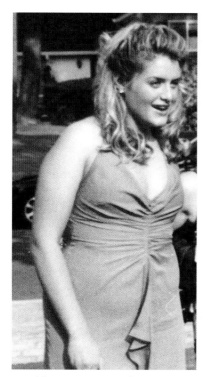

Me at my prom: Seventeen and 180 pounds.

I wanted to explore, it was all right there in the kitchen just waiting to be discovered. Talk about a coinciding of culinary cultures! Weekly menus at our house were like an eating tour at Epcot.

We ate perfect *pomodoro* sauce over delicate strands of angel hair; a lentil soup spiced with cumin and cardamom, served with dried dates and garlicky yogurt with dill; homemade bread spread with fresh butter and jam or loaded up with smoked salmon, capers, and cream cheese; whole baked fish stuffed with rosemary, garlic, and lemon wheels; pickles and stews and chowders out my ears; and the very occasional meatball that jumped between Swedish, Turkish, Italian, and soy/seitan/tempeh (my mother raised us almost entirely pescatarian, with rare exceptions made for when we visited family or foreign countries or somehow procured gifts of meat from friends who were hunters and gatherers of the modern age). And that was just Monday.

Though we ate mostly healthful food, the quantity of my portions did not stop at adequate. Instead, I would happily steal bites from the cutting board, sampling from every dish and pot on the stove, snacking my way through an afternoon of homework on the kitchen stool conveniently within arm's reach of the refrigerator, and then tucking into a heaping helping of whatever delicious meal I'd been sneaking tastes of all afternoon. I spent every free moment thinking about either what I wanted to eat or how I shouldn't be thinking about eating.

At seventeen, I weighed 180 pounds. The food I loved was making me fat, not because it was unhealthful—almost everything was homemade or procured from local, conscientious producers, and my mother and grandmother were way ahead of the game with an eye for organics and limiting excessive animal products and processed foods—but because I let food have control over me.

As the only heavy girl in a family full of health nuts, I was constantly aware of the fact that food could be a force for healing or a force for harm, a force for feeling totally empowered or desolately insecure. Somehow I kept finding myself landing on the losing side of that coin.

I associated the sensation of enjoying wonderful food with the feeling of belonging and love I got from cooking and creating a meal as part of a shared social experience with my

GET A GREEN THUMB

With a row full of green plants on a sunny windowsill, you can add cheer to your kitchen and help recycle carbon dioxide in your home into fresh oxygen, and you'll never find yourself without that essential addition of fresh herbs in your next meal. These five favorites are easy to grow and maintain, and just a snip of your kitchen shears will offer garden-fresh flavors to any dish or libation year-round. Not to mention, it'll give a little life to your living space—feng shui bonus points!

It looks pretty to grow your herbs all in one pot, and you can certainly figure out an easy pattern to make it possible. But since different herbs like different sunlight and watering conditions, I find it's easiest to contain them in individual pots. It's also a good idea to start each pot with a layer 1 to 2 inches deep of small planting pebbles or rocks under the layer of soil. This will help ensure good drainage—mold will kill your herbs fast!

Basil

Care for it: Basil should be kept in full sun and watered when it begins to wilt. Stress is bad for you, good for basil. When the plant is stressed from not enough water, it produces more essential oils, which give it more basil-ness when you eat it. And here's another tip: Don't water basil on a day you plan on using it, because it dilutes the flavor in the leaves.

Devour it: Tear it into green salads, tomato sauce, or with fresh mozzarella and tomato.

Chives

Care for it: Chives are really hardy, so you can grow these onion relatives in partial shade or partial sun. Water only when the soil feels slightly dry. Choose a pot with good drainage so you don't get fungus buildup. As a bonus, chives blossom into beautiful flowers you can eat, so you get to enjoy the taste and sight.

Devour it: Chives work well in herb vinaigrettes, mixed greens, egg dishes, potato salads, pastas, and as a colorful garnish.

Mint

Care for it: Mint should be kept in partial shade or partial sun and watered often; the soil should stay moist to the touch. Make sure you keep it well drained, though, because too much water will rot the root system. Mint will grow like a weed if you let it, so prune it back and use it often—not hard to do considering how easy it is to use! It also dries well, but remember that dried herbs have twice the flavor of their fresh counterparts, and this is especially true of herbs that have a lot of water in them when fresh (such as mint and basil), so cut back quantities in recipes if you're going to go the dry route.

Devour it: Julep, anyone? Mint is also lovely in summer salads—think watermelon and feta!—and in iced tea, steeped in hot tea, with fresh fruit, and paired with lemon, rosemary, and garlic for flavorful fish.

Parsley

Care for it: Parsley should be kept in the sun, and the soil should be kept moist but not soaked. Flat-leaf parsley is a little bit hardier, and I think it's prettier and has more flavor, so choose that if you have the option—otherwise, curly parsley is fine!

Devour it: Just chewing a leaf will freshen your breath after meals! Plus it's a natural diuretic, meaning it helps the body flush toxins plus is chock-full of powerful antioxidants itself. Parsley is a staple in Mediterranean dishes, where'll you find it chopped finely into tabbouleh with bulgur wheat, tossed with lemon and pine nuts for a beautiful garnish, or added on its own to give a dish a boost of color.

Thyme

Care for it: Thyme flourishes in bright sunlight and needs minimal water, so keep soil well drained and only slightly damp. Give it a couple months of growing time (if you're planting from seeds) before you start snipping—if you can resist! The pretty buds are also edible.

Devour it: Cut the stems and dry by hanging upside down in trussed bundles to use all year. Store it in airtight containers away from bright sunlight and heat or freeze. Use it fresh for roasting veggies and proteins, flavoring vinaigrettes and soups, or infusing delicious cocktails! Just make sure you get rid of the woody stem ahead of time—not fun to bite into.

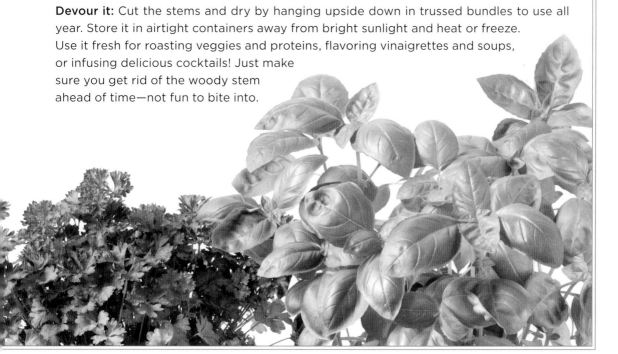

family, but I also feared food and its power over me. I knew that once I got into the kitchen, surrounded by loved ones and caught up in the moment of enjoying time and food with them, I would not be able to resist the charms of so many delicious dishes. The eater had fallen prey to the eating.

I tried fad dieting over and over and failed miserably (as nearly everyone does). The result was that all throughout high school I accepted being overweight—and gave myself permission to underachieve, because I felt held back and incapacitated by being so heavy. I would get picked for varsity sports teams and then sit the bench for the season because I didn't have the endurance to play. I was lucky to have lots of friends, but I didn't feel socially secure. I felt stuck—and just a bit underwhelmed by myself. I needed a change.

I became uncomfortable with how comfortable I'd become settling for a second-rate me, and it was a wake-up call. I wanted to get my health back and regain a body that felt empowered to achieve anything. Most important, I wanted to do it in a way that also allowed me to rediscover my love of food, so my food could start loving me back.

LEARNING TO EAT HAPPY

When I went off to college, I developed a healthful lifestyle that let me shed over 30 pounds permanently and without having to give up any of the foods I craved. How did I do it after all those years of trying and failing to strike a healthful relationship with food? I decided to shift the balance of power so that the eater—me—could get back in control.

The whole premise of this lifestyle shift was to quit thinking about some foods as good and others as bad. The truth—and a much simpler categorization—is that the difference between healthful and unhealthful is the difference between moderation and excess. This meant learning how to pay attention, savor bites, and portion appropriately—and it also meant never feeling deprived.

We seem stuck on the idea that to be healthy, we have to be struggling, deprived, and constantly absorbed by our pursuit of the size 0. This is just not the case! As with everything in life, balance is key. I can eat whatever my little heart desires—freedom!—as long as I quit chomping once I've had enough rather than keep indulging a guilt-fueled binge. I had to learn how to get back in tune with my body, listen to what it was telling me. And I had to keep reminding myself that every bite after the first tastes the same.

Being able to eat whatever I wanted came with the responsibility of also needing to moderate myself. If there are no rules, what I say goes. If something is out of bounds, it's because I put it there—and I have the power to bring it back if I want. To have that freedom, I had to trust myself to be able to make the smart choice, the one that would serve me best long term. I had to stop eating based on instinct or emotion and start eating with awareness.

Once I stopped letting it have control over me, food and I could get back to loving one another.

Out of this love, I developed my very simple, very successful, very balanced approach to eating well for life: *Eat happy!* For me, this means eating food that gives me vitality, experience, joy—or all three! Whether it's a gorgeous fresh veggie juice loaded with phytonutrients, a rare house specialty at a fabulous restaurant or my favorite ultra-decadent glazed Coconut Pecan Pound Cake that's a Christmas staple (page 322), my food now serves one purpose and one purpose only: to enrich my life. And the best part is that happy eating sets up the foundation for a happy home, which makes it possible to have more fun and a happier life overall. Sound simple? It is!

When I eat happy, I'm making health a priority, not an obsession. I'm letting go of all the neuroses, confusion, and anxiety that plague people who think about food in terms of isolated

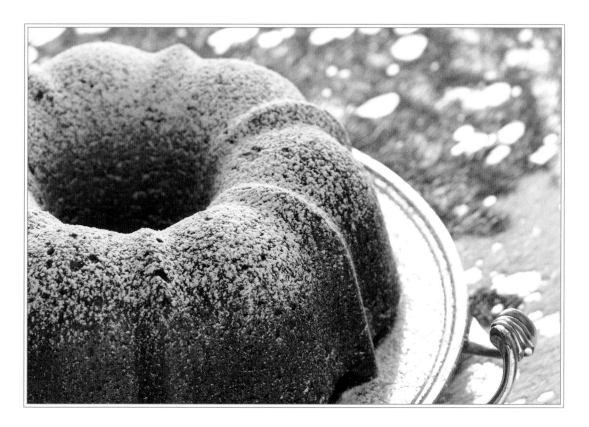

nutrients or specific numbers (grams of fat, calories, sodium). I'm also letting go of being controlled by food, the way that people who are addicted to fast, processed junk food become slaves to the caffeine, sugar, and simple carb fix. I'm letting go of the desperation of being "stuck" in a situation where there's "nothing I can eat" because of how restrictive my eating guidelines are. I'm letting go of the "need" to have meat (or soda . . . or dessert) at every meal. But I can totally have these things if I *want*!

In sum, I'm getting to truly enjoy food as *part* of my life rather than letting it define my life. And you know what? It's working.

Guess who loves to eat? Me! Guess who gets to eat whatever she wants? This girl! Guess who never has to worry about saying, "No thanks, I'm on a diet," ever again? That'd be *moi*. And guess who knows when it's time to have one less bite of pie because her pants are a little snug—but still gets to have a taste if she thinks it's worth it? Me, again. And it could be you! Now, doesn't that sound fun?

HEALTHY AND HAPPY

Yes, there are healthful habits that take getting used to. But the idea behind long-term health is that it should be something you settle into, like a favorite sweater, not a painted-on dress you need a shoehorn and a tub of Vaseline to get into. It should be easy, confidence-building, and fun!

The irony is that the more healthful living becomes second nature for you, the more likely it will be that you'll be wearing that painted-on dress, looking (and feeling!) like a million bucks, reaping all the benefits of an eating plan that fits you like a glove. Okay, enough with the clothing metaphors for now.

Every bite you take becomes part of your biochemistry. In other words, you really are what you eat. The more you learn, the more you'll find yourself naturally making healthier choices every time your mouth waters. The effortlessness is the best part. Okay, I lied: The best part is finally, truly, freely *loving* every tasty bite. And that painted-on dress looking so freaking awesome isn't bad either.

PANTRY PRIMER

To help make the best eating choices possible, I keep a supply of certain pantry and fridge essentials on hand at all times. These are the items that let me live my daily life better by giving me everything I need to make delicious everyday recipes like the ones in this book. From healthy staples to decadent indulgences, readily available ingredients are the ultimate must for on-the-go menu planning. And if there's one thing I've learned through many years of figuring out how to eat happy, it's to set yourself up for success and go from there!

The list below shows my favorite fresh foods, staples, and specialty items, all of which are used throughout the recipes in this book. It's not a short list, but don't worry—you don't need all of it right away. Some of the staples you might invest in right now—things like oils and vinegars that will keep well for a while. The fresh produce items you'll purchase as you need them. And as you try more of the recipes in this book, you'll accumulate the specialty items I use to add a ton of flavor to dishes without much work at all. So don't fret about having to go out and fill three shopping carts immediately!

There are some things that are absolutely indispensable in my kitchen, and you'll see them pop up again and again in the following recipes. These include **sea salt**, **olive oil**, **vinegar** (of all kinds), **organic coconut oil**, **yogurt**, **maple syrup**, and **honey**. As you read through the list of pantry items, you'll see that some of them are printed in bold, like the ingredients I just listed. That's because this is two pantry lists in one: a preview of what you'll be seeing more of coming up in the recipe chapters, and my kitchen staples that I think every happy home cook should have on hand, all the time, no matter what the season or meal might be.

DAIRY AND EGGS

Butter	**Eggs**	Sour cream (full fat or low-fat)
Buttermilk (or see my trick on page 3)	Heavy cream	**Yogurt** (Greek, regular, goat's milk)
Cheese (feta, cheddar, pecorino, Parmesan, low-moisture mozzarella, Monterey Jack, mascarpone)	Milk (whole or 2%)	

FRUIT

Apples (Gala, Pink Lady, Granny Smith)	Grapes	Oranges
	Lemons	Pomegranate seeds
Bananas	**Limes**	Raspberries
Blueberries	Melon (watermelon, cantaloupe)	Strawberries
Grapefruit		

VEGETABLES

Artichokes

Asparagus

Avocados

Beets

Broccoli

Carrots

Cauliflower

Celery

Chile peppers
(habañero, jalapeño)

Corn on the cob

Cucumbers (Persian,
English seedless)

Garlic

Ginger

Green beans

Haricots verts

Kale

Leeks

Lettuce (romaine,
mesclun greens, iceberg)

Onions (Vidalia, yellow, red)

Potatoes (russet,
small new red)

Purple cabbage

Red bell pepper

Scallions

Shallots

Shiitake mushrooms

Snap peas

Snow peas

Spanish olives

Sweet potatoes

Tomatoes (plum,
heirloom, cherry)

Turnips

Yellow squash

Zucchini

HERBS

Basil

Chives

Dill

Mint

Parsley (curly, flat-leaf)

Tarragon

Thyme

THE REFRIGERATOR DOOR

Capers

Ketchup

Mayonnaise or **Vegenaise**
(vegan mayonnaise made
from oil)

Mustard (Dijon, grain)

Olives (Niçoise, green,
oil-cured black)

Sriracha hot sauce

Tahini (sesame paste)

Wonton wrappers

BEVERAGES

Almond milk	Ginger ale	Seltzer
Apple cider	Pineapple juice	Tomato juice
Coconut milk		

FREEZER

Bananas, peeled, in zip-top bags	Organic chicken breasts/thighs	Spinach
Blueberries	Peaches	Strawberries
Cookie dough (roll as a log for convenient slicing and baking)	Soups/stocks/sauces, for easy weeknight meals	Whole grain or whole-wheat bread, sliced

COOKING AND BAKING BASICS

Active dry yeast	Brown sugar	**Pure vanilla extract**
All-purpose flour	Cornstarch	**Raw honey**
Baking powder	Good-quality cocoa powder	**Salt** (sea, kosher, flavored)
Baking soda	Granulated sugar	Whole-wheat flour
Brewer's nutritional yeast	**Pure maple syrup**	

SALT

I'm a big fan of salt—it wakes up your taste buds and actually helps you enjoy all flavors better, which is why salty and sweet makes such a nice pairing. Some people—especially those with hypertension—need to be wary of having too much, but for most, salt is a vital part of a healthy body and, when used correctly, a happy mouth. I use iodized salt for most of my cooking and baking, because iodine is absolutely crucial for thyroid health and iodized salt is one of the few places North Americans can get it (seaweed is an even better source, but not quite as versatile).

When it comes to presenting and finishing a dish, though, flaked sea salt is my standby. It's a little bit more expensive, but way worth it for the delicate, saline explosion it provides. Sea salt comes in beautiful crystalline formations and is rich with minerals. Crush it between your fingertips and sprinkle on everything from salads to cookies right before serving for an extra burst of salty flavor.

Though I do occasionally use cane sugar (dehydrated cane juice), granulated sugar, and brown sugar in my recipes, I typically rely on raw honey and 100 percent pure maple syrup for all my sweet needs. The less refining, the better in my book.

Maple syrup does go through some refining processes, but pancakes call for it and if you opt for Grade B Pure Maple Syrup, it's still dark and rich with mineral goodness from the tree's sap. Honey is even better—this sticky-sweet, liquid gold is an antibacterial, antiviral, antioxidant-, vitamin-, and mineral-loaded powerhouse. But only if you're eating the real deal.

The issue is, a lot of honey available at the supermarket is ultra-filtered, meaning it's been heated and treated to remove the pollen (the only way to truly identify the quality and source of your honey), denaturing enzymes and removing valuable health benefits. The best way to guarantee that you're reaping all the benefits honey has to offer is to opt for raw, unfiltered versions that have not been heated above hive temperatures and therefore still contain all the potent, bioactive compounds and enzymes you want. You can find the good stuff at farmers' markets and health food stores, or online!

OILS, VINEGARS, AND SAUCES

Extra-virgin coconut oil

Extra-virgin olive oil

Flaxseed oil

Hot sauce (Tabasco, Cholula, or your favorite!)

Low-sodium soy sauce or Shoyu

Sesame oil

Umeboshi paste (plum paste)

Vinegar (apple cider, balsamic, champagne, red wine)

White truffle oil (I like Urbani Truffles)

Worcestershire sauce

SPICES

Bay leaves

Cardamom, pods and ground

Chipotle powder

Cinnamon, ground

Coriander, seeds and ground

Cumin, seeds and ground

Dried chile flakes

Dried mint

Dried oregano

Fleur de sel or flaked sea salt

Fresh-cracked black pepper

Garlic powder

Nutmeg

Onion powder

Paprika

Powdered mustard

Smoked paprika

DRY GOODS (GRAINS, SEEDS, LEGUMES)

Amaranth

Brown basmati rice

Brown rice

Chia seeds

Flaxseed (keep in the fridge)

Hemp seeds
(keep in the fridge)

Lentils (red, green, Puy)

Millet

Quinoa

Raw sunflower seeds
(keep in the fridge)

Rolled oats
(not quick-cooking)

Sesame seeds
(keep in the fridge)

CANNED GOODS

Beans (black, pinto, cannellini, kidney, garbanzo/chickpeas)

Canned tomatoes (whole, crushed, and pureed; I like the San Marzano variety)

Chipotle chiles in adobo sauce

Peaches (canned in fruit juice only!)

NUTS AND DRIED FRUITS

Dried currants

Hazelnuts

Medjool dates

Pecans

Pine nuts

Pistachios

Prunes

Raw cashews

Slivered almonds

Smoked almonds

Sultans or raisins

Unsweetened shredded coconut

Walnuts

BREADS

Baguette

Ciabatta

Corn tortillas

Pullman loaf

Whole-wheat bread (with whole grains)

Whole-wheat pita

SUNDRIES

Almond butter

Applesauce

Barlean's organic greens powder

Chai tea bags

Chicken or vegetable stock

Chile jam

Dried lavender

Green tea

Italian bread crumbs

Pasta (linguine, capellini, spaghetti, orecchiette, penne, or your preferred shape, made with semolina or alternative flours)

Psyllium husk powder

Semisweet chocolate chips

Unsweetened coconut milk

Wheat germ

THE LIQUOR CABINET

Bourbon

Bright white wine (I like Spanish Verdejos, Italian Verdicchios, and dry Napa wines—most of these are about $10 a bottle)

Champagne, cava or prosecco

Cognac

Full-bodied red wine (I like Super Tuscans, Chiantis and Malbecs; Pinot Noir if I want something a little more bitter—most of these come in at about $15 a bottle)

Gin

Light rum

Tequila

Vodka

Whisky

Now that you're armed and ready for a kitchen coup d'état, it's time to sound the trumpets and tell the powers that be that you're through settling for overprocessed, overpriced, under-delicious fare.

Long live the home-cooked meal!

THREE

JARGON SLAYER

navigating the supermarket like a pro

Eat food. Not too much. Mostly plants.
—MICHAEL POLLAN

IF YOU'VE BEEN IN A GROCERY STORE LATELY, CHANCES ARE the items that ended up in your shopping cart were as much the result of a clever marketing strategy employed by supermarkets to force you to spend money where they'll stand to make the most profit as they were a product of the meals you're planning to eat that week.

Think about it: You got some produce on sale, and it probably wasn't organic or grown anywhere you could drive to; the things you got organic probably cost you an arm and a leg. Then you went to get your pantry essentials and you had to reach to the top shelf to grab them, but while you were up there on your tippy-toes, you noticed some expensive gourmet items that just happen to be on special this week—conveniently placed at eye level.

The cheapest things you got were some family-size, prepackaged "foodlike substances." Ironically, these are the items that take the most time and money to produce because they have to be processed down from real food into barely recognizable bite-size pieces. Add in a few premade convenience meals for those days when you're constantly on the run and your grocery bill is not only pushing the max but also loaded with stuff you probably didn't really need in the first place.

Part of eating *consistently* healthfully is learning how to navigate the food system as a smart shopper and fill your plate with the right balance of ingredients without letting these goals sap the joy out of eating great meals. Figuring out how to get the best nutritional bang for your buck is understanding the facts and then figuring out what actually works for you so you're not constantly obsessing over whether you're supposed to get cage-free or free range or whether you have exactly four ounces of protein on your plate.

The point is to first empower you with the smarts and then to make the process simple and strategic. You don't need one more thing adding stress to your life, right?

As it happens, reading up on food politics, the latest nutritional research, labeling laws, and factory farming are among my favorite pastimes. I know, I know, it doesn't sound glamorous. But guess what? It may just save your life. The easier it is for everyone to have access to affordable, nutritious food, the easier it will be for everyone to make healthful choices. The better we feed ourselves, the better our quality of life will be—and the less likely it will be that we end up on an operating table or dealing with the chronic lifestyle-related diseases so many struggle with today.

Think about quality food as an investment toward a long, happy, healthful life. If you're a gambling gal, the safest bet you can make is to spend the money now and avoid depositing it at the hospital down the road.

I'm going to spend a little time outlining what I think are the key things to keep in mind when it comes to incorporating healthful habits into everyday life easily, from portion sizing to navigating the supermarket successfully so you can make it second nature for yourself.

PLAYING THE NUMBERS

How we think about healthful eating boils down to numbers: calories in versus calories out. Basically, if you're constantly taking in more energy (calories) than you are spending, you'll pack on the pounds. Reverse the scales, and you should start shedding. But calorie counting isn't so simple anymore, because a lot of the food we're eating on a regular basis isn't "real food." Instead of the nutrient-rich energy your body expects to find in real food, a lot of our meals are full of "empty calories," energy that comes without the valuable nutrition it would have if it hadn't gone through complex chemical processing (essentially, digestion by a machine) before reaching your mouth—think of all your partially hydrogenated, sugar- and sodium-loaded, "part of me used to be a real food, I swear!" packaged foods. You never really feel satisfied, even after you've scarfed the whole bag and are fiending for another. And neither does your body.

Part of the reason we can't just pay attention to calories anymore is that food is not the same as it was one hundred—or even twenty—years ago. In order to provide huge quantities of food at an affordable cost that also pays hefty profits, our food suppliers have had to cut a few corners (that's an understatement) to deliver the goods. Within the meat and dairy industries, this may mean that animals are raised in dire conditions with no room to move around, given feed that historically they might never have eaten and that their bodies have no way to process (like feeding corn to fish and fish to cows), and that they are regularly dosed with antibiotics and hormones that get passed directly to us through their meat, eggs, and milk. As a result, we get a much lower-quality product that's been sapped of many of the basic nutrients that food is supposed to deliver.

When it comes to fruits, veggies, and grains, we've witnessed a surge in genetically modified foods—plants whose genes have been scientifically altered in labs and through crossbreeding to create an entirely new gene with a new set of properties, whether it's to grow faster, be weed resistant, or self-destruct at the end of every year so farmers are forced to buy new seed the following spring. Then again, maybe you haven't witnessed this, since the United States still does not have uniform labeling laws requiring producers to adequately label their products so that consumers know whether they contain genetically modified ingredients or not. Sound fishy? Well, given that your tomato just might have a cold-water fish gene spliced into it to make it frost resistant so it can grow in the snow, it might be tasting a little fishy, too. (No, that's not a joke.)

Why does any of this stuff matter? It matters because for ten thousand years, humans have been relying on an incredibly evolved and complex system of digestion that has served us well. As our food choices and food quality changes almost overnight, our bodies cannot keep pace. If our bodies don't know how to adequately extract nutrients from our food—or if the food doesn't have many of these nutrients to begin with—we're the ones who suffer, everything from depleted immune systems to chronic lifestyle-related diseases. There are plenty of people in this country who are both obese and malnourished because their bodies are missing key nutrients they need to function properly, even after enjoying an "extra value" meal. That goes for anyone who eats most of her meals out of a box or wrapper.

In fact, when our bodies are in constant overdrive—when we're chronically deprived of the vital nutrients we need to function optimally—they eventually begin to break down. We get sick more often. We get tired more easily. So we dose ourselves with medicines to mask the sickness and consume more sugar and caffeine to give us fake energy, which only adds to the problem. The result is an increasing number of people who struggle with obesity, diabetes, heart disease, and other lifestyle-related diseases who are treating the symptoms but not the root cause of their sickness.

These diseases can often be entirely reversed and/or prevented by supplying our bodies a chance to heal naturally with high-quality, wholesome foods—those that arrive in our kitchens looking much the same as they do when they come out of the ground. Our bodies are self-cleaning, self-operating machines! They know how to heal themselves, how to function optimally—we just have to give them the raw materials, then get out of the way and let them work their magic.

In general, I try to keep industrial meat and dairy, genetically modified produce, and processed foods as far away from me as possible. Now, I've been known to keep a boxed cake mix on hand for dire emergencies—surprise dinner parties, impromptu birthday celebrations, and of course, those "I just *need* to eat cake batter with a spoon" scenarios, but these are very rare and desperate occasions. That's because I have learned that if I have ten minutes and the right ingredients in my pantry, it's just as easy to whip up something great from scratch and avoid all the unnecessary chemical additives, toxic sweeteners, and processed fats. The point is not that you can *never* eat this stuff. It's that you'll be doing yourself a huge favor if you see how it isn't your best choice and how easy it is to do without, whether you make the stuff from scratch or find a healthier alternative.

Still, it can be tempting stuff, and since food producers are going to keep creating junk food until we the consumers demand otherwise (and vote with our wallets for better options), we've got to stay one step ahead for now and equip ourselves with the knowledge to successfully navigate today's food scene.

Essentially, we've got to get smarter to keep pace with our constantly evolving food system, and this comes down to thinking about portion sizes rather than calorie crunching, understanding how to interpret labels and staying alert to some tricky advertising, and figuring out the easiest, most delicious ways to make cooking at home a part of our regular lives.

"JUST RIGHT" PORTIONS AND SERVINGS

Play Goldilocks for a minute. Instead of obsessing over calories, I'd like you to start thinking about portion sizes. Not too big—too much food leads to weight gain no matter how healthy it is. Not too small—too little food means lowered metabolism, not to mention constant, nagging hunger. Just right is what we're going for: enough food to keep you energized, not so much that you overeat yourself right into an afternoon nap.

The simplest way to manage your portion sizes is to learn what they actually look like in the real world. By supersize standards, it's too easy to imagine that beverages should be served in bathtubs and that popcorn comes in vats, not bowls. And it's no surprise that the bigger the portion you take on your plate or get with your meal, the more food you're likely to eat. Let's get back on track with a few quick, simple tricks you can use to make sure you understand what true portions look like.

First, gather your tools. No, you don't need to go anywhere. Choose a hand—it's all you'll need to measure with.

Carbohydrates

Carbohydrates are the fuel (sugars) our bodies run on. Without them, we would be tired, cranky, slow-firing messes, and eventually . . . dead. Fortunately, they're delicious, and you should be at no loss for easy ways to incorporate them into your diet, especially after working your way through the recipes in this book!

Carbohydrates are traditionally broken down into two categories: complex and simple, and the easiest way to remember which is which is to think about whether it will be "complex" or "simple" for your body to extract the sugars it needs from the food you're eating.

Imagine carbohydrates as the pot of gold at the center of an obstacle course. With complex carbohydrates, your body first has to conquer hurdles like fiber, and sometimes protein and fat, before it can claim its prize. This extra work helps slow down digestion and keep you full for longer. Complex carbohydrates are generally left in their whole form or are minimally processed. They include whole grains (like oats, amaranth, quinoa, millet, and even whole-grain bread), beans, and legumes. Fruits and vegetables fall into this category, too, but we'll keep those separate for now.

Simple carbohydrates, on the other hand, have gone through mechanical and chemical processing to break down whole grains such as wheat, corn, and rice and create products like white-flour bread, crackers, bagels, and other baked goods, all of which are loaded with refined sugar. Essentially, these products have already been digested for you. When this is the case, the obstacle course becomes nothing more than a quick slide down a jungle gym before your body has all the sugar it can handle. Instead of a slow and gradual replenishing of sugar in the bloodstream the way complex carbohydrates are digested, you get a sudden sugar spike all at once. The shock forces your body to immediately go into overdrive to bring your blood sugar levels back to normal, but the spike and then dive in blood sugar catalyzes a chain reaction that sets your body up for carb cravings all day—bad news for you and your waistline! When it comes to carbohydrates, the harder your body has to work to break them down, the better they are for you.

A single portion of complex carbs is about the size of your palm or a deck of cards, and you're aiming for three servings a day. Even though they're absolutely essential, you can go overboard: If your complex carb portions up to now have been the size of, say, a kitten, you may be seeing the results in a little extra padding around your midsection. Your body loves the fuel it is getting from these types of foods and needs it to function properly (everything from cell renewal to brain firing works on carbohydrates, so don't go cutting them out entirely!), but it will store extra reserves in all the wrong places if you don't give it some good ways to put that energy to work. If you've been overindulging in the CCs, quick, get thee into your sports bra and spandex and break a sweat—or risk kissing those skinny jeans good-bye for a while.

Please note that I'm not including any daily serving recommendations for simple carbohydrates. In stripping away the fiber and many of the nutrients that naturally occur in a whole food, all you're left with is something that's going to spike your blood sugar and leave you on a carb-craving binge all day. These types of items—think of all your boxed cookies, cakes, crackers, and snacks plus processed breads and baked goods—are really best left for special occasions, tasty though they may be.

Piling your plate high with simple carbs tonight is a surefire sign that you'll be frowning at the scale tomorrow (and probably sporting a few more pimples and wrinkles to boot, since refined sugar not only feeds bacteria throughout your body and weakens the immune system but also speeds the aging process along—yikes!). Simple carbs are loaded with empty calories, meaning energy/sugar that enters the body without a ton of nutritional value. Because your brain is smart and knows to look for nutrients, not just calories, coming in, simple carbs don't satisfy its needs, so the brain signals you to keep eating. Even worse, a diet high in refined, simple carbohydrates saps your energy by distorting normal hormone production. All good reasons to keep the simple carbs to a minimum.

Fruit and Veg

Fruits and vegetables are an essential part of a good diet because they're loaded with a wide array of vitamins, minerals, amino acids, and antioxidants we need to feel and look our best. For optimum results, and to make sure you're getting the full benefit of nutrient-rich, fiber-loaded produce, you need to stick with the real deal: Eat raw as much as possible, cook lightly as needed, and avoid fruits and vegetables that have been fried, candied, drowned in cream sauce or syrup, or are otherwise no longer recognizable. And though all fruits and veggies are great choices, some are better than others when it comes to watching sugar intake. Ideally, you want to limit starchy vegetables like corn and potatoes (except for sweet potatoes) in favor of cruciferous ones (broccoli, cauliflower) and colorful options such as peppers and leafy greens (kale, spinach). For fruits, the lower the sugar content the better, so berries, melons, and citrus are your best bets, while sweeter fruits like bananas, cherries, and grapes should be eaten in smaller portions. But any vegetable or fruit is preferable to a highly processed alternative.

Now loosely touch the tips of your four fingers to your thumb to form a circle. See the size? Your hand should look more or less like a tennis ball. That's your basic measurement for fruits and vegetables. And you'll want five to eight tennis ball–size servings of these a day, mostly vegetables and some fruit for sweet treats.

Cheese and Dairy

Now touch the tip of your pointer finger to your thumb to form a circle about the size of a golf ball (or, for those of you not into golf, imagine it's about the size of a nail polish bottle without the cap). The golf ball is a good indicator of how much cheese makes up a serving. For milk and yogurt, ¾ cup is usually the right amount—that's about as much liquid as you can cup in both hands. In both cases, pay attention to how many servings a given package contains by checking the nutritional label to help you hit your target. Try to stick with two servings or fewer of dairy daily. And if you're not a fan of dairy, you can get calcium and vitamin D elsewhere, such as from cod liver oil, leafy greens, and supplements.

Red Meat

When it comes to red meat, you'll want to keep it to a minimum—we're talking less than two palm-size (4-ounce) servings a week. Even lean cuts are fatty, and new research is showing that consumption of red meat contributes to colon cancers, because our bodies have trouble digesting and excreting meat products and wastes efficiently. Red meat is, however, a great source of B vitamins, iron, and valuable protein (though, in general, Americans need way *less* protein than most of us are getting—some of us are getting up to five times too much each day!). The most important thing to keep in mind is that when you do choose to enjoy red meat, enjoy a little less of it and make it a really high-quality piece. The last thing you want is something that came out of a factory farm, where the steer was loaded up with feed that made it sick and fatty, hormones to make it grow faster, antibiotics to ward off the many diseases it was exposed to, and so on. Bottom line: When you can, spring for the best-quality meat at the grocery store, farmers' market, or farm. And when you're enjoying your favorite burger at that restaurant you love, maybe go halfsies.

Nuts and Fats

Fats have gotten a bad rap over the years, but they're finally being granted redemption as we come to understand how crucial good fats in the diet are to overall health. They add lubrication to all parts of the body—from lustrous skin and nails, to properly functioning joints, to efficient nutrient absorption, and even to help balance hormone production to keep you naturally healthy and happy—and are an integral part of every cell membrane. But best of all, fats carry flavor and help us feel full, so adding a bit of fat to a meal not only helps it taste better but may also help you eat less overall. Score!

However, not all fats are created equal. Some are highly processed, low-quality, altered versions of the original—these are the ones you typically see on ingredient labels as "hydrogenated" or "trans fats." And saturated fat, like the kind in butter (any fat that is solid at room temperature), should be enjoyed in moderation, and the less processed the better. The exception to this is extra-virgin coconut oil, which, though a saturated fat, is a medium-chain triglyceride—basically, just a fancy way of describing a fat formation that's very easy for your body to metabolize. Cultures where coconut oil is the predominant fat have a low incidence of heart disease and obesity, and some research indicates that fats like coconut oil may even help us *lose* weight by speeding up metabolism. This news is doubly exciting, because coconut oil tastes divine!

The best kinds of fats come from natural sources such as nuts and seeds, olive oil and coconut oil, and avocados and fatty fish. These contain essential fatty acids (EFAs), which are basically the fats your body cannot synthesize on its own, so you need to get them through your diet. There are three types of essential fatty acids: omega-3, omega-6, and omega-9 (technically, the body can produce a small amount of omega-9 but only if the other essential fatty acids are present in the diet).

Of course, even though these are great fats, you still want to keep them in balance and relatively small amounts. Most Americans get plenty omega-6 EFAs because they can be found in vegetable oils like those used in many store-bought, shelf-stable goods, so focus on the omega-3 and omega-9 essential fatty acids—ideally, you want to get a 1:1 ratio of omega-6 to omega-3, but even 4:1 is great. You can do this by limiting vegetable oil consumption, and instead of settling for the vending machine snack at the office, throw a fistful of raw nuts in a baggie for on-the-go snacking, slather a little organic coconut oil on your toast, add a dash of olive oil and a sprinkle of hemp seeds on your salad, take a spoonful of cod liver oil in the mornings (shots! shots! shots! with orange juice), or simply opt for an avocado or two and a few servings of fatty fish such as salmon, mackerel, and anchovies each week. You'll be glossed up in no time!

Let's recap:

DAILY SERVING CHECKLIST*

☐ Complex carbs: 8 to 11 servings
    – Complex carbs from grains, beans, legumes: 3 servings
    – Complex carbs from fruits or veggies: 5 to 8 servings

☐ Dairy: 2 servings (a golf ball–size serving of cheese or ¾ cup milk or yogurt; check the package to confirm serving sizes)

☐ Protein: 2 to 3 servings

☐ Red meat: no more than 2 palm-size servings *per week*

☐ Nuts and fats: 2 teaspoon-size servings (check the nutritional label for measurements)

* The servings above were computed for a five foot five woman who weighs 125 pounds. Hand sizes change with height and weight, so chances are if you're working off your own hands as a measure you're in good shape. But keep in mind that if you're smaller, you may want to eliminate one serving of complex carbs or one from fat or dairy. If you're taller or an athlete, you'll want to increase your food intake by increasing servings of complex carbs or proteins—not fats.

WHAT IN THE WORLD IS A GMO?

It's easy to see the world has become obsessed with health-food labeling, or at least advertising. Sure, we all want to eat heirloom tomatoes, and seeing the words *free range* on the menu next to your chicken club sandwich is exciting—even if the twenty-five-dollar cost is not. But what do all these phrases mean? Is there really a difference between organic and conventional? Which labels should we care about, and which are designed only to part us from our dollars as quickly as possible? Here is my breakdown of the whole kit and caboodle:

rBGH-, genetically modified-, and antibiotic-free. Always look for meat and dairy products from animals that were *not* given rBGH (recombinant bovine growth hormone, used to artificially boost milk production), genetically modified food, and/or antibiotics. The easiest way to do this is to buy organic options or find a local farm where you can go and check out how the animals are raised. Many local farms can't actually afford organic certification since it is an expensive, taxing process—but because they are smaller scale and can give their animals individual care and attention and space to run around, they don't need to rely on tons of medications to keep the animals alive. If you can take a weekend trip out to see what an actual running farm functions like, chances are you'll be much more comfortable with their business practices and want to take home some fresh meat and dairy that will not only taste better but will likely be more nutritious, too. Maybe you'll even make friends with the farmer. Field trip!

The bottom line: Spend your money buying higher-quality in smaller portions and/or less frequently. That way, you'll get the great flavor and taste you crave without going overboard (on money or portions) and without exposing yourself to toxic chemicals and additives in low-quality products that could wreak havoc on your health.

Organic. Fruits and vegetables labeled *organic* were grown without the use of toxic pesticides, synthetic fertilizers, genetic modification, or sewage sludge (sounds delicious, huh?). So if you wouldn't order a side of toilet water with your broccoli, buying organic is the way to go. There's a ranking system of those fruits and veggies it's most important to buy organic versus those you can get away with having conventional because they won't absorb as much of the toxins from pesticides/fertilizers (see page 69).

When it comes to meat and poultry, the U.S. Department of Agriculture (USDA) insists that in order to be called organic, animals must not be given hormones or antibiotics, and they must have room to exercise, sleep, and be outdoors, at least for part of the time. Organic farming is good for the planet as well as your body since it limits the amount of toxic chemical runoff that flows from farms into our water supplies, and it keeps workers from being exposed to potentially hazardous materials. Good news all around!

Free range. Free-range poultry get some access to the outdoors, although there's no USDA specification for what this means precisely—it could just be a single open door at the end of a huge factory that the chickens never actually find. Egg-laying hens may not get any time outdoors at all. It's not necessarily a label to take a lot of comfort in.

MYTH BUSTER

Healthful foods are not always more expensive! Most comparisons that claim healthful food is significantly more expensive look at cost per calorie, so if you divide the 300 calories in a candy bar by the $1.00 it costs you to buy, you get 3 calories to a penny, whereas 70 calories in a banana that also costs you $1.00 equals about .7 calories per penny. But when it comes to health, the ideal isn't necessarily to get tons of calories on the cheap. Not to mention the fact that the calories in that candy bar are pure fat and sugar, while the banana is going to give you some fiber with that sugar, and tons of vitamins and minerals to boot. What you're not paying for upfront with the candy bar is the potential health-care costs of obesity, diabetes, heart disease, and even cancer down the road that go hand in hand with a highly processed diet.

So shake that faulty logic next time you try to convince yourself that fast food is the economical choice. To save money on the good-for-you goods, buy in season and local to save on shipping and middleman costs. And if organic really is outside the price range, skip pricey, perishable items like berries and opt for frozen or canned veggies and hardy fruits like bananas, apples, and pears. At the end of the day, I would rather see you eat conventional produce frequently than organic produce once a week. Buy dried lentils, beans, and brown rice in bulk and save a fortune. Be practical and see what fits your lifestyle.

Grass fed. Animals that have been allowed to graze are considered grass fed, although it doesn't mean that they were raised on a pasture or that they haven't been exposed to growth hormones and antibiotics (unless it says so on the label). Cows were designed to eat grass, but the ballooning global demand for beef is such that producers have had to get crafty in raising cattle on the cheap to get them fatter faster so they're ready for slaughter sooner. Instead of grass, they're fed grain, which they can't digest. The result is animals get sick easily because they're not getting the nutrients they're used to (and are often living in horrible conditions, crammed together with no room to move, exposed to each other's sickness), so they're also constantly receiving antibiotics along with growth hormones. This is not even getting into the environmental toll of growing enough grain to feed all the cows being bred today. *Pasture fed* is a better indication that producers are thinking about the health of their animals and a likely sign that the cows actually spend a good deal of time outdoors in a field.

Certified humane. This gold standard indicates that animals have lived as they would on a regular farm, under "normal" circumstances: with open space for wandering, shelter from the elements, no confinement in tiny crates. Likewise, they are not given artificial growth hormones or antibiotics and must be butchered quickly and as painlessly as possible. Certified humane eggs come from free-nesting hens. This is the best of the best of product labeling when it comes to wholesome food!

Local. Local means that your product was grown, well, locally—generally by neighbors in a hundred-mile radius. More than one hundred miles and you may not be able to call yourself a locavore; but an apple grown five hundred miles from your door is still better for you—and the planet—than one shipped to your door from, say, New Zealand.

Something more to think about: While there are primary safety standards kept throughout the United States, imported goods are an entirely different ball game. All imports are labeled, processed, and exported at the whim of their own local governments. In Mexico and Chile, for instance, where many of the grapes we eat are grown, it's not illegal to use human feces as fertilizer. If that sounds gross to you, it's an even bigger argument for becoming a locavore . . .

Non-GMO. Genetically modified organisms (GMOs) are those in which the genome of a given plant or animal was altered by adding genes or components of genes from another genetic structure. We want to pay attention to the development of genetically modified foods because we don't yet know the long-term effects of eating them. There is suspicion that changing the genetic makeup of plant and animals, while in some cases delivering immediate results—like fast-growing animals and bug-resistant crops—could yield less nutritious products with unknown long-term problems. Think about the genetically modified fish that are engineered to grow faster with less food—the net result is a possible hazard to their health because they're being forced to grow at too rapid a pace and a decline in their overall nutritional quality when we consume them. And we have no way of knowing the possible resulting health detriments they could pass on to us when we eat them.

The big fight right now is to compel producers to at the very least label foods when they contain genetically modified ingredients and to let us know if an animal was raised on genetically modified feed. It's interesting that Europe has almost unanimously rejected large-scale genetic modification in food, despite the claims that it would "help feed the world" (this is largely bogus, especially once you start analyzing the way genetically modified crops kill heirloom seed crops that farmers have cultivated for years, how they're actually programmed to self-destruct after a year so that farmers must keep repurchasing seeds, and how they only

BE A LABEL JUNKIE

When it comes to clothes, being too focused on labels isn't always a good thing. When it comes to your fruits and vegetables, it's exactly what you should be doing. You know those little stickers you're always peeling off before you bite into a supermarket apple? Next time, take a closer look.

Those codes are called PLU codes, which stands for "price lookup." They were introduced in 1949 to help grocery stores use new technologies more efficiently, but these days they're good for much more than just pricing. If the fruit you're about to enjoy has a four-digit PLU code, it's just a conventional piece of fruit, likely grown with pesticides and possibly in depleted soil. If it has a five-digit code beginning with the number 8, it's a GMO and contains genes not put there by nature. The best option is produce with a five-digit code beginning in 9, which was grown to organic standards.

If you want to do even more research on where the food on your table originated, check out www.plucodes.com, which lets you look up PLU codes so you can Nancy Drew where your banana was grown. You smarty-pants overachiever, you.

work with the addition of a specialized fertilizer or pesticide that, conveniently, is also made by the seed's producer, and so on). Maybe they know something we don't.

AVOIDING PESTICIDES

We need to eat plenty of fresh fruits and vegetables every day, but not all produce is created equal. Produce that isn't organic is often grown with the help of toxic fertilizers and pesticides, which means that all of those vitamins and minerals we're eating to be healthier can come with a side helping of health issues. According to government agencies, pesticides have been linked to cancer, hormone disruption, and more. Think about it: Pesticides are *designed* to kill living things such as bugs and worms! Imagine what they're doing inside your body. Moreover, pesticides that are used on crops get washed away by rain and irrigation into our water supply, ruining natural habitats, which disrupts life cycles at a much more basic level.

The ideal is to buy everything organic because these foods will have had the least exposure to pesticides, but that can certainly get expensive. My best policy is to shop as often as possible with small, local producers—the closer my produce was grown to my home, the more intact the nutrients are and the fewer preservatives are needed to make sure the fresh food reaches me looking great. Moreover, small producers generally don't need to use the extremely efficient (and toxic) pesticides that industrial farms do.

Get to know your farmers at a farmers' market and ask the right questions: What do they think is perfectly ripe right now? Any particularly great crops you should try? Join a CSA (community supported agriculture) farm, and you'll have access to fresh, seasonal, local produce at a great price. Use the experts who are all around you—your grocers, your butchers, your fishmongers—to learn which are the safest, healthiest, most delicious, best-quality ingredients you can purchase, and then see what your budget will allow!

The Environmental Working Group does research to check out threats to the environment

EASY PRODUCE WASH

This is a great all-natural, homemade produce wash to help remove any remaining waxes, residues, or dirt from your fresh produce. It's great to use on any hard fruit or veggie with skin you'd like to eat—think apples, pears, cucumbers, and zucchini. You can also use this for citrus fruits so you don't bring toxins from the skin into the flesh when you're cutting into them.

For potatoes, I find it's easier just to get a scrub brush and scour the skin well under warm water before baking—ideally, buy organic if you like to eat the skin. As for berries and more absorbent fruits, it's important to buy organic because they can only tolerate a quick dunk under running water to get off any dirt or they'll soak up a ton of extra liquid and dilute their beautiful berry flavor.

1 cup water
1 cup white vinegar
1 tablespoon baking soda
Juice from ½ lemon

1. Combine all the ingredients in a bowl and stir to combine. Pour into a spray bottle and generously spray all over produce just before using. Let sit for 5 minutes, rub with a clean towel, rinse with cool water, and enjoy!

2. I like to make fresh batches, but you can keep the water, white vinegar, and lemon mixed together, covered in the fridge for up to 3 days, and just add baking soda right before using.

and to your health. Every year, it publishes a list of the fruits and veg that pose the biggest risks, and the ones that are the safest. Copy these lists and keep them in your wallet for convenient reference while grocery shopping:

OBSESS ABOUT ORGANIC FOR . . . "THE DIRTY DOZEN"

Apples	Strawberries	Lettuce
Celery	Nectarines (imported)	Cucumbers
Sweet bell peppers	Grapes	Blueberries (domestic)
Peaches	Spinach	Potatoes

BE COOL WITH CONVENTIONAL FOR . . . "THE CLEAN 15"

Onions	Cabbage	Eggplant
Sweet corn	Sweet peas (frozen)	Kiwi
Pineapples	Asparagus	Cantaloupe (domestic)
Avocados	Mangoes	Sweet potatoes*

SPEAK UP

Clearly, I could talk (write) for hours about this stuff, but don't worry—I'm done for now!

I just get so excited about what a huge difference our generation can make and how important it is that we do! Which brings me to my next point: Now it's your turn to use your voice to start pushing for a healthier food source we can all enjoy.

The most important thing food producers need to hear is that we care about the quality of our food and will buy better if they make it available. Tell everyone you know to ask for organic at their favorite restaurants; to approach their grocery managers about getting non-GMO meat and fish; to talk to local schools about protecting kids by giving them adequate school lunches that aren't loaded with toxic chemicals, sugars, and additives; to demand that we get to know—and feel good about!—what we're eating because our country upholds strong labeling and growing standards. It's up to educated consumers like us to focus on making the system better—we all deserve it.

All right, kids—it's lunchtime!

* www.ewg.org/foodnews

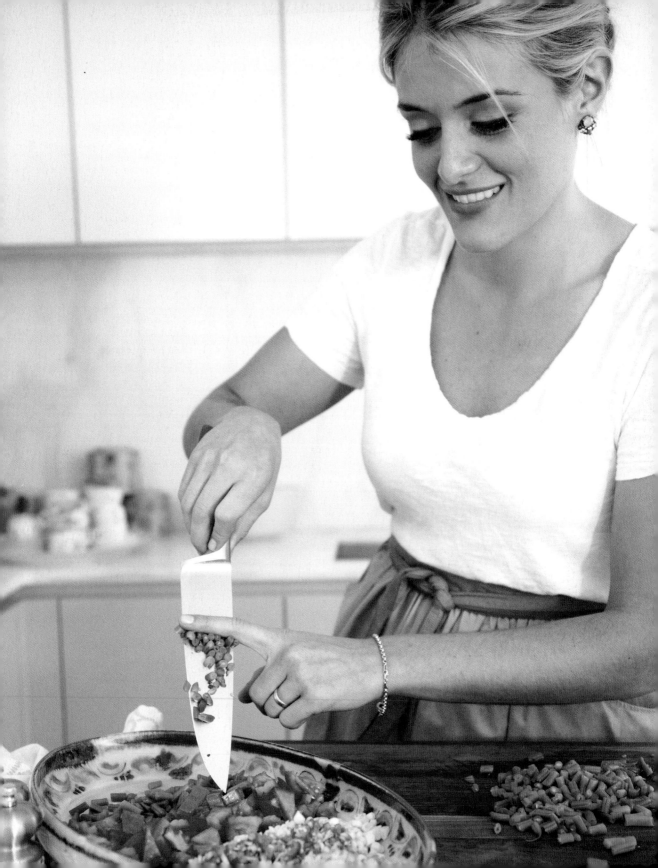

FOUR

LUNCH BREAK

soups, salads, and sandwiches

Ask not what you can do for your country. Ask what's for lunch.
—ORSON WELLES

SAME SALAD, DIFFERENT DAY. RIGHT? WRONG! LUNCHTIME ISN'T a reason to bore your taste buds into submission with another take-out order from the place down the block or the white bread sandwich on . . . well, white. It's an excuse to remind your mouth just exactly how transcendent your lunch break can—and should—be. After all, this is time just for you—to escape the office, the desk, the meeting, and make time for your mouth.

Relishing life is about never settling for second best, and that includes your midday meal. So invite some new spices in. Give in to the season by adding grilled cantaloupe to your vegetable salad. Get inspired by the Incas, who called quinoa "the mother of all grains"—and bonus: It's *much* easier to make than the rice you might have used instead. In this section, lentil soup goes Moroccan. Good old gazpacho gets a hot new makeover with watermelon and jalapeño. Sandwiches go rogue with pita pizzas, shrimp toast, and the best damn veggie burger . . . ever. Because it's lunchtime—and anything can happen.

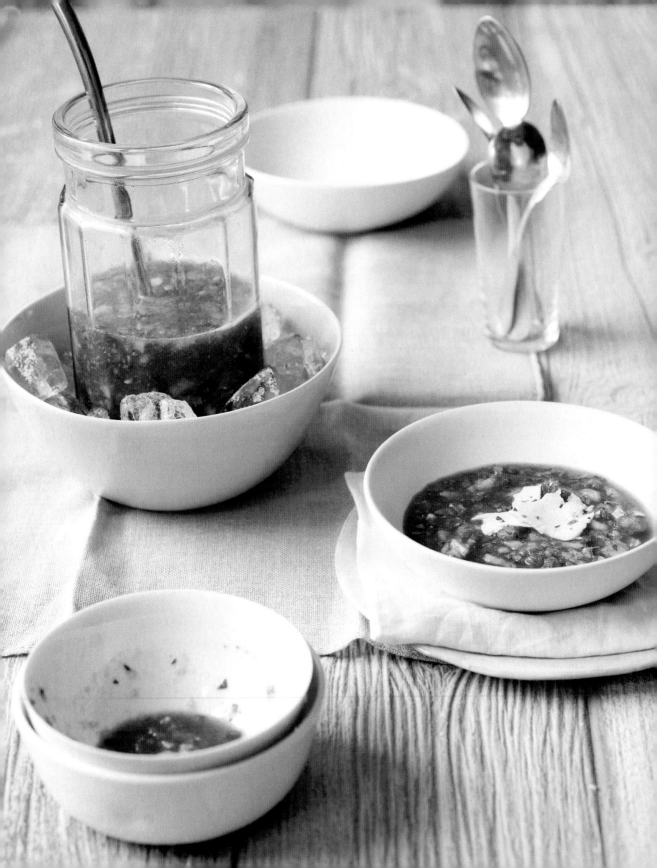

WATERMELON-JALAPEÑO GAZPACHO WITH FETA

serves 4

ALL THIS SOUP NEEDS to wow is a blender and a willing audience. It's especially delicious on a hot summer's day when it helps take the edge off with a healthful dose of sweet, cooling watermelon and spicy jalapeño!

In a blender or food processor, blend the tomatoes, watermelon, cucumbers, onion, jalapeño, garlic, herbs, vinegar, lime juice, and tomato juice until the desired consistency is reached (I like to leave mine slightly chunky). Season to taste with salt. Pour the soup into serving bowls and garnish each with 2 tablespoons of the crumbled feta. Serve with hot sauce or Worcestershire sauce on the side, if desired.

6 ripe plum tomatoes, chopped

2 cups cubed seedless watermelon

2 medium seedless or English cucumbers, peeled and chopped

¾ cup diced sweet Vidalia onion

½ jalapeño, minced (discard the seeds and ribs if you want less heat)

1 garlic clove, peeled and minced

¼ cup chopped fresh flat-leaf parsley leaves

¼ cup chopped fresh mint leaves

¼ cup red wine vinegar

Juice of 2 limes

1 cup tomato juice

Kosher salt

½ cup crumbled feta cheese for garnish

Hot sauce or Worcestershire sauce for garnish (optional)

GRILLED CANTALOUPE AND VEGETABLE SALAD

serves 4

2 ears sweet summer corn, in their husks

Olive oil for the grill or grill pan

2 medium zucchini, sliced lengthwise into ½-inch strips

1 bunch of asparagus, woody ends removed

1 medium cantaloupe, halved, seeded, skin removed, and cut into 1-inch-thick wedges

1 head of romaine lettuce, finely chopped

3 Persian cucumbers, sliced into ¼-inch rounds

1 avocado, pitted, peeled, and cut into ½-inch dice

1 cup cherry tomatoes, halved

12 fresh basil leaves, shredded

½ cup Red Wine–Shallot Vinaigrette (recipe follows)

Lemon wedges for serving

WHEN I VISIT FAMILY in Los Angeles, my lunch break—after a guava-cheese pastry at Café Tropical in Silverlake for breakfast and an appetizer of grilled artichokes at the Newsroom—is spent eating my favorite salad of all time at the Ivy. This is my best approximation, and I took the liberty of adding some sweet cantaloupe to the mix. Perhaps a Nobel Prize for flavor is too much . . . but I don't think so.

1. Soak the corn (in husks) in cold water for 30 minutes.

2. Prepare a gas or charcoal grill to medium-hot, or heat a stovetop cast-iron grill pan to medium-high. Brush the grill lightly with oil (and apply again before grilling new items).

3. Husk the corn, discarding the corn silk and husks. Grill the corn, rotating in quarter turns for 20 to 30 minutes until all the kernels are cooked and tender and some have blackened and charred.

4. Grill the zucchini until tender, about 5 minutes per side. Grill the asparagus until tender, about 8 minutes. Grill the cantaloupe on each side until heated through and grill marks develop, 2 to 3 minutes per side. Chop the zucchini, asparagus, and melon into bite-size pieces, and cut the corn kernels from the cob.

5. Lay a bed of lettuce on each serving plate and top with the grilled items and the cucumbers, avocado, and tomatoes. Tear fresh basil over the top. Drizzle with the vinaigrette (about 2 tablespoons per serving). Serve the salad with fresh lemon wedges.

RED WINE-SHALLOT VINAIGRETTE

makes 1 cup

1. In a blender or using a whisk, combine all the ingredients and blend until emulsified.

2. Keep any remaining dressing in the refrigerator in a clean, airtight glass jar for up to 1 week. I like to save and sanitize (simply boil in hot water for 5 minutes and dry) old mustard or jam jars for just this.

½ cup extra-virgin olive oil

¼ cup red wine (or apple cider) vinegar

2 tablespoons minced shallot

2 teaspoons Dijon mustard

2 teaspoons raw honey or pure maple syrup

1 tablespoon fresh lemon juice

½ teaspoon ground coriander

Salt and fresh-cracked black pepper

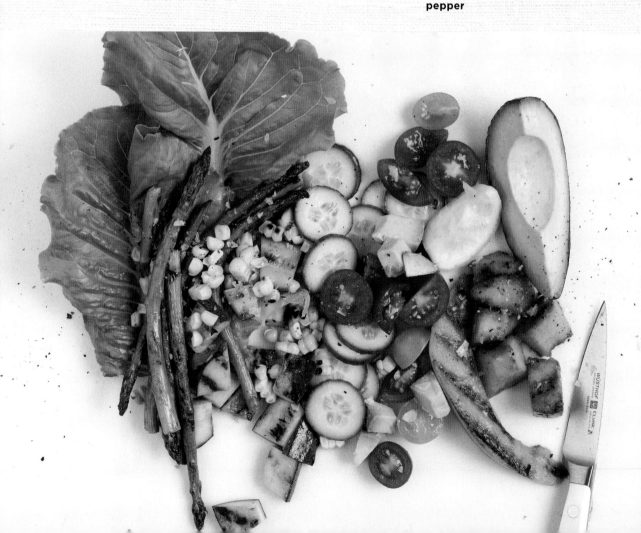

PIZZA PITAS

makes 4 mini-pizzas

¼ cup olive oil

½ tablespoon dried chile flakes

4 whole-wheat pitas, 4 to 6 inches in diameter, pocketless works best

¾ cup Staten Island Special sauce (see page 258), pureed

1 cup shredded low-moisture mozzarella cheese

¼ cup grated pecorino cheese

Fresh basil leaves

Sea salt (flaked salt is great for this—little bursts of salinity with every bite!)

THESE ARE AN EASY APPETIZER or snack for anytime you're craving pizza but don't feel like breaking out the real dough or ordering in—literally, they're ready in 10 minutes. Beat that, delivery boy! They're easily customizable with whatever toppings you feel like—I love mine traditional with just tomato sauce and cheese, then made spicy with crushed chile flakes and garnished with fresh basil, flaked sea salt, and a drizzle of olive oil right before serving.

1. Place the oil and chile flakes in a small glass bowl and set aside to infuse for 20 minutes or up to 2 hours, covered with a plate or plastic wrap to keep dust out.

2. Preheat the oven to 375°F. Place a baking sheet in the oven to heat (or—even better—if you have a pizza stone, use that).

3. Spread each pita bread with 2 to 3 tablespoons of the sauce, leaving a ½-inch rim around the edge. Top each pita with ¼ cup mozzarella and 1 tablespoon pecorino cheese. Place the pitas on the baking sheet and bake for 6 to 8 minutes, or until the cheese has melted and the bottoms of the pitas are crispy and beginning to brown. Remove the pitas from the oven, drizzle them with some chile-spiced olive oil, and top with a few freshly torn basil leaves. Add a sprinkle of salt, cut each pita into 4 wedges and serve.

═══════════ DASH ═══════════

HOT PIZZA! **Heating your baking sheet—or pizza stone— for a few minutes in a preheated oven before putting the pizzas in to bake will help give them crispy, evenly cooked crusts. Don't forget this if you ever decide to bake a pizza from scratch. (Store-bought dough counts, too!)**

KALE SALAD WITH HEMP SEEDS & PARMESAN

serves 4 generously

PRACTICE YOUR MASSAGE SKILLS on this easy salad. Everyone's favorite green is just as great raw as it is cooked. Even better, the longer this salad sits, the more flavor it picks up—I like to make a big bowl to enjoy for dinner and then pack the leftovers for lunch at work the next day. Keep covered in the fridge for up to 3 days, giving it a toss now and then to make sure the bottom layer doesn't get soggy. Then again, if I make it when my husband is around, there isn't ever much left over . . .

Place the kale in a large bowl. Pour the oil on top and sprinkle with coarse sea salt. Using your fingertips, massage the kale thoroughly for 5 minutes, until the leaves start to soften; the kale will reduce to about half its original volume—it will keep reducing the longer you massage. Drizzle it with fresh lemon juice, top with the bell pepper and hemp seeds, and toss to combine. Just before serving, sprinkle with grated Parmesan.

1 large bunch of kale, thick stems removed, washed, and cut or torn into bite-size pieces (about 12 cups)

3 tablespoons olive oil

Large pinch of coarse sea salt

Juice from ½ lemon

½ red bell pepper, cored, seeded, and finely diced

¼ cup hemp seeds

¼ cup grated Parmesan

=== DASH ===

If you like the idea of a little sweetness in your kale salad, try swapping in dried currants and pine nuts for the red pepper and hemp seeds in this recipe!

MOROCCAN LENTIL SOUP WITH SWEET POTATO

serves 6

2 tablespoons olive oil

2 medium carrots, peeled and cut into ⅛-inch rounds (about ¾ cup)

2 medium celery stalks, cut into small dice (about ¾ cup)

1 medium yellow onion, cut into small dice (about 1 cup)

Pinch of iodized or sea salt

½ teaspoon chipotle pepper flakes or dried chile flakes

½ teaspoon ground cumin

¼ teaspoon ground cinnamon

½ teaspoon dried oregano

3 garlic cloves, coarsely chopped

2 cups dried red lentils

½ medium sweet potato, peeled and cut into small dice (about 1¼ cups)

7 cups water or vegetable or chicken stock

1 cup dry white wine or 1 additional cup water/stock

2 bay leaves

Fresh-cracked black pepper

Fresh chopped parsley for garnish

4 Medjool dates, pitted and chopped, for garnish

1 lemon, cut into wedges, for garnish

I ADDED BITS OF SWEET POTATO and chipotle chile flakes to lend some sweetness and spice to the traditional Turkish lentil soup I grew up eating. It's just what I crave on a chilly autumn afternoon, and it's filling enough to be a meal on its own or equally nice as an appetizer.

1. Heat the oil in a medium soup pot over medium heat. Add the carrots and celery and sauté until softened, about 4 minutes. Add the onion, salt, pepper flakes, cumin, cinnamon, and oregano and sauté 3 minutes. Add the garlic and sauté until fragrant, 1 to 2 minutes, stirring constantly to prevent burning.

2. Add the lentils, sweet potato, water, wine, and bay leaves and bring to a boil. Reduce the heat to medium low and simmer, partly covered, stirring occasionally, for 20 to 30 minutes, or until the soup is creamy and the lentils and sweet potato are cooked through. As the soup cooks, skim any foam that rises to the top and discard.

3. Season to taste with salt and pepper. Remove the bay leaves. Garnish with chopped parsley, dates, and a squeeze of fresh lemon before serving.

=== DASH ===

To add a boost of green and tons of healthy antioxidants, stir in two cups kale, cut into ribbons (chiffonade), 10 minutes before you're done cooking, or two cups fresh baby spinach just before serving.

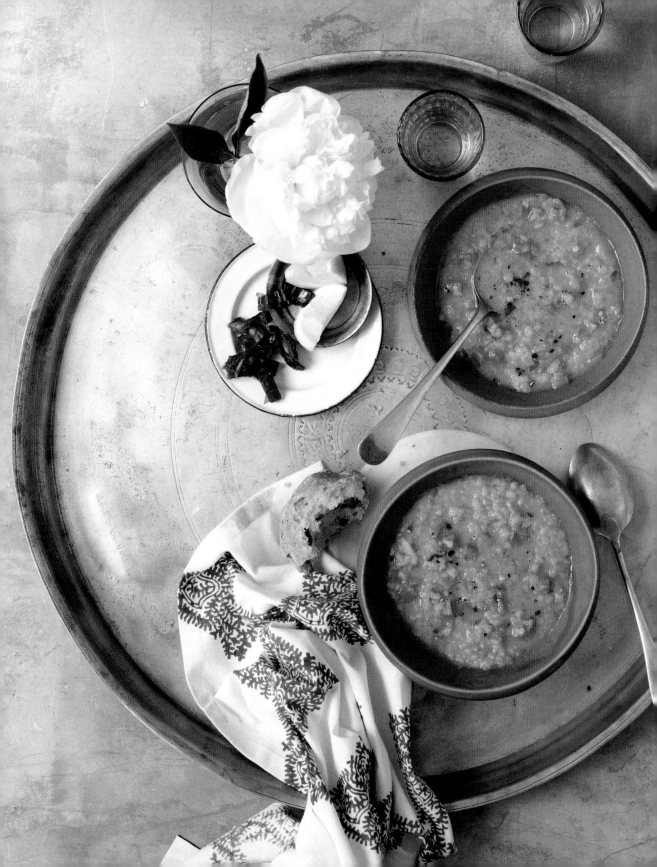

QUINOA WITH CHICKPEAS, CURRANTS, AND FRIED SHALLOTS

serves 6 (approximately 7 cups)

1 cup uncooked quinoa

1 large handful string beans, trimmed

6 tablespoons olive oil

1 large shallot, peeled and thinly sliced

2 garlic cloves, peeled and minced or pressed

About 2 cups canned chickpeas (garbanzo beans), drained and rinsed

About ¾ cup canned kidney beans, drained and rinsed

3 tablespoons dried currants

3 tablespoons apple cider or other light vinegar

1 teaspoon ground coriander

½ to 1 tablespoon raw honey

Sea salt and fresh-cracked black pepper

¼ cup slivered blanched almonds or toasted walnuts (optional)

QUINOA IS A VERSATILE SEED that deserves your love and appreciation for its virtually gluten-free, fiber- and protein-packed goodness. It makes the perfect backdrop for sweet porridges and savory salads, and it's a cinch to make! My eighteen-year-old sister, Zoe, is the pickiest of picky eaters, and every time I'm with her, this is what she asks for because she craves the tart-sweet savory flavor. If you've never cooked with quinoa, this is a great place to start—you'll fall in love.

1. Soak the quinoa in water for 5 minutes (this will help it cook evenly). Rinse well and place it in a medium saucepan and add water to cover by 1 inch (about 2 cups). Cover the pan and bring to a boil over medium heat, then reduce the heat to low and cook, covered, until all the water has been absorbed, about 15 minutes. Remove from the heat and let sit, covered, for 10 minutes. Fluff with a fork and let sit another 5 minutes. Fluff again.

2. While the quinoa cooks, in a separate medium pot of boiling water, blanch the string beans for 1 or 2 minutes, until just tender. Dunk the string beans in a bowl of ice water to stop the cooking process. Cool, drain, and chop into bite-size pieces.

3. Heat 3 tablespoons of the oil in a skillet over medium-low heat. Add the shallot and reduce the heat to low. Cook for 3 minutes, stirring frequently, then add the garlic and continue stirring, until the shallot has crisped slightly and garlic has turned golden brown, about 2 minutes. Remove the pan from the heat.

GARLIC BE GONE To get garlic smell off your fingertips, rinse with soap and warm water and then rub your hands well on anything stainless steel—like your sink! Want to get the same smell off your breath? Eating raw parsley can help mute the smell of garlic and freshen your breath and your stomach (where the smell continues to come from even after you've brushed).

4. In a large bowl, combine the warm quinoa, string beans, chickpeas, kidney beans, and currants. Add the shallot, garlic, and the oil from the pan and toss. Add the remaining oil, the vinegar, coriander, and honey and toss again thoroughly. Season with salt and pepper. Let the salad rest for 5 to 10 minutes before serving to give the currants time to plump up. Serve, sprinkled with the almonds, if desired.

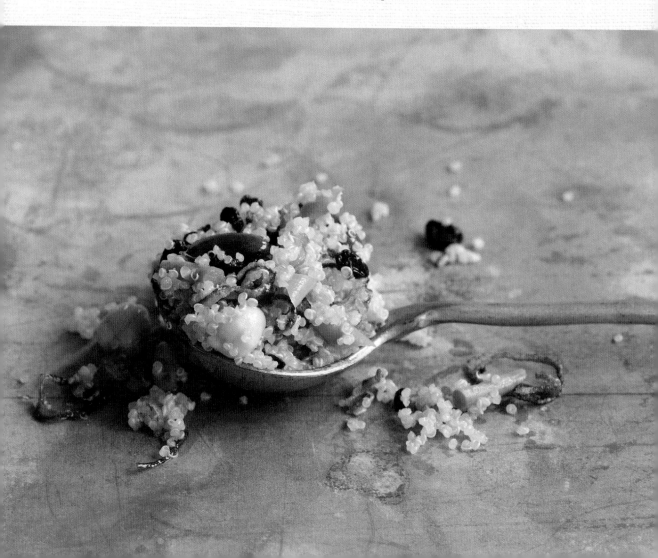

ITALIAN TUNA SALAD WITH APPLES AND OLIVES

serves 4 to 6

Two 4-ounce cans water- or organic olive oil–packed high-quality albacore tuna (I order mine from Vital Choice, www.vitalchoice.com)

One 15-ounce can cannellini beans, drained and rinsed

¼ cup diced red onion

½ red bell pepper, cored, seeded, and diced (about ½ cup)

2 celery stalks, sliced thin

1 Granny Smith apple, peeled, cored, and diced

3 scallions (white and light green parts only), sliced thin

¼ cup green olives, pitted and sliced thin

2 tablespoons capers, drained

¼ cup coarsely chopped fresh flat-leaf parsley

1 cup Italian Dressing (recipe follows)

4 cups mesclun greens, washed and dried, or 8 to 12 lettuce cups

4 tomatoes, cored and sliced into thick wedges

Tomato Toast (page 105) for serving (optional)

EQUALLY GOOD AS an entrée, appetizer, or hors d'oeuvres (thank you, lettuce cups), this tuna salad, with the addition of sweet crunchy apple and Italian seasoning, leaves school lunches in the rearview. Pronto!

Use a fork to break the tuna into small pieces. In a large bowl, combine the beans, onion, bell pepper, celery, apple, scallions, olives, capers, parsley, and dressing. Toss the tuna salad and set aside to marinate for 10 to 15 minutes. Serve the tuna salad over a bed of the mesclun with the tomato wedges and a slice of toast, if desired.

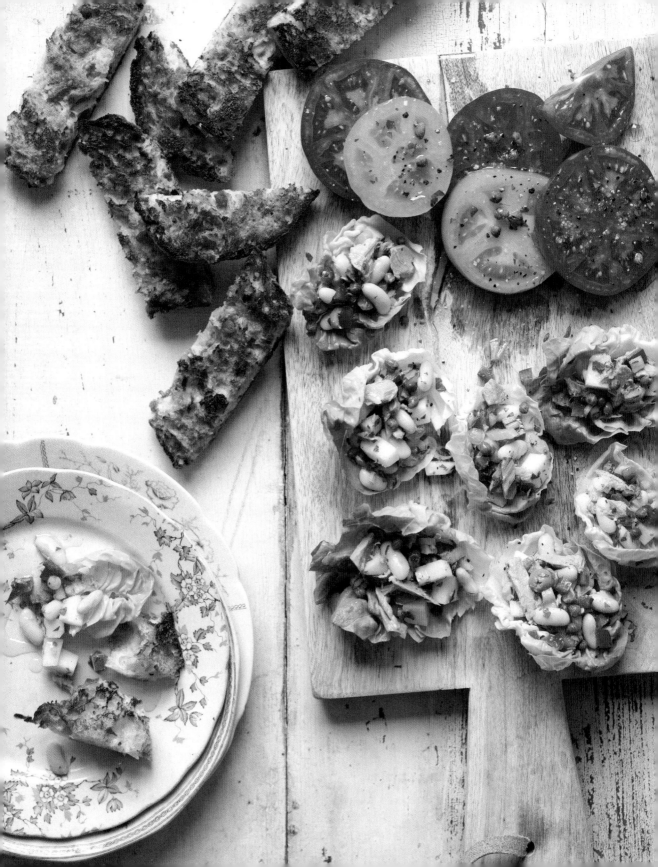

ITALIAN DRESSING

makes 1 cup

½ cup olive oil

⅓ cup red wine vinegar

3 teaspoons Dijon mustard

3 teaspoons dried oregano

1 red-hot chile pepper, thinly sliced, or ½ to 1 teaspoon dried chile flakes

½ teaspoon sea salt

Fresh-cracked black pepper

In a small bowl, whisk all the ingredients together. Taste for seasoning and adjust as needed.

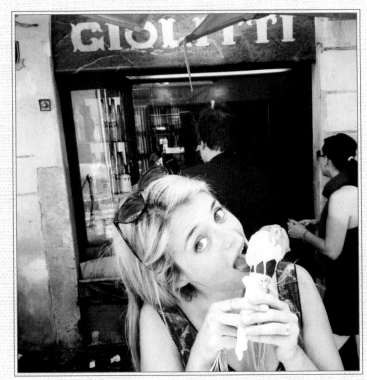

When in Rome, do as the Italians do and enjoy a daily gelato! I never skip dessert on vacation.

SALMON NIÇOISE SALAD WITH DIJON VINAIGRETTE

serves 4

IN TYPICAL FRENCH FASHION, this recipe looks really complicated but is actually just a bunch of easy steps that get you to a miraculously delicious—and very elegant—final product. The French eat their Niçoise with tuna, but salmon makes a perfect understudy, especially if you're watching your mercury levels. So go fish!

3 tablespoons olive oil

1 tablespoon fresh lemon juice

½ cup chopped fresh dill

1 garlic clove, peeled and minced

Two 8-ounce salmon fillets

4 to 6 small new red potatoes

1 tablespoon salt

½ pound haricots verts (skinny green beans), trimmed

4 eggs

1 head romaine lettuce, torn into bite-size pieces

4 ripe tomatoes, quartered

½ cup Niçoise olives or marinated black olives, drained

½ red onion, thinly sliced

1 cup Dijon Vinaigrette (recipe follows)

1. In a small bowl, whisk together the olive oil, lemon juice, dill, and garlic. Place the salmon fillets in a glass dish and pour the marinade on top. Cover the dish with plastic wrap and refrigerate for 20 minutes (up to 1 hour) before cooking.

2. While the salmon marinates, place the potatoes in a medium saucepan, add enough water to cover them by 1 inch, and bring the water to a boil over medium heat. Add the salt and cook for 12 to 16 minutes, or until you can easily insert a fork into the potatoes. Use a slotted spoon to remove the potatoes from the water. Cool the potatoes, then slice each one in half.

3. Reuse the boiling water to cook the haricots verts for 1 to 2 minutes, until crisp but tender. Drain the beans in a colander, then plunge them into an ice bath to stop the cooking. Drain the beans, then lay them on paper towels to dry.

4. Preheat the broiler. Heat a large oven-safe skillet over medium heat and place the salmon fillets skin side down in the pan. Cook for 2 to 3 minutes, depending on the thickness of the fillets. Place the skillet under the broiler and broil for 2 to 4 minutes, or until the top of the salmon is browned and the salmon is cooked to the desired doneness.

LESS FISHY FISH

- Shocking though it may seem, you will find that the less you cook fish, the less fishy it will taste, so if you're not a big fan of that real "taste of the sea," cook your fish until it is just heated through and still quite oily in the center rather than dry.

- A good rule of thumb is to cook fish for 10 minutes for every inch of thickness.

5. In a small saucepan over medium heat, bring the eggs and enough cold water to cover to a boil. Turn off the heat and let the eggs sit in the water, covered, for 12 minutes. Rinse the eggs under cold water, then peel them. Let the eggs cool, then cut in half lengthwise.

6. For each serving, lay a bed of lettuce on a large plate. Arrange the tomatoes, potatoes, eggs, haricots verts, and olives in separate sections around the plate. Scatter the onions on top. Arrange half a salmon fillet in the center of each serving. Serve the dressing on the side.

DIJON VINAIGRETTE

makes 1 ⅓ cups

½ cup fresh lemon juice (from about 4 lemons), or 6 tablespoons white wine vinegar

1 medium shallot, peeled and chopped

1 garlic clove, peeled and chopped

1 tablespoon Dijon mustard

1 teaspoon raw honey (optional)

½ teaspoon salt

¾ cup extra-virgin olive oil

¼ cup chopped fresh flat-leaf parsley

MAKE EXTRA AND store the leftovers in a glass jar for up to a week for fast salads on the go. Ooh, this is so good! Thinking about all the chopped veggies I'll use it as a dipping sauce for . . . in place of mayonnaise on sandwiches . . . as a marinade . . .

In a blender, combine the lemon juice, shallot, garlic, mustard, honey (if using), and salt. Turn the blender on high and slowly drizzle in the oil until the dressing is rich and creamy. Stir in the parsley.

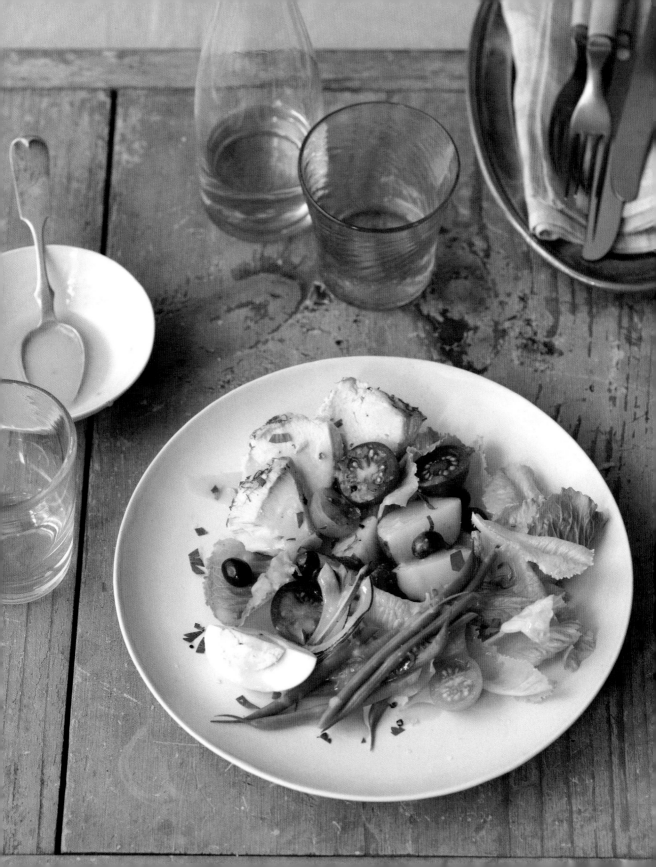

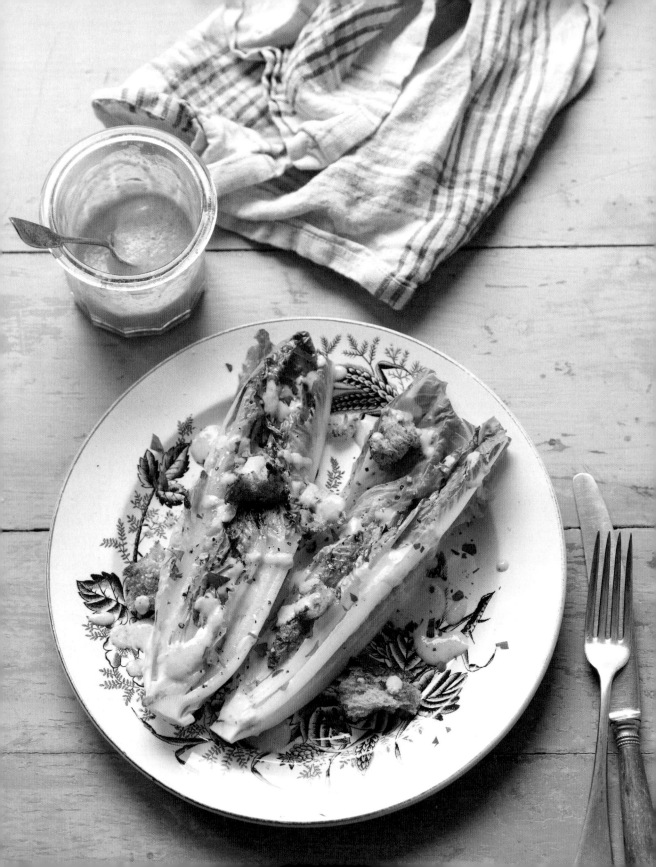

GRILLED VEGAN CAESAR SALAD

serves 4

YOU DON'T NEED ANCHOVIES or Worchestershire sauce to make a Caesar worth its weight in gold. This vegan Caesar dressing works like a charm every time—and paired with grilled romaine and homemade garlic croutons, it makes for a special weeknight or weekend affair.

2 tablespoons olive oil

3 romaine lettuce hearts, cut in half lengthwise

Sea salt

1 cup Homemade Garlic Croutons (recipe follows) or store-bought croutons

¼ cup chopped fresh flat-leaf parsley

1 cup Vegan Caesar Dressing (page 91)

1. Preheat a grill or grill pan over medium-high heat.

2. Drizzle the oil over the surface of the lettuce, sprinkle it with salt, and place cut side up on the grill or grill pan for 30 seconds, just until grill marks form. Flip and grill the lettuce cut side down for 1 minute, until it is heated but not cooked and good grill marks have formed. Remove the lettuce to serving plates and top each with a portion of croutons, some parsley, and a drizzle of the dressing.

HOMEMADE GARLIC CROUTONS

makes 2 cups

1 head of garlic

4 tablespoons olive oil

Sea salt

2 cups day-old bread (preferably whole wheat), torn or cut into bite-size cubes

1. Preheat the oven to 400°F.

2. Use a sharp knife to cut off the top quarter of the garlic bulb. Place it in the middle of a square of aluminum foil large enough to wrap around the garlic. Drizzle the garlic with 2 tablespoons of the oil and a sprinkle of sea salt. Gather the foil into a packet, leaving a small chimney vent at the top. Roast the garlic for 30 minutes, then check to see if all the cloves are tender. Use a fork to remove each clove or cool the bulb slightly and squeeze from the bottom to remove all the cloves at once. Leave the oven on.

3. In a large bowl, mash half of the roasted garlic with the remaining 2 tablespoons of oil and a pinch of sea salt. (You can use the remaining roasted garlic in the Vegan Caesar Dressing—2 roasted cloves for every 1 raw clove—or use it to flavor toast, purees, soups, and so on.)

4. Toss the bread in the oil and garlic mixture to coat all sides. Spread the bread in an even layer on a baking sheet and bake for 10 to 15 minutes, tossing periodically, until all sides are golden brown. Set the tray aside to cool the croutons.

VEGAN CAESAR DRESSING

makes 1 ½ cups

Combine the garlic, lemon juice, capers, mustard, Worcestershire sauce (if using), sunflower seeds, almonds, nutritional yeast, salt, pepper, and sugar (if using) in a blender or food processor and blend on high until well combined. With the machine running, slowly drizzle in the oil and blend until creamy; the nuts and seeds will remain slightly grainy to give the dressing texture. Refrigerate the dressing, covered, for 40 minutes. Blend again, and if needed, mix in ¼ to ⅓ cup water, to reach the desired consistency.

4 medium garlic cloves, peeled

¼ cup fresh lemon juice (from about 2 lemons)

2 tablespoons capers plus 1 tablespoon caper brine

1 tablespoon powdered mustard

A dash of vegan Worcestershire sauce (optional)

⅓ cup raw sunflower seeds

⅓ cup slivered almonds

3 tablespoons nutritional yeast (see DASH)

½ teaspoon sea salt

½ teaspoon fresh-cracked black pepper

½ teaspoon sugar (optional)

¾ cup extra-virgin olive oil

DASH

Nutritional yeast is a supplement often used by vegans and vegetarians as a valuable source of B complex vitamins, including B_{12}, and protein. (Brewer's yeast is very similar to nutritional yeast in B complex content except that it does not contain B_{12}.) Because of the lack of meat and animal products in a strictly vegan diet, the addition of these vital nutrients through supplements is crucial to cell health and energy production. Even if you aren't vegan, nutritional yeast is an excellent way to supplement your diet. I sprinkle it on popcorn and use it in this dressing to achieve a delightful nutty, cheesy flavor and rich, creamy consistency.

ROASTED BEETS WITH GOAT CHEESE, GRAPES, AND HAZELNUTS

serves 4

4 medium beets, scrubbed

2 tablespoons olive oil

Sea salt

¼ cup hazelnuts

2 ounces goat cheese

2 teaspoons finely chopped fresh chives

2 teaspoons finely chopped fresh flat-leaf parsley

Fresh-cracked black pepper

4 cups mixed baby greens or arugula (optional)

16 red grapes, cut in half lengthwise

½ cup Balsamic Vinaigrette (recipe follows)

BEETS GET A BAD RAP because they smell so awful when they're cooking, but they're incredibly good for you and sweet as can be. I actually love them shaved raw or cooked in this salad—boiled is the traditional way to go, but we're roasting in this recipe to keep all the nutrients locked in. As they cook, the beets turn tender and ultra-sweet and make the perfect pairing to tart, herbed goat cheese and crunchy toasted hazelnuts. I throw the grapes in for good measure. If you can find them, beets come in all different shades of red and gold, and the bright, jewel tones make for a gorgeous presentation.

1. Preheat the oven to 400°F.

2. Place the beets on a sheet of aluminum foil inside a glass baking dish or on a cookie sheet. Drizzle the beets with the oil and a sprinkle of salt and gather the ends of the foil into a tent, leaving a small chimney at the top of the packet for steam to escape. Roast the beets for 45 to 50 minutes, or until you can easily insert a fork into the center of each beet. Set the beets aside until cool enough to handle.

3. Lower the oven temperature to 200°F and place the hazelnuts on a dry baking sheet to toast for 10 minutes, shaking the pan intermittently, just until insides are lightly golden brown when broken open. Rub the hazelnuts together in a clean dish towel to remove any skins. Set the hazelnuts aside to cool, then coarsely chop them.

4. Meanwhile, combine the goat cheese, chives, and parsley in a small bowl and mash to combine. Season with salt and pepper.

5. Gently peel the skin from the beets and slice them into ½-inch-thick rounds. Lay the beet slices over a bed of baby greens (if using) or arrange them on salad plates. Crumble the goat cheese mixture on top and sprinkle the grapes and hazelnuts around the plate. Drizzle with vinaigrette.

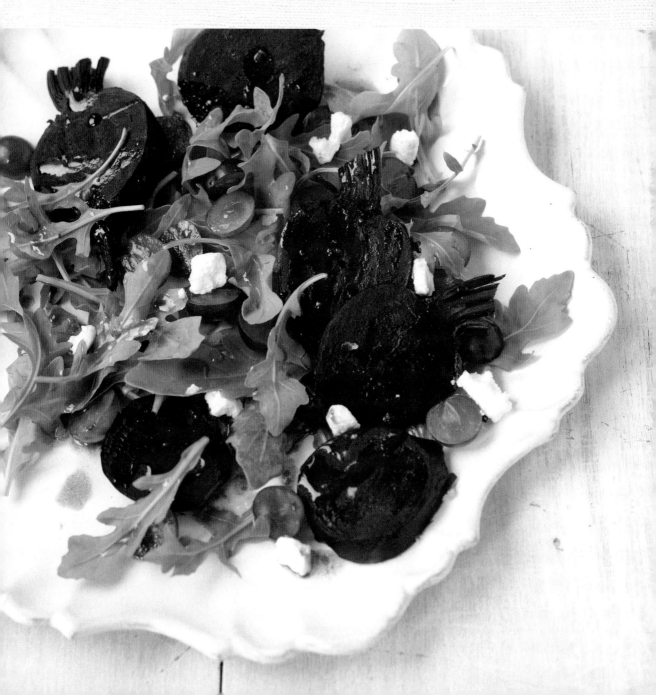

BALSAMIC VINAIGRETTE

makes a generous ⅓ cup

1 small clove garlic, peeled and smashed

2 tablespoons balsamic vinegar

2 teaspoons Dijon mustard

½ teaspoon raw honey

1 teaspoon fresh lemon juice

Sea salt and fresh-cracked black pepper

¼ cup olive oil

THIS IS A GREAT RECIPE to make in bulk and keep in a glass jar in the fridge for quick salads. The blender method will yield a thicker, creamier version. Store in the fridge in a sanitized, airtight glass jar for up to 1 week.

Place all the ingredients in the blender and blend on high until emulsified and creamy.

If making by hand, mince the garlic clove and place it and all ingredients except the oil in a bowl. Using a whisk, incorporate the olive oil into the mix in a slow and steady stream until creamy.

TURKISH KÖFTE "BURGERS"

makes 4 sandwiches (from ten to twelve 2-inch köfte)

EVERY SUMMER, we go to visit family in Turkey. Though I grew up mostly pescetarian, I couldn't resist the fragrant köfte, *or Turkish meat patties (like a flattened meatball). They're served all over the country, but are especially delicious in the southern town of Bodrum after a long day of swimming and sunning. The authentic ones are made with lamb and beef, flavored with all the aromatics of that region—oregano, parsley, garlic!—and served up alone or with spiced yogurt. This recipe is an easy way to experience their great flavor at home, without a passport.*

1. In a small bowl, combine the oregano, mint, cardamom, coriander, cumin, cinnamon, smoked paprika, and salt and mix thoroughly.

2. In a large bowl, combine the beef, onion, parsley, and egg. Squeeze the bread to remove most of the milk and add the bread to the meat mixture; mix thoroughly with clean hands to combine, squeezing the mixture to incorporate. Add the spice mixture to the beef mixture and use your hands or a wooden spoon to combine well.

3. Wet your hands with water and form 10 to 12 loosely packed patties about 2 inches in diameter, rolling the mixture into a ball between your hands and then gently patting each down to flatten to ½ inch thick. Place the patties on a parchment-lined baking sheet, pressing a thumb into the center of each patty to form a small indentation. Cover with plastic wrap and refrigerate for 1 hour.

BURGERS

1 teaspoon dried oregano

½ teaspoon dried mint

½ teaspoon ground cardamom

½ teaspoon ground coriander

1 teaspoon ground cumin

½ teaspoon ground cinnamon

½ teaspoon smoked paprika

¼ teaspoon salt

1 pound lean ground beef (or combo ground beef/lamb)

1 large sweet Vidalia onion, grated or minced

¼ cup chopped fresh flat-leaf parsley

1 large egg, lightly beaten

1 slice day-old bread, soaked in ¼ cup whole milk, just to wet

Olive oil

4 whole-wheat pita pockets, ¼ top trimmed off to make a pocket

salt

WHIPPED FETA-DILL SPREAD

4 ounces whole or 2% Greek yogurt

6 ounces feta cheese

2 teaspoons chopped fresh dill

CUCUMBER-TOMATO SALSA

2 medium plum or heirloom tomatoes, chopped

1 small seedless cucumber, chopped

¼ cup minced red onion

½ bunch of fresh flat-leaf parsley, chopped

4. To grill the köfte, preheat a grill to medium heat and brush the köfte liberally with oil. Grill the burgers about 4 to 5 minutes on each side for medium doneness, or to the desired preparation. To cook the köfte in a skillet, heat 1 or 2 tablespoons oil in a skillet over medium heat and cook the patties for about 4 minutes, or until a golden crust forms. The patties will release themselves from the pan when they have cooked, so don't move them too soon. Flip the patties and cook them for 2 to 3 minutes. The köfte should be springy to the touch.

5. Lightly drizzle both sides of the pita with oil and a sprinkle of salt and toast them in a warm oven or on a grill or grill pan until warm but not crisp.

6. To make the feta-dill spread, combine the yogurt, feta, and dill in a food processor and blend until smooth, or combine in a medium bowl and whip until smooth with a hand whisk or mixer.

7. To make the salsa, combine the tomatoes, cucumber, onion, and parsley in a medium bowl.

8. Spread each pita pocket with a quarter of the whipped feta mixture. Add 2 or 3 köfte to each, top with the cucumber-tomato salsa, and serve immediately.

DASH

You could absolutely use this recipe to make regular-size hamburgers. This mix would yield about four ¼-pound patties. Grill or pan-fry as you would regular burgers, making sure to give the köfte enough cooking time to release themselves from the pan before you flip them. Flip and cook to desired doneness, usually until only the center of the burger is a light pink (medium-well doneness).

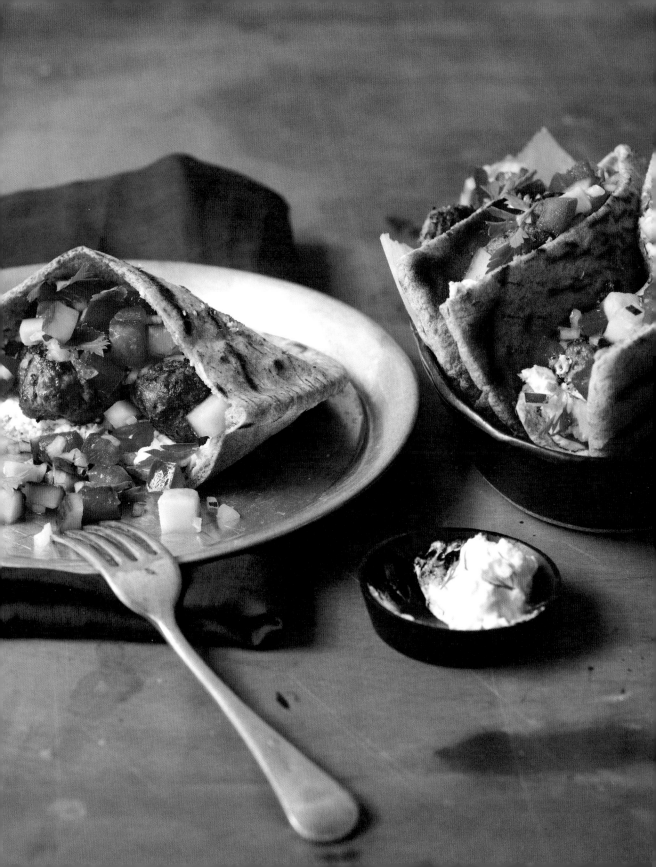

SWEET CORN SUCCOTASH

serves 4

3 ears sweet summer corn, shucked

3 cups water

Salt

½ pound green beans, rinsed and trimmed

¼ cup white wine or champagne vinegar

1 tablespoon Dijon mustard

1 teaspoon raw honey

½ teaspoon sea salt

Fresh-cracked black pepper

¼ cup olive oil

2 large shallots, peeled and minced

¾ cup chopped fresh flat-leaf parsley

1 medium tomato, seeded and chopped

¼ cup raw or smoked almonds, chopped

½ jalapeño, minced (discard the seeds and ribs if you want less heat)

1 large ripe avocado, pitted, peeled, and diced to ½-inch cubes

SUCCOTASH IS A SOUTHERN FAVORITE meant to harvest all the glory of sweet, fresh produce. This raw version lets you enjoy the same great flavor minus the time at the stove. Plus you get a ton of veggies without feeling like a rabbit. Let the Southern bells ring—and belles rejoice!

1. Remove the corn kernels by laying each cob on a flat surface and slicing down each side with a sharp knife as near to the cob as possible. Discard the cobs. Reserve the kernels in a large bowl. You should have about 2 cups.

2. Bring the water and large pinch of salt to a boil. Create an ice bath by filling a large bowl three-quarters full with ice water (2 parts water to 1 part ice). Blanch the green beans by boiling them for 1 to 2 minutes, uncovered, until tender but still crisp. Drain or scoop the beans out of the boiling water and plunge them into the ice bath to stop the cooking process. Remove the beans from the ice bath and drain them on a clean dish towel. Chop them into bite-size pieces and add them to the bowl with the corn.

3. In a separate bowl, combine the vinegar, mustard, honey, sea salt, and pepper. Slowly pour in oil, whisking vigorously to form a smooth vinaigrette. Stir in the shallots and ¼ cup of the parsley. (Alternatively, add the shallots, parsley, oil, vinegar, mustard, honey, salt, and pepper to a blender and blend until smooth and creamy.)

4. Add the tomato, almonds, jalapeño, and vinaigrette to the bowl with the corn and beans. Serve the salad garnished with avocado and the remaining ½ cup parsley.

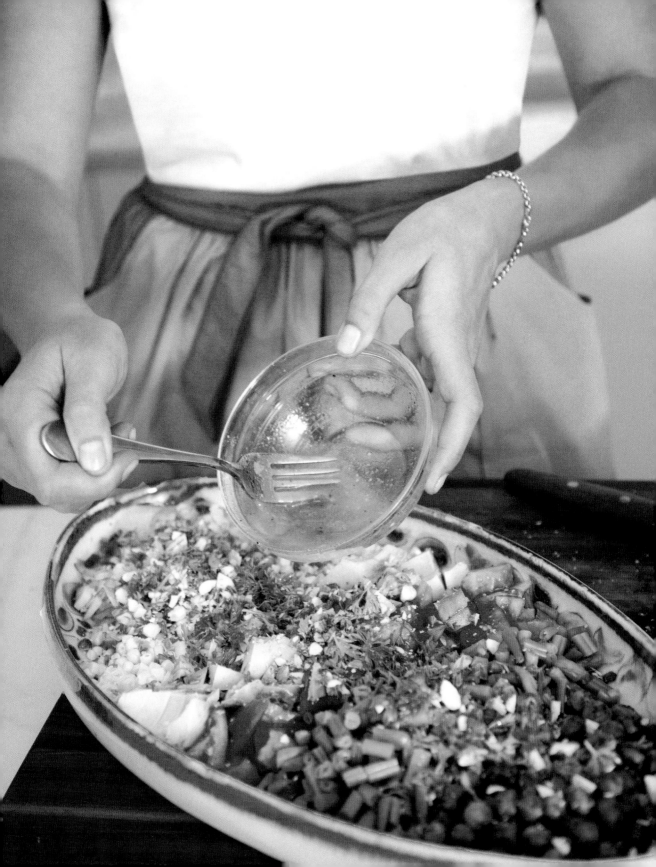

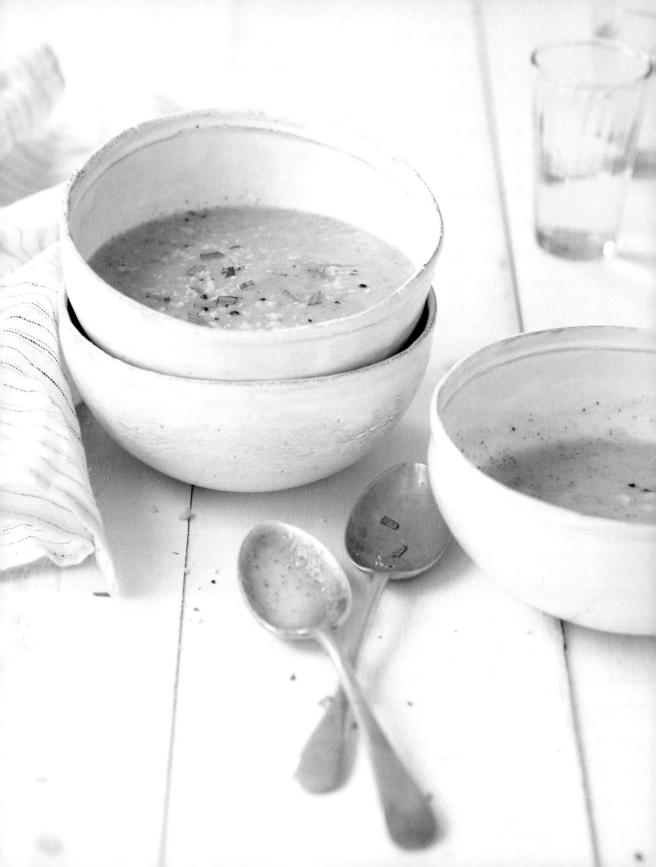

CREAMY ZUCCHINI-TARRAGON SOUP

serves 4

YUM. THIS SOUP practically makes itself, and I'm always amazed by how creamy it comes out, even when I don't add the heavy cream, which makes it even more velvety. A drizzle of white truffle oil to finish and you're verging on the spectacular.

White truffle oil is one of my extravagances that, though some will disagree, I think pretty darn near gets me the sinful sensation of eating $500 worth of white truffles for under a buck a serving. Sounds worth the purchase to me! I like one from Urbani Truffles, but any high-quality version will do.

2 tablespoons olive oil

2 garlic cloves, peeled and chopped

1 medium sweet yellow onion, chopped (about 1½ cups)

4 small to medium zucchini, chopped (about 5 cups)

2 tablespoons fresh tarragon leaves

2 cups vegetable or chicken stock or water

Sea salt

¼ cup white wine

Fresh-cracked black pepper

⅓ cup whole blanched almonds, chopped

¼ cup heavy cream (optional)

White truffle oil for garnish (optional)

1. In a large soup pot, heat the oil over medium heat. Add the garlic and onion and sauté until the onion is translucent, 2 to 3 minutes. Add the zucchini, 1 tablespoon of the tarragon leaves, 1 cup of the stock, and a pinch of salt. Bring to a boil, then reduce the heat to low and simmer, covered, for 15 to 20 minutes, or until the zucchini is soft.

2. Transfer the soup to a blender and puree until smooth, or use an immersion blender. Return the soup to the pot, add the remaining cup of stock and the wine, and return to a simmer. Cook, uncovered, for 5 minutes. Season as desired with salt and pepper and garnish with the remaining tablespoon of tarragon leaves and the blanched almonds. If you feel like living on the edge, stir in the cream and drizzle with a swirl of white truffle oil.

THE CARNIVORE'S VEGGIE BURGER

serves 6

BURGERS

3 tablespoons organic coconut oil

1 onion, diced small (about 1¼ cups)

2 raw beets, peeled and grated (about 1¼ cups)

1 zucchini, grated (about 1 cup)

3 garlic cloves, peeled and minced

About 1 cup canned pinto or black beans, drained and rinsed

1 tablespoon umeboshi paste (optional)

1 tablespoon balsamic vinegar

1 tablespoon fresh lemon juice

1 canned chipotle in adobo sauce, finely sliced, plus 1 tablespoon sauce from the can

3 prunes, chopped

1 teaspoon salt

1 teaspoon ground cumin

Leaves from 3 fresh thyme stems

(list continues)

CALLING ALL YE meat eaters! Open wide. This one's for you.

And psssst, vegetarians: You have struggled through flavorless, frozen texturized wheat gluten patties long enough. There's a new meatless burger in town. This recipe calls for umeboshi, a plum paste that adds an incredible earthy hit of umami *flavor to veggie burgers. You may omit it, but it is well worth finding at a local Asian supermarket or online! Just make sure the kiddies' ears are covered when you sink your teeth into this mouthwatering mess: Exuberant, euphoric expletives have been known to fly.*

1. To make the burgers, heat 2 tablespoons of the oil in a large skillet over medium heat and sweat the onions with a pinch of salt until they are translucent, 2 to 3 minutes. Add the onion, beets, zucchini, and garlic and stir to combine; cook 2 minutes, until softened and onion is translucent. Add the pinto beans, umeboshi paste (if using), balsamic vinegar, lemon juice, and chipotle and sauce and stir to combine. Use a fork to gently mash some of the beans as they heat. Add the prunes, salt, cumin, and thyme and stir to combine. Remove from heat and set aside to cool slightly. In a large bowl, combine the mixture with the rice, almonds, oats, egg, and bread crumbs. Cover and refrigerate the mixture for 1 hour.

=== DASH ===

Nonstick skillets won't give you the crispy crust you want here, so opt for a cast-iron or stainless steel skillet.

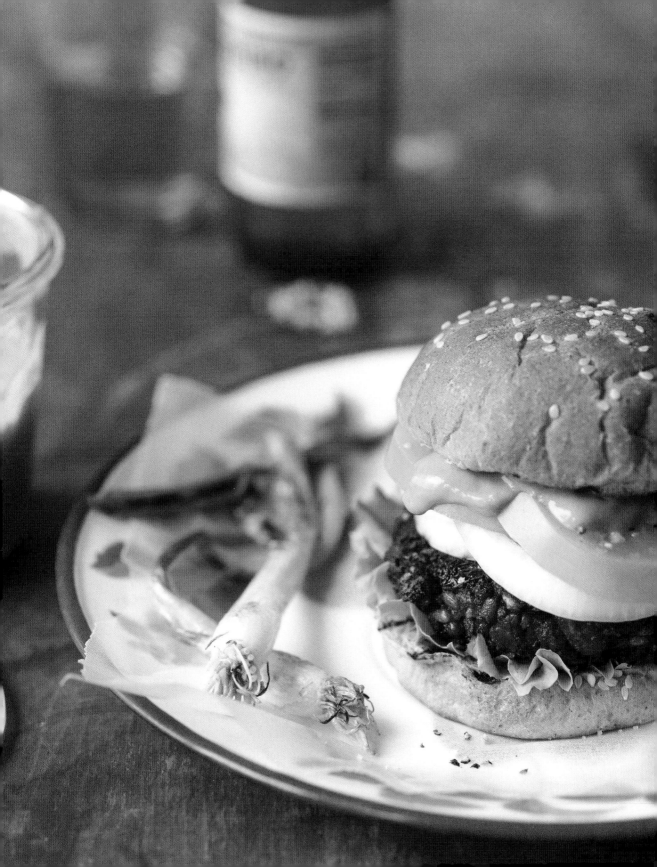

1 cup cooked brown rice
(day old is best)

¼ cup hickory-smoked
almonds, pulsed in food
processor

½ cup quick-cooking rolled
oats, pulsed in a food
processor or chopped fine

1 egg, whisked

2 tablespoons fine bread
crumbs

6 to 8 slices sharp cheddar
or Monterey Jack cheese
(optional)

HONEY-JALAPEÑO
SPECIAL SAUCE

¾ cup ketchup

¼ cup Dijon mustard

¼ cup Vegenaise or
mayonnaise

½ jalapeño, minced
(discard the seeds and
ribs if you want less heat)

1 tablespoon honey

6 whole-wheat buns

Fixings of your choice
(such as crisp lettuce,
tomato, and sliced onion)

2. Form the burger mixture into four 4-inch patties. Use your palms to shape the patties, but don't compress them. Reheat the skillet over medium-high heat with the remaining 1 tablespoon of oil. Place the patties in the skillet and cook 3 minutes. Flip, top with cheese (if using), and reduce the heat to medium. Cover the pan and cook another 2 to 3 minutes, or until a golden-brown crust forms on the bottom of your burgers.

3. To make the honey-jalapeño sauce, in a food processor, blend the ketchup, mustard, Vegenaise, jalapeño, and honey. If you prefer a chunkier mixture, you can simply combine these ingredients in a bowl.

4. Toast the buns in a warm oven. Spread the buns with the honey-jalapeño sauce and add the fixings of your choice. Top with the burgers and serve.

TOMATO TOAST

serves 4

THIS BREAD PREPARATION, *called* pa amb tomàquet, *is used all over Barcelona to make sandwiches, crostini, and tapas. This is a really simple technique for flavoring your toast and doctoring up bread that might be a little drier than you'd like. If you were at a loss for fresh ripe tomatoes, I'd bet you could make this with pureed tomato sauce. Use as bread for a sandwich of salted Parma ham and cheese like the Barcelona locals would, or let it carry a delicious bed of grilled veggies, fresh basil, and mozzarella.*

1 ciabatta, Pullman loaf, or baguette

2 garlic cloves, smashed

2 very ripe medium tomatoes

¼ cup olive oil

Sea salt

1. Split the loaf in half lengthwise and place on a sheet pan under the broiler until the top is just turning golden brown. Rub each half thoroughly with a garlic clove. Cut the tomatoes in half, and gripping one tomato half so the opening faces away from palm, rub the inside of the bread loaf thoroughly with tomato. Use all the tomato halves, making sure to squeeze plenty of tomato juice to soak the insides of the loaf. Place the toast under the broiler again, crust side down, and allow to warm through and crisp slightly (some areas can get a little bit dark, but avoid lots of black char).

2. Cut the toast into serving sizes and plate. Drizzle with oil and sprinkle with salt.

SPICY GARLIC BUTTERED SHRIMP TOAST

makes 4 sandwiches

SHRIMP

3 tablespoons unsalted butter

2 tablespoons olive oil

5 garlic cloves, peeled and chopped

1 tablespoon dried chile flakes

24 medium shrimp, peeled and deveined

⅓ cup dry white wine

Juice from ½ lemon

2 tablespoons chopped fresh flat-leaf parsley

SANDWICHES

1 avocado, pitted, peeled and thinly sliced

4 pieces Tomato Toast (recipe follows)

1 cup mixed greens, washed and dried

Sea salt

½ cup fresh pomegranate seeds (optional)

1 lemon, cut into 4 wedges

EVEN READING THIS recipe makes my mouth water. My husband and I took an overnight trip to Barcelona on the way home from a family vacation, and I made him take me to a restaurant called Paco Meralgo three times in two days so I could enjoy their take on garlic shrimp with traditional Barcelona tomato toast called pa amb tomàquet. *When I got home, I was still fiending, so I invented my own version.*

1. To make the shrimp, in a large skillet over medium heat, heat the butter and oil until oil glistens. Add the garlic and chile flakes and cook for 1 minute, stirring frequently with a wooden spoon so that the garlic doesn't burn. Just as garlic begins to turn golden, add the shrimp and cook 2 minutes on one side. Flip the shrimp and add the wine; cook, uncovered, 2 to 3 minutes, or until the wine has reduced. The shrimp are cooked when they are pink all over and the centers have just turned from translucent to opaque. Be careful not to overcook them, or they will be rubbery.

2. Toss the shrimp in a medium bowl with a squeeze of lemon juice and the parsley.

3. To assemble and serve the sandwiches, layer the avocado slices over each piece of tomato toast. Top with a small bed of mixed greens and 6 shrimp. Spoon some of the garlic butter on top, season with sea salt, and sprinkle with pomegranate seeds if desired for a burst of sweetness. A squeeze of fresh lemon juice will brighten the dish just before serving.

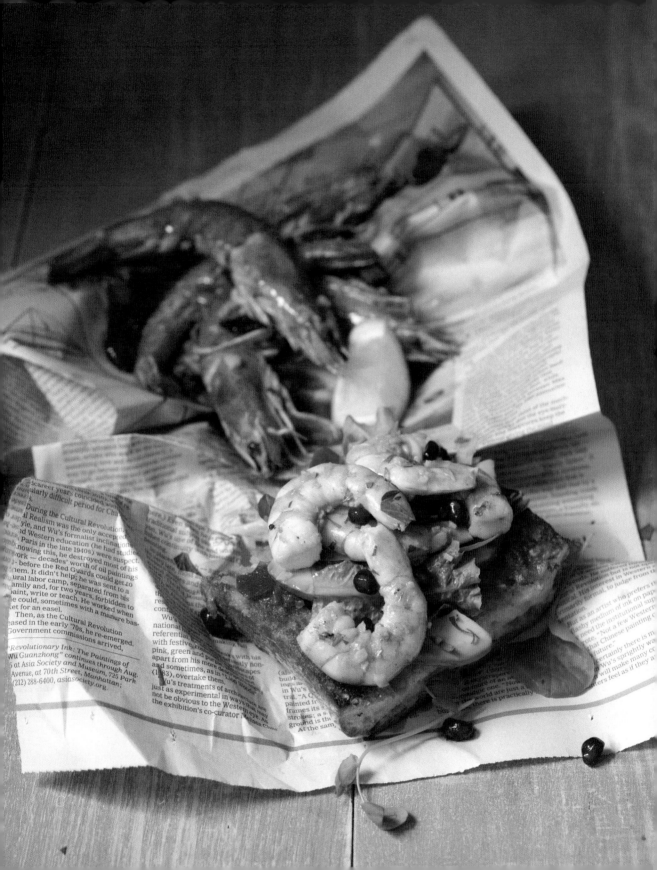

ROASTED CAULIFLOWER GRILLED CHEESE WITH JALAPEÑO AIOLI

makes 1 sandwich

1 medium onion, sliced into ¼-inch-thick rounds

3 tablespoons olive oil

¼ small head of cauliflower, sliced into flat, ⅜-inch-thick pieces

Sea salt and fresh-cracked black pepper

2 slices whole-grain or favorite bread

2 ounces aged cheddar cheese, shredded (about ¾ cup)

¼ cup baby arugula, washed and dried

½ tablespoon butter

AIOLI

1 tablespoon mayonnaise

1 small garlic clove, peeled and minced

¼ to ½ medium jalapeño, minced (discard the seeds and ribs if you want less heat)

Pinch of sea salt

YES, THIS IS AS GOOD as it sounds. Yes, you'll be writing to tell me how much you liked it. Even better, send me an Instagram of you eating it! I'm @daphneoz.

1. Preheat the oven to 425°F.

2. Add the onion and 1½ tablespoons of the oil to a medium sauté pan and cook over medium-low heat, stirring frequently, until the onion is softened and caramelized, 20 to 25 minutes. (You'll have about ½ cup of onion.)

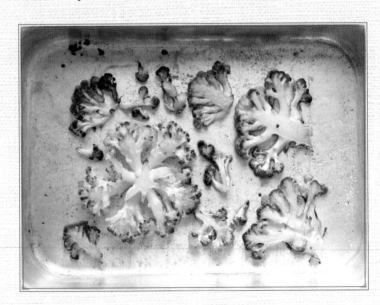

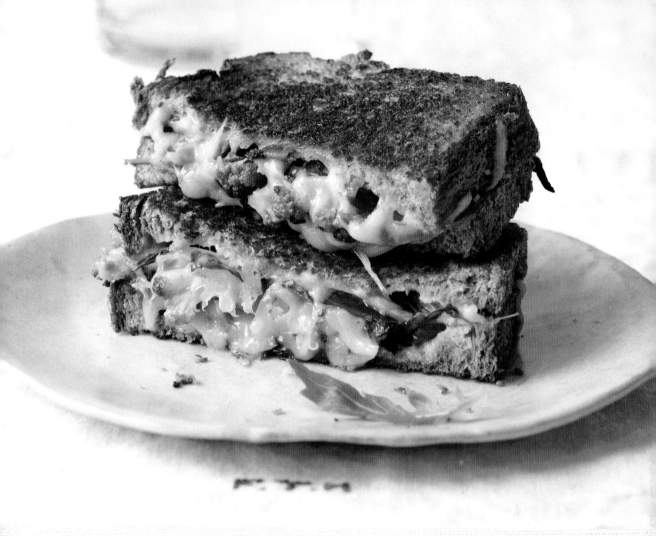

3. Gently toss the cauliflower pieces with the remaining 1½ tablespoons of oil, sprinkle with salt and pepper, and spread the cauliflower in a flat layer on a baking sheet. Roast for 10 minutes, or until lightly browned. Use a rubber spatula to flip the cauliflower, then roast another 5 minutes, or until golden brown, watching carefully to make sure the pieces don't burn.

4. Combine all the aioli ingredients in a bowl and mix well. Spread both slices of bread with aioli. Layer 1 slice with caramelized onions, roasted cauliflower, shredded cheese, and arugula. Top with the other slice of bread. Add the butter to the pan used to caramelize the onion (fewer dishes for you!), heat the pan over medium-low heat, and add the sandwich (the bread closest to the cheese layer should be on the bottom). Cook the sandwich for 4 to 6 minutes, or until the bottom is golden brown and the cheese is melting, applying pressure to the top of the sandwich with your spatula or a weighted plate. Flip the sandwich and brown the other side, about 3 or 4 minutes. Slice the sandwich in half before serving.

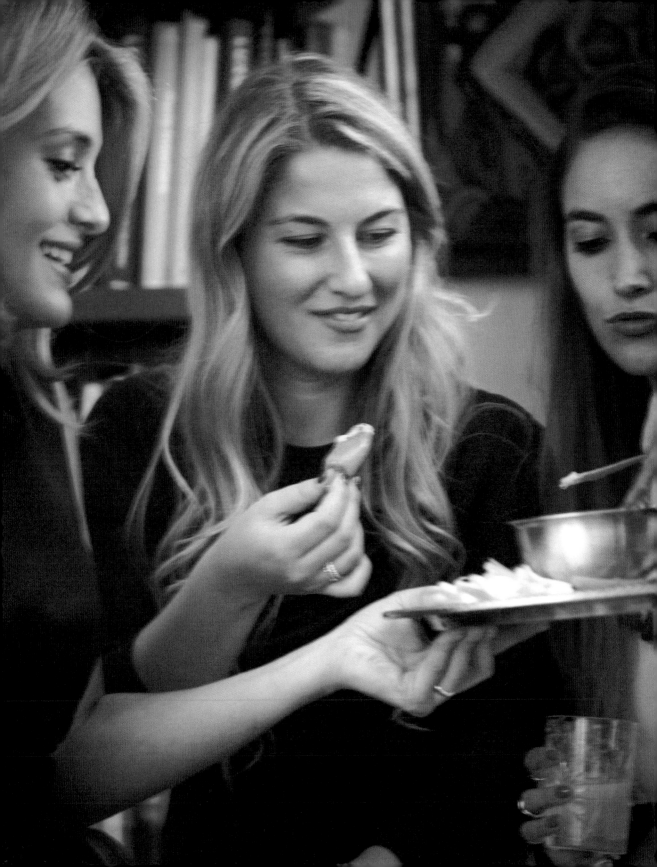

CRUDITÉ WITH DIP

I AM BIG ON SNACKING, and I like to keep flavorful, healthful items close at hand so I don't go reaching for the pretzels and chips. One of my favorite options is vegetables with dip. Simply choose your favorite vegetables, slice them up neatly, and serve them with any of the dressings from this chapter or with one of these delicious and nutritious homemade accompaniments for an instant flavor boost. Some veggies to consider: carrots, cucumbers, zucchini, peppers, radishes, snap peas, cauliflower, and broccoli.

GARLIC YOGURT DIP
Makes about 2 1/2 cups

1. Cover the walnuts in cold water and refrigerate 8 hours or overnight.

2. Drain the walnuts and chop them fine. In a medium bowl, combine the walnuts, garlic, dill, mint, oil, salt, and pepper. Mix in the yogurt, cover, and refrigerate 30 minutes to overnight to allow the flavors to combine. Or, if you prefer to use a food processor, add everything but the oil and yogurt and pulse to a mealy consistency. Drizzle in the oil and pulse to incorporate, then add this mixture to yogurt, stir to combine, and refrigerate as above.

1 cup walnut halves

4 garlic cloves, peeled and minced

3 tablespoons finely chopped fresh dill

3 tablespoons finely chopped fresh mint

2 tablespoons extra-virgin olive oil

Pinch of salt

Grind of fresh-cracked black pepper

2 cups Greek yogurt

CUMIN AND CORIANDER HUMMUS

makes 3 cups

½ tablespoon coriander seeds,
or 1 teaspoon ground

½ tablespoon cumin seeds,
or 1 teaspoon ground

Two 15-ounce cans chickpeas
(garbanzo beans), drained and
rinsed

4 medium garlic cloves, peeled

2 tablespoons tahini
(sesame paste)

1½ to 2½ tablespoons fresh
lemon juice

¾ to 1 cup olive oil

½ cup fresh flat-leaf parsley
(optional)

½ teaspoon paprika (optional)

1. To take the flavors in this hummus to the next level, use fresh-ground toasted spices. Toast the coriander and cumin seeds in a dry pan over medium-low heat, constantly moving them in the pan, until the oils release and you get a beautiful aroma, about 2 minutes. Remove the spices from the heat and cool 5 minutes. Use a spice grinder to pulse the spices to a powder.

2. Combine the chickpeas, garlic, tahini, and lemon in a food processor and blend until smooth. Turn the processor on and slowly add oil to the mixture. If using parsley and paprika, add them now and blend to incorporate. Add the coriander and cumin and blend until smooth.

3. Scoop any leftovers into an airtight container, press plastic wrap over the surface of the hummus, and cover with cap. Store in the fridge for up to 1 week.

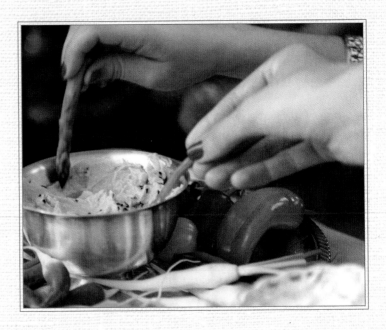

FIVE

HEAD IN THE GAME

focus, fitness, and purpose

As for the future, your task is not to foresee it but to enable it.
—ANTOINE DE SAINT-EXUPÉRY

MENS SANA IN CORPORE SANO. IF THE LATIN ISN'T RINGING A bell, the translation should. "A sound mind in a sound body" is the foundation for maximum enjoyment of food, life, love, and laughter. Relishing every moment requires keeping your mind sharp and your body strong so you can experience every moment fully. When our minds are easily distracted, when our bodies are weak and tired and prone to illness, we cannot possibly achieve our biggest—or smallest—dreams.

So are you sharp and alert, ready to pounce on every opportunity? Are you strong and fit, able to leap small curbs in a single bound, in towering stilettos no less? Or are you too stressed and busy to even think about how you're do-ing, how you're feeling, let alone answer the tougher existential questions: *Who are you? Who do you want to be? What's your purpose?*

This chapter is all about seizing the future by being totally present, alert, and aware in the now. To focus our minds, take care of our bodies, and commit to finding our purpose is to set ourselves up for the success we want. First we invest in ourselves; then we take on the world.

PRACTICING HOW WE PLAY

The way we feel influences everything inside us and around us, from our thoughts and be-havior to our work and relationships. The attitude you take toward the rest of your life starts with how you feel about yourself: a belief that your ideas are good, your feelings are valid, your work is top-notch, and you are a catch all play into the complete being you present to the world. How you see yourself also affects the way you interpret the world's response to you. In other words, self-confidence can be your greatest asset or your most debilitating missing piece.

Cultivating self-confidence doesn't—and shouldn't—happen overnight. You earn it from and for yourself by experiencing things that build you up—achievements, success—and things that might rattle you, such as disappointment and failure, growing through them and coming out stronger on the other side. Being confident is about being aware of your strengths and your weaknesses, and looking to get better rather than just more comfortable in what you're already good at.

Life is full of ups and downs, victories and disappointments, both small and large. It's also full of free will, and we make our own choices that either keep us paralyzed in unproductive patterns or propel us forward to bigger and better things. The goal is to stay focused on the positives, be fit to take on the challenges, and keep our purpose in mind so that we're always moving toward the light rather than wading in the doldrums of self-doubt.

With the right game plan, every moment can be one that brings us closer to happiness. And sometimes the right game plan is to let go of the plans you made, live off-road, and un-derstand that life is full of opportunities to jump forward or fall back without really knowing the outcome. Living in the moment, making your best bet, tapping into your subconscious, and paying attention to what we think will make us truly happy are the only guides we really have, but they're also the only ones we need.

This time in your life is not just about experimenting. It's time to make choices that define us. Create space for abundance. Practice an attitude of gratefulness and emanate self-confidence that is founded on real experience. Then if we play how we practice, we'll be in it to win. And winning is fun!

FIND YOUR FOCUS

What if I told you that you could relieve stress, relax, sharpen your mind and intuition, and fight the common cold just by doing nothing? Wouldn't you want to know how? Or would you say that you're too busy to waste your time?

Most of us spend our time doing *something*, even if it's a mindless and totally unproductive something. We have a cultural aversion to taking time to do nothing, so we keep ourselves busy. We run from here to there, entertaining others or being entertained. When was the last time you sat still without instinctively reaching for your phone in the first minute to provide distraction? Even when we're being lazy, we don't let our minds enjoy a moment of quiet.

Today I'd like to invite you to schedule in some time for nothing. The kind of nothing that takes only around ten minutes. The kind that you can do anytime to feel better and perform better with no advance planning or special equipment. The kind that proves true the old adage: The best things in life are free.

What kind of nothing am I talking about? Meditation. Meditation is an ancient practice with a lot of modern benefits. Focused thinking and breathing has been shown to help with a wide range of physical and psychological conditions, so if you're stressed by work, fatigue, or chronic pain; if you're prone to binge eating, insomnia, anxiety, or depression—all of these can be helped by daily meditation.

If you've never meditated before, not to worry. You won't have to hang upside down from a Banyan tree or sweat it out in a hot room fumigated with incense next to forty chanting bodies. You'll simply pick a comfy position in a cozy place and sit still for a few minutes, relaxing into a pure, unadulterated experience and enjoying a true break.

Whether I'm seeking problem solving, inspiration, or equanimity (otherwise known as learning how to be comfortable in uncomfortable situations), meditation is where I go to take a moment and give my mind a chance to recalibrate so I can try out a new way of thinking and seeing myself and the world. Sure, if you need a break, you can certainly pay for a day at the spa. But you might also consider taking a comfortable seat and a few deep breaths in the comfort of your own living room to achieve the same benefits.

Waiting to Exhale: Breathing Technique

Breathing techniques are your always-available, portable relaxation tool. I call this breath work "balancing breath" because it encourages you to pay attention to your breathing patterns so that you can find a steady rhythm of inhalation and exhalation. Not too fast . . . not too slow . . . just right.

1. Sit comfortably. You can sit on a chair or on a cushion with your legs crossed. If you're sitting on the floor, you'll want to make sure that your hips are above your knees. Trust me: If you aren't comfortable, you won't be focused on your breathing; you'll be thinking about your back or your neck or your butt instead. Decidedly *un*relaxing.

2. Just breathe. Begin by breathing normally to get a sense of your natural rhythm.

3. Increase your inhale. Count to four as you breathe in slowly. Count to three as you breathe out. Breathe with a long inhale for thirty seconds to a minute—but don't pass out! Work up to longer inhales and exhales *slowly.*

4. Increase your exhale. Now reverse, and breathe in slowly to a count of three, breathing out to a count of four. Breathe with a longer exhale for thirty seconds to a minute.

5. Breathe in balance. Now you'll progress to a four-count inhale, breathing to the count of four on the way in, followed by a four-count exhale, counting to four as you breathe out.

6. Extra credit. You might also try pausing for a moment with your lungs full and pausing for another moment when your lungs are empty. How does it feel to have your lungs full? How does it feel when they are empty? One might feel more or less comfortable for you. Don't judge the feelings . . . just observe them. And keep breathing!

Sitting Still: Meditation Technique

I took a course in transcendental meditation after reading about the positive effects it was having on hyperactive schoolkids who were now suddenly able to focus, excel, and cope with stress. I do have a really hard time quieting my mind, so when I meditate I keep it short and sweet: ten minutes max, lying flat on my back or in a comfy chair.

While I'm sitting or lying down, I repeat one word over and over again until I lose track and drift off. It might not be the "correct" way to do it, but I think "correct" kind of contradicts what meditation is all about anyway. Those ten minutes I carve out and take for myself to remove everything that's generally racing through my brain so I can relax, center, and calm myself are so much more valuable to my well-being than stressing to sit still for an extra ten minutes. I don't try to overthink what I "should" be feeling or thinking when I'm sitting there, and I don't "try to think of nothing" (all right, now I'm thinking again!)—I just relax and get comfortable.

Even just the act of sitting still without distraction is an incredibly calming experience. So do yourself a favor and print out the following note and tape it to your fridge or bathroom mirror, wherever you'll see it regularly:

Dear [Your Name],

Please join me this morning/afternoon/evening in the park/backyard/living room for five/ten/twenty minutes of meditation. Wear something comfortable. Drink some water. And don't forget to take a bathroom break first.

Love,
[Your Name]

Find a quiet, clean place to sit. Unless you're a really experienced meditator, the subway is not the right place to practice. Nor is a boring meeting. Letting your eyes glaze over is not meditating. Meditation is not about escaping: It's about being fully present.

Chill out. Your phone is buzzing, you've got a ton of work to do, that guy hasn't called yet, and you don't know what you're going to wear later. I get it. Hectic schedules have a way of putting us on overdrive and making everything feel dramatic and desperate. That's why you're learning to meditate—so you can see how transient all of that stuff is and reclaim your quiet confidence. Your friends can leave a message, you'll get your work done, he'll call or he won't, and you'll look great tonight. Meditating shouldn't up the frequency; it should slow it down. So let it.

Don't go from zero to sixty. If you've never meditated before, don't feel as if you have to sit there for an hour. Start with five minutes. That's right—five minutes. Set a timer, then hide your watch or your phone so you're not tempted to watch the clock. When you get really comfortable with sitting still, you can increase your meditation time.

Use your breath as an anchor. You can use the "balanced breathing" exercise above to begin your meditation. When you're breathing evenly and steadily, use the breath as a metronome to keep yourself present. Many people think that the trick to meditating is to stop thinking. That's no trick—it means you're in a coma. Our brains are working all the time. When we meditate, we're slowing down so that we can learn to watch the incessant flow of thoughts instead of reacting to them. Your synapses are always telling you a story. Listen to the story, but don't let it carry you along. I know it sounds wacky, but you'll understand once you're drifting in that dreamy, liminal space between consciousness and subconsciousness, which, by the way, is where your supreme creativity kicks in!

Be consistent. The key to a meditation practice that has long-lasting impact is to make it a regular part of your life. We all have our daily rituals: coffee with breakfast, tea in the afternoon, a glass of wine in the evening. Add a daily meditation ritual to that list, and you will ultimately reap benefits that will make you feel as good as that morning cappuccino—maybe better.

Finding Your Inner Child: Yoga Technique

I know, I know: meditation *and* yoga? Trust me on this: There's a reason all the cool (that is, fit, relaxed, glowing) kids are still doing it—and have been for centuries. Even if you've never been to a yoga class, you've likely spent time in child's pose. This relaxing position encourages reflection and focus and is an amazing way to hit pause at home, in a hotel room, in a conference room, or wherever there's enough room to get on the floor and not be stepped on. This little bit of simple yoga can help you get more centered and more creative; calmer and more peaceful. Like deep breathing, it's a free, accessible way to connect to yourself on a daily basis.

1. Begin by kneeling on a clean mat or carpeted floor, then widen your knees to shoulder width, and sit back on your heels.

2. Leaning forward, walk your hands out in front of your knees as you drape your torso over your legs until your arms and fingertips are completely outstretched.

3. Let your forehead touch the ground or a pillow.

4. Relax your hands and let your butt sink down toward your heels.

5. Breathe deeply to expand your rib cage, allowing your neck, back, and shoulder to get a nice, long stretch.

FIND YOUR FITNESS

Yoga. Pilates. Cycling. Weights. Tennis. Swimming. Whatever your favorite workout is, you've got to stick with it if you want to stay energized and alert. In your twenties, you have a lot of natural energy and your metabolism is still working with you instead of against you. All the more reason to find a workout you have fun with and give Mother Nature a helping hand in delivering you the body of your dreams. As you get older, though, things will start to shift, mostly downward—and if you want to fight gravity, keep your mind sharp, and stay strong and fit, you've got to set up a routine that keeps you limber, and stay with it. Aging gracefully is entirely up to you in this regard.

When I was figuring out how I was going to healthily, permanently shed 30 pounds in college, a lot of it boiled down to learning how to be conscious of when my body was full rather than eating with my eyes and my emotions. I also resolved to make daily exercise fit into my schedule by starting every morning with an easy, ten-minute stretching and cardio routine to limber up and get my heart pounding. It helped perk me up for 8:00 a.m. class then, and gets me off to the studio bright and early these days. By making it something short and sweet that I (almost) always have time for—sometimes the snooze button gets the better of me—I guarantee myself at least this quick calorie-burn each morning. But it also gets me thinking about my body, how I'm feeling, and what my energy level is like, and lets me consciously recommit to making health a priority in my life even if it's not an obsession. When I start my day with this routine, I'm that much more likely to make choices that prioritize my long-term health, not just my immediate satisfaction.

With this in mind, I'm always looking for ways to work easy activity into my day.

I take the stairs whenever possible. Basically, anything under ten stories I walk. I rely on walking as my primary mode of transportation (a lot easier in a city than in the suburbs but still doable for anyone!)—anything under two miles I walk, and I usually get in four to five miles a day between all my errands, walking to and from work, and strolling home after dinners out. Upping my basic daily activity helps in two ways: (1) It allows me to burn calories even on the days I can't get in a "real" workout without my even having to make a conscious effort to do it, and (2) it relieves a ton of stress and chronic pain that comes from sitting still and being trapped indoors all day.

Of course, active bodies also need to break a real sweat—ideally three to five times a week for at least thirty minutes. I've never been a gym rat, and I hate pounding away on treadmills, so I had to hunt for some workouts that gave me a thrill.

It turns out that even though I have no coordination, and some would say (ahem, my *Chew* cohosts) I'm a terrible dancer, I absolutely love spinning classes because they are basically dance parties on a bike. It's a killer forty-five-minute routine that I can fit in two or three times a week and feel really good about. Because it's a fairly aggressive workout, I like

TEN-MINUTE STRETCHING AND CARDIO ROUTINE

1. First things first: get your heart pounding. One minute of jumping rope in place. Go.

2. Next, 10 push-ups, then 15 sit-ups. Repeat 4 times.

3. Get into upward facing dog position (hold for 15 seconds), glide through upper pushup position (hold for 15 seconds) to downward facing dog (hold for 15 seconds). Glide back through upper push-up position to upward facing dog. Repeat for 2 to 3 minutes. These are very well-known yoga poses with tons of great tutorials available on YouTube if you want some pointers!

4. One more minute of jump rope!

5. Fifteen deep lunges with your left leg in front, stepping your feet back together in between each lunge. Fifteen deep lunges with your right leg in front, stepping your feet back together in between each lunge.

6. Lie on the floor with your eyes closed for 1 minute (or however long you have!) and breathe deeply, letting vital oxygen fill your lungs completely with each inhale and emptying them completely with each exhale. Start your day centered and ready.

to balance it out with more calming yoga or strengthening and toning routines other days of the week. I still get that dreadful "I don't want to work out today!" feeling every time I'm putting my workout clothes on, but I tune out that voice, march myself over, and walk out riding high on the endorphin buzz.

Taking time to sweat gives you an opportunity to zone out while still feeling productive. For me, working out clears my head and often gives me the break I need if I've really been chewing a problem over to the point that I'm just not seeing any new perspectives. Working out boosts blood flow to the brain, endorphins (our happy hormones so you get the real-deal high), and the immune system, and it obviously kills calories, which is of course the reason we schlep over there even when it's the last thing we feel like doing. It's funny, but even though I generally hate the idea of having to work out, once I get the clothes on, I love how I know I'm going to feel immediately after it's done.

So which one will it be, ladies? Are you an "intends to" or a "does" kinda gal? Building fitness into a routine creates habit—the kind of habit we all want and need. A body in motion stays in motion! So if you want to feel energized instead of lethargic, lean instead of puffy, amazing instead of *ehhh*, grab a friend, get off that couch, and hit the courts, the street, the field. Anything that gets you moving fits the bill as long as you stop intending to go and start actually going.

After your workout, you'll be primed to go after whatever it is that your little heart desires. Here are some tips for getting started and maintaining your schedule over the long run:

Choose something you enjoy. If you absolutely hate running, jogging should not be your go-to workout. Same goes for anything that you don't look forward to: If you don't like it, you won't stick with it. So make it fun and make it convenient! What do you enjoy? If it's hiking, go hiking. If it's yoga, find a studio with teachers you like and respect. I adore my indoor cycling workout, but even that can be hard to get into when I'm totally exhausted, so I mix it up with yoga or strength training or even just a long walk. When exercise is fun, it makes it more likely that you'll opt for the sweat instead of the sweets.

Make sure it's easy to get to. Do you like hiking, but you live in the middle of a big city where mountains and forests are two hours away? Then hiking can be a hobby, but it cannot stand in for your fitness routine, unless long-distance driving is another thing you love. Save the hiking for when the opportunity arises, but a regular routine requires something you can access on the regular without major travel time, expense, or other barriers.

Create a schedule. Just like you'd never see your best friend if you didn't make plans to meet for brunch or visit your dentist without an appointment, you'll never get to yoga class if you don't put it in your calendar. Between your smartphone and your laptop and your desktop and that daily planner your aunt got you for Christmas, there's no excuse not to type it in, pencil it in, and set an alarm to make sure you get up and at 'em when the allotted time arrives. Building positive habits requires doing things more than once, more than twice, more than three times . . . If you can get yourself out the door in your sneaks regularly for a few weeks, you'll know that you are on the path to positive habits that become second nature rather than a regular battle with yourself of to go or not to go. The key to replacing poor habits with good ones is to make them fun, practical, and regular.

Don't overdo—or underdo—it. Working out is crucial; working out too much is a crisis waiting to happen. Sprains, muscle tears, and exhaustion are side effects that none of us needs. So plan your fitness according to your fitness levels, and save the heroism for Superman. Once a week, of course, is not enough. Do you sleep once a week? Do you eat once a week? Exercise is a bodily need, so make sure you sweat it out three to five times a week. Do it for you. Do it for fun. Do it so you can feel the burn, get over it, and feel incredible afterward . . . And for those of you who work out so you can eat what you like, do it for the love of a great meal!

Keep it interesting. Your body is smart, and doing the same workout over and over again bores it to tears, and when it loses interest, you stop getting the results you want. Different fitness routines offer different benefits and keep your muscles engaged so you keep getting stronger and leaner. Like you'd do with a date: Leave your muscles guessing and you'll have them giving you their best and wanting more.

GET YOUR ZZZZZS

Want to have the energy you need to slam through your to-do list? Get enough sleep. Schedule a nap instead of a lunch date, or pick a morning to sleep in. Even a twenty-minute nap can be restorative, so steal a little shut-eye when you need it.

If you get your six to eight hours, you'll feel—and see—the difference. Studies show that people who get plenty of sleep have an easier time maintaining healthy weights, are better able to cope with stress, can tap into their creativity more easily, and most important, don't get dealt the hideous under-eye bags so many of us are running around with! Plus sleep is the major way we increase growth hormone, the main stimulant to staying vibrant as we age.

Extra credit: Whenever you can, go to bed early (sleep before midnight is twice as rejuvenating as sleep after Cinderella's carriage has turned back into a pumpkin again).

Relax. Try lavender essential oil before bed on temples and bottoms of feet, mixed with a small amount of carrier oil like jojoba or coconut, to induce relaxation. You could also try an easy-dispensing hydrosol: These are floral waters that are steam distilled to create a less-concentrated form of the essential oil. They have antiseptic, soothing properties, so a quick spray over your face before bed has the double benefit of gentle skin toning while perfuming you with a delicious, calming scent like rose geranium or chamomile cucumber. I especially like the ones from Mountain Rose Herbs (www.mountainroseherbs.com).

Snuggle up. Research shows that people sleep best in cool rooms with warm blankets, so open the windows or kick up the AC and get comfy with your comforter. You may also find that keeping your extremities warm helps you sleep deeper, so put some socks on those pedicured piggies! Even better, slather on some richly hydrating cream and cover them up with white cotton socks for a DIY pedicure while you sleep.

DOCTOR, DOCTOR

Even if you always wake up early to get a run in, it's still a good idea to see the doctor now and again. I asked my dad, Dr. Mehmet Oz, what his baseline recommendations would be for doctor's visits for women in their twenties and thirties. Here's what he had to say:

Internal medicine. As long as you see your gynecologist annually, doctor's visits are not officially necessary, though it makes sense to have a relationship with an internist who can keep track of any chronic illness or pain and ensure everything is running smoothly. Seeing him or her once a year is plenty.

Ob/Gyn. Go every year. This is an absolute must. Once a year, you should be getting a pelvic exam (with periodic pap smears) to check for infection, make sure your cells look healthy, and keep an eye on any potentially irregular ones that could indicate a more serious condition. For most women, their ob/gyn is their primary care physician, so he or she should be up to date on any medications you're taking, any recent surgeries or illnesses, and the rest of your medical and family history. If your ob/gyn thinks another expert should take a look at you, you'll be referred to a specialist, but the ob/gyn is a great first line of health defense and a resource for all your health questions.

Dermatologist. Choose one of your more detail-oriented friends to check you for new spots and dots once a year—and make sure they get an eyeful. Your whole body, please! And then be sure to return the favor. Take a picture of any new moles next to a coin to help you gauge size changes in the future. You should see a dermatologist if you believe you have a disease of the skin, hair, or nails, or if you find any unusual or suspicious-looking moles, marks, or spots on your skin. You should also see a dermatologist if you have risk factors for skin cancer, such as a family history of the disease or fifty or more moles on your skin. And if a mole or spot that used to be circular suddenly gets larger than the size of a pencil eraser or becomes irregularly shaped or bordered and darkened, get thee to a dermatologist!

Dentist. Get those snappers professionally cleaned and shined up every 6 to 12 months. A good dentist will check your teeth for tumors, cavities, and any particular staining or wear down that could mean you're grating your teeth in your sleep (often a sign of stress). And remember to floss daily, and brush twice a day for 2 minutes (sounds like a long time, but no one says you can't be watching *Game of Thrones* while you're brusha-brusha-brushing!).

Eye doctor. If you have any issues, make an appointment immediately. If you get frequent headaches, it may be a sign you're putting too much strain on your eyes, so it's a good idea to go for an exam once every couple of years even if you don't wear glasses or contacts.

Listen close. I loved listening to books on tape as a kid. Zoning out and listening to a familiar story—not a new one or a thriller so you're tempted to stay awake to hear the shocking ending—helped stop the racing trains going through my head. And it still works today. Especially when I'm traveling, books on tape are my go-to soporific.

Take notes. Keep a pen and paper or documentation device by the bed so you can jot down to-dos you remember just as you're dozing off—relieving your brain of all the managerial work it does during the day will help you both catch some zzzzzs.

Try this sleeping aid. If you find yourself tossing and turning, melatonin and calcium-magnesium supplements can

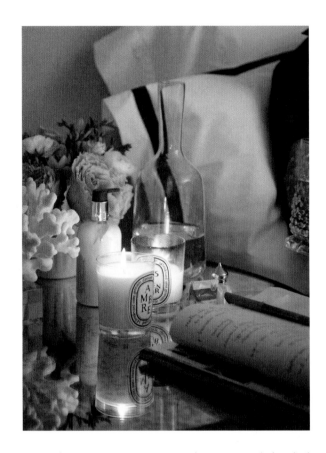

help you relax and regulate sleep cycles. Or give this sweet, warm smoothie a try! It's loaded with calcium, magnesium, and potassium, and the warm milk is sure to have you drifting on cloud nine in no time.

SWEET DREAM SMOOTHIE

½ cup warm milk
½ banana, at room temperature
¼ teaspoon ground cinnamon
½ teaspoon pure vanilla extract
1 teaspoon pure maple syrup or raw honey (optional)

Combine the milk, banana, cinnamon, vanilla, and syrup (if using) in a blender and whirl until frothy and smooth. Drink before going to bed.

FIND YOUR PURPOSE

Taking care of the physical body is only part of taking care of yourself. Making sure you're mentally and emotionally nourished, too, is equally important, especially for a lady relishing her life! To feed your interior life, you have to first figure out who you are, what you stand for, and what your purpose is so you can live a life with meaning. But how does one do this exactly?

Here's what I do know. You don't have to go to Africa to find yourself. You don't have to quit your job, live out of a van, and drive cross-country to get in touch. You don't have to share a flat with François in Paris for a season, painting still lifes of croissants (even though they're delicious and certainly worthy of such adoration) to be artistic. You don't have to go to church or synagogue or mosque to be spiritual. These kinds of experiences can be helpful because, by totally uprooting or giving structure to our lives, they help us reorganize, prioritize, and make sense of everyday life. But you don't need these things to find center. You can achieve the same results sitting in the comfort of your living room if you're willing to do the self-work it takes to cut through the clutter in your life.

You just have to commit to an experience, a value, and a path. Once you have these things, you're living with purpose. Purpose is about feeling useful, valuable, and important. People with purpose know what they want, what they wake up for every morning, what gives their lives meaning—and they don't waste time on things that don't somehow feed this big-picture life.

They also recognize that purpose is flexible. Right now, your purpose might be to volunteer at an orphanage in Tibet, or it might be to get the promotion at work you've been gunning for, or it might be to study the poems of Mary Oliver, or it might be to be a better wife/mother/lover/friend in x, y, and z ways. But that could change overnight! Your purpose does and should adjust as the goals of your life do—and as the lessons you need to learn evolve with you, so will the experiences you have to go through to learn them.

Sometimes it's those very situations that we most want to escape that are pointing us directly toward our purpose. In my case, my struggle with weight led me to learn and research easy, practical health solutions I desperately needed. Applying these principles in my own life, and learning how to balance wanting to love my life and enjoy great food with wanting my health back, led me to write *The Dorm Room Diet*. Doing a book tour gave me an opportunity to see the world and practice sharing usable, fun health information that people could incorporate to make their lives better every day.

The media exposure and experience I got as a result of doing book publicity landed me an audition for my job on ABC's *The Chew*! And the fact that I personally knew exactly how difficult it can be to find a healthy balance when you love food (perhaps a bit too much) and that I'd succeeded in doing just that because I loved figuring out how to make the smart, healthy choices easy for myself and for others got me the gig of a lifetime.

Instead of continuing to feel inadequate because I'd been overweight, I was able to reframe the process as one in which I fought a personal battle and triumphed, which is often the hardest (but most rewarding) kind of win. Even better, here was my purpose, waiting for me to start living it. The only thing I'd had to do was was run with opportunities and be open to good things coming out of difficult situations.

Our life's journey teaches us lessons and strips away layers of ourselves so it's easier for us to see what's going on inside. But you might be able to spare yourself some of that searching—and the angst, pain, boredom, and anxiety often associated with it—if you figure out where to look for the answers, learn the lessons early on and quickly, and keep pushing forward. All of these self-discovery experiences only exist to teach you more about yourself—if you like who you are, it should be fun!

To get going, start with a mission statement: At their founding, most companies outline why they exist, what they hope to create, and, in some cases, how they plan to do it. So treat yourself like a successful business and, as part of your New Year's resolutions—or today—write out your mission statement: What is your life's purpose, what are your goals, and how do you plan to accomplish them? Once a year, update this statement to reflect all the new developments of your life. Then invest fifteen minutes one day a week to considering and putting down finite goals that will help you live out the purpose you've set for yourself. There should be some goals you can accomplish within the week and some goals that are a bit more long-term on your list. But put your brain in the mind-set of thinking meaningfully about your life and bring yourself back to this place each week. Here are some great ways to start finding your purposeful path:

Take a gut check. Own your mind and you own your fate; let it control you and you'll wind up under the covers with a pint of ice cream. Start thinking about what really matters to you. Why do you get out of bed in the morning? What do you want to accomplish while you're here on this planet? I want you to think identity, not image; purpose, not paycheck; partner, not pretend boyfriend. Figure it out in your head and get that self-confidence going because you are exactly who you tell yourself you are, so be kind, be honest, and be ambitious—life is too short to aim low.

Pull the plug. How many hours a day do you spend reading through social media online? The more time we spend looking at other people's lives through a screen, and living in other people's universes, the more we're tempted to wish we had their lives, could go to their parties, knew their friends. The less time we spend reading other people's gloating social media missives, the more time we have to actually be creating tweet-worthy lives for ourselves!

Why are we so quick to make comparisons? Who cares what everybody else is doing? Take your life back. Throw your own parties. Quit feeling like you're living on someone else's totem pole. Create your own totem pole, offline, in your Real Life. Trust me, people are *way* more curious about what they don't know than what they do, so deactivate, go rogue, and see where it takes you! It might be hard to sum up what happens in 140 characters.

Ask questions. Give yourself space. Try things. Get outside your comfort zone. And then pay attention to that tiny voice inside that says, *This feels right.*

Choose your values carefully. There are plenty of successful people who will tell you that in the long run it was the struggle getting there that gave them the most satisfaction. When they were up-and-comers, they had a goal to focus on: They were getting better, learning new things, keeping life interesting. Some manage to hold on to these things—curiosity and humbleness—even after they've had success, and they're probably much happier than the ones who let things fall by the wayside (relationships, introspection) in the effort to make green mountains—and now, they have a gold-plated toilet seat to keep them warm at night.

Those who managed to balance family, work, and personal growth perfectly did this by choice and effort, not accident, and there are only so many hours in the day, so you can rest assured they had to make their share of compromises, too. Make sure you choose wisely where you pour your energies, because the fruit you plant today is the juice you'll be drinking tomorrow. So make it sweet!

MAKE IT HAPPEN

Whatever "it" is, "it" can be yours. So make a decision. Take a chance. Trust yourself! Quit waiting for things to happen to you or for your life to make perfect sense! Moving forward begins now, today, not tomorrow in some imaginary future. There's no such thing as the "perfect moment," which means the perfect time to start making anything happen is now.

TURNING CHALLENGES INTO TRIUMPHS

Life feels most overwhelming when we see circumstances as only ever happening to us, when the reality is that you are not the first person to struggle with your problems, and you (sadly) won't be the last. If you can see challenges as learning opportunities instead of roadblocks, you're already ahead of the curve. Try to experience these momentary disappointments in your life as growth spurts rather than crushing defeats. If you don't let negatives in your life define you, they won't. Even better, if you can turn them into positives, they actually can help you.

The truth is that sometimes situations that seem as if they'll drag us down ultimately pull us up. You got dumped by that crappy toad boyfriend, and it freed you up to get swept off your feet by Prince Charming. You didn't get the job you thought you wanted, so you had the free time to join a friend's road trip and ended up finding your new home and a new life altogether. You flunked chemistry, so you became an English major and won a Pulitzer Prize, or maybe you just decided to write novels in a cottage by the shore. And you're happy!

Take, for instance, the years I spent feeling like the heavy girl in the room even after I'd lost the weight. Being overweight as a kid, and my struggles first with failing to lose weight and then ultimately with being successful and regaining my health, defined a major part of my identity when it no longer had to. I was still hung up on the insecurities I felt before I succeeded in getting back on track. Holding on to those hang-ups was just like wearing a mental fat suit.

Realizing that I was self-sabotaging when I should have been celebrating was a big turning point in my relationship with myself, and in my ability to be comfortable and happy in my relationships with other people. Instead of feeling insecure and needy, I learned to come to the table feeling abundant and complete, which made me a better friend and partner and a happier individual.

Of course, this wasn't an overnight process. As I visited college campuses around the country on the book tour for *The Dorm Room Diet*, I told my story again and again: How I let food control my life, felt overwhelmed and frustrated by constantly failing to lose weight, and overate to help myself feel better. Everywhere I went, I found people who were in exactly the same situation as I had been. Instead of seeing it as a shortcoming, I realized that my own struggle with weight gave me the tools I needed to help others establish a new happy relationship with food.

Over the course of your life, you're going to encounter many unexpected challenges—it's what you do with them that matters. Do you feel overwhelmed and paralyzed by them, or do they motivate you to see the silver lining in every scenario?

The best thing to do: Live in love, not fear. Embrace failure, try anyway, and do it better next time. And remember: Nothing is stronger than you are. You are part of a bigger picture. Life is good. You can make it great.

Be a self-starter. If you want to maximize this moment, it's up to you. If you want to find happiness, it's up to you. Searching for happiness is not greedy or selfish; it's an inalienable, human right. Frankly, no one else can ever make you happy; it's your attitude, your choices, your hard work that's going to get you there. If you're not going to prioritize this pursuit, who will?

Be productive. I'm a list maker. I get some sick pleasure out of writing lots of one-line directives for myself and then crossing them off one by one. I have lists for things I have to do at home, things I have to do at work, things I have to do in life. Sometimes I even make lists of things I've already completed, just so I can tick them off. I also make lists of fun things, like restaurants I want to eat at and stores or exhibits I want to visit, hotels I like, and any inspiration blogs or websites—I take playtime very seriously.

So imagine my joy in discovering that one of the key underlying habits of successful people is that they write down things if they want to remember them! They don't trust their frazzled brains to remind them at eleven o'clock at night as they're fitfully trying to get some shut-eye. If they care about something or it's important, they put it on a list and make sure it gets done. They are *organized* about the things they care about. And they give themselves a break from having to remember by putting it down on paper, in a phone, on a computer, in an email, or wherever suits them best. A more productive you means more efficient work time and more relaxing playtime!

Congratulate yourself for what you've already done. As a society, we're always looking for ways to get better—our constant capacity for self-improvement is beautiful! But it's equally important to prize our natural abilities, praise ourselves, celebrate our strengths. So make a list of your proudest accomplishments, and then admit that you're kind of freaking awesome. Being aware of your achievements and successes and being able to express them clearly to others is a big part of "stumbling" across new opportunities.

Quit worrying. When people ask me my greatest regret, it's all the time I wasted worrying. No one has ever solved anything by festering over possible outcomes, past events, or great unknowns they have no control over. So now, when I catch my brain stuck in a loop of pity-party Muzak, I ask myself if I can think myself toward a solution. If it's in my control to change something, I do. If not, I let it be and move on.

If you fall down, get back up. Sometimes the road to utopia has a few potholes. None of us is in control of the world around us! Not every résumé gets a callback. Not every relationship turns into a walk down the aisle. Not every friendship lasts forever. Disappointments abound, from little things (a broken heel) to major flops (a broken heart) to the really sad stuff (the death of a loved one).

We can't *stop* things from happening, but we can *accept* that they happen and that they happen to *everyone*. Many of these are part of the human experience, and watching ourselves becoming wiser and more empathetic from these events helps us manage life's challenges and all the emotions that come with them. Then we can start to process things a little better each time. We learn from our mistakes, look for the silver lining, and keep moving toward a happier place.

Identify your values. When one of the great mentors of my young adult life passed away when I was just out of college, I thought about him and his impact a great deal. After his death, as his family went through his belongings, they discovered an incredible essay he'd written as a high school student. He wrote about the pursuit of happiness and listed the things he hoped to achieve if his life was to be considered a success: great love, great loss, great gifts to others, great accomplishment for himself.

Well, his life was indeed a great success, and his words found me at a time when I was just beginning to search for the tools to create a rich, vibrant life myself. They struck me as incredibly insightful and probing, especially given that he was only seventeen when he wrote them. Most impressive was his wisdom to know that a life woven with passion and purpose—for experiences of every kind—would always be rich and vibrant. I strive to live with these principles in mind every day.

Be grateful. Being grateful is free, it's easy, and it's something that, ironically, benefits you more than anyone else. Practicing an attitude of gratefulness—for every little experience and thrill and heartbreak and triumph that build your life into something worth remembering—is the greatest gift you can give yourself. Even better if you can give this gift to others. Being of service and sharing your happiness is sure to bring more smiles all around!

When people talk about having a happy attitude, what they mean isn't that these people only ever have good things happen to them. They mean that these people only focus on the good in things. So make this your life's motto: Live happy. You deserve it. Now take a deep breath and get ready to show your best face to the world, pretty bird!

SIX

ALL DONE UP

*expert tips to help you
look good and feel great*

Over the years I have learned that what is important
in a dress is the woman who is wearing it.
—YVES SAINT LAURENT

NOW THAT YOU'RE FEELING IT ON THE INSIDE, WHAT ABOUT owning it on the outside? Women want to look good. Ever since Cleopatra smeared some crocodile dung on her face to brighten her complexion, women have been rubbing oils in their hair, slathering on the lotion, and pinching their cheeks to do the most with what their mommas gave them. And you know what? All that effort to try to get glowy, youthful, and superpretty may pay off, because sleek hair and glowing skin make women appear to be fertile, which subconsciously attracts men. We're still just animals! And modern research shows that people who are considered attractive tend to do well at work and have success dating. So that extra five minutes in the mirror may be time well spent after all, as long as you don't go all Narcissus on me.

It only takes one glance at a magazine rack to realize what a national obsession our attractiveness is. Keep hair frizz free! Look great in a bikini! Make your boobs look bigger (or smaller)! Make your butt look smaller (or bigger)! Take years off your face! But it's not just about always looking like you've just left the salon. All this focus on looks negates the most important part of being as gorgeous as you are: how you feel on the *inside.*

Don't think feeling gorgeous matters? Think again. There's an idea called the self-fulfilling prophecy that's been floating around for a little while now. A Stanford University social psychologist named Elliot Aronson posited that the way we see ourselves, complemented by the responses we get from the people around us, is a major factor in personal and professional success. That means, in essence, other people will see us the way we see ourselves and will treat us accordingly. Basically, it's one big mind game—but the first person you have to convince is yourself.

So yes, eat right and work out because you like the way it makes your muscles feel and your clothes fit. But also take time to appreciate the results, and give yourself a pat on the back for making it happen. Dress up and doll up because you can, not because you have to. Focus on, embellish, and appreciate your best qualities, because the more you like what you see in the mirror, the more you'll emanate that confidence and sparkle to others, and the more they'll treat you like the crown jewel you are!

Before you leave home for the day, make sure that you feel comfortable in your clothes and that your makeup is highlighting your natural beauty, not hiding your face. And then relax! Quit worrying about whether your blemish is totally hidden, whether your dress looks tight, whether you're wearing too much—or too little—makeup. I promise: It's how you feel that really registers when you walk into a room. Whatever you're thinking about, that's what you're projecting—no one will even notice your gorgeous new do if you're not owning it from the inside out. Once you've arrived at your destination, check your self-consciousness at the door and radiate the serene grace you want other people to see. Even if it's not there yet, as they say: fake it 'til you make it. Because beauty is only skin deep, but *confidence* goes all the way through.

Let's start with a blank canvas: You in your pajamas, fresh out of bed. Make feeling beautiful part of your daily ritual by creating time to invest in yourself at the start and finish of each day. Tresses first . . .

PRETTY HAIR

Don't be a washout. Wash your hair as infrequently as possible. It might sound gross, but shampoo can strip your hair and make it dull. Since grease is best for French fries, avoid it by using a dry shampoo powder in between scrubs (which also gives hair great texture and body). Curly girls: try "shampooing" a few times a week with conditioner only for soft, fresh waves.

Go deep. Once a week, you'll want to use a deep-cleansing shampoo to get all the styling gunk off your scalp and strands and follow with a deep conditioning hair mask, especially if you color your hair and often use styling tools. Color and heat can strip your hair of vital oils and ultimately leave it looking dull and brittle. A weekly hair mask is a must for swimmers, beach lovers, bottle blondes, and anyone who uses a blow-dryer or a straightening or curling iron.

Soften up. This is an expert tip from my very clever hairdresser, Jeanna, that never fails to get my tresses happy and healthy. Run melted coconut oil through your hair and sleep in a shower cap. The next morning, shampoo, condition, and style as usual for ultrahydrated, protected locks!

Warning! Never touch the nose of a hair dryer to the surface of your hair—it gets searing hot and can burn it right off, leaving you with frayed ends and flyaways.

Embrace casual chic. Updos and blowouts are beautiful, but we can't be perfectly coiffed every single day. If there's a morning where you're on the run, learn how to dress up a casual do—a bun or pony or braid style—in a way that works for you. I'm a big fan of the ballerina bun or French braid. That way, if you oversleep and you have a meeting in five, you can get there in time and still look pulled together.

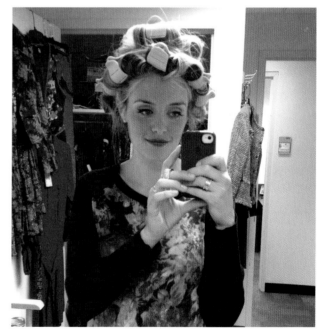

Getting ready in my dressing room at *The Chew*. Not exactly a casual hairstyle, but hot rollers are the best way to give my hair bouncy body and style memory—meaning I get a great hairdo for days!

PRETTY NATURAL

When it comes to getting pretty, natural is always my first choice. I hate the idea that most common cosmetics are loaded with artificial dyes and fragrances, not to mention tons of toxic chemicals and silicones you do *not* want to be slathering on your skin day after day—remember, it's your biggest organ and will absorb everything! Here are a few of my tried and tested, all-natural homemade substitutes for a radiant face, silky hair, soft skin, and pampered toes!

RADIANT SKIN MASK

½ ripe banana, mashed

½ cup Greek yogurt

2 tablespoons ground flaxseed or ground almonds

1½ teaspoons raw honey

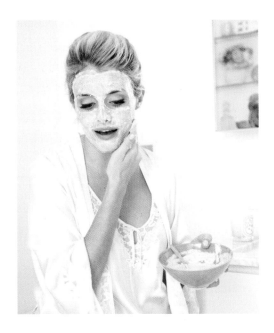

Combine all the ingredients in a bowl. Apply to clean skin in a circular motion to help the ground flaxseed or almonds exfoliate dead skin cells. Allow to sit 10 minutes, then remove with a warm, wet washcloth. The minerals in bananas help to fortify your skin cells, while the lactic acid in yogurt smooths and softens. Honey is a natural antibacterial and moisturizer, helping to keep your skin hydrated and breakout-free. Remove with warm water and a washcloth and follow with toner (I like an all-natural witch hazel with lavender since it comes alcohol-free and refreshes my skin without overdrying it) and a moisturizer for your skin type. A few nights a week, I'll use a dime-size amount of good-quality flaxseed oil in place of or added to my moisturizer to give my skin an extra dose of omega-3 essential fatty acids.

SILKY SMOOTH TRESSES HAIR MASK

Beautiful hair starts at the scalp. To promote healthy hair follicles and balance the scalp's pH (necessary for optimal luscious hair growth), you need to exfoliate your scalp. Once a week, rinse your hair with a solution that is 1 part apple cider vinegar to 2 parts water. Allow it to sit on your scalp for 2 to 3 minutes, then rinse and pour ¼ cup olive oil over your hair, using fingers to massage it throughout your hair and over your scalp. Allow this conditioning treatment to sit on your hair for up to 30 minutes; to boost penetration of the hair follicle, don a shower cap and wrap your head in a warm towel. Rinse well and shampoo, condition, and style as usual. Olive oil rubbed through dry hair is a great way to protect it from drying out in the sun and sea, and a small amount can also be rubbed between palms to seal ends and smooth flyaways—it's the secret of Mediterranean women that works like a charm!

ENERGIZING CITRUS BODY SCRUB

½ cup sea salt
½ cup melted organic coconut oil or olive oil
2 teaspoons citrus zest (lemon, orange, grapefruit, or lime)
4 dashes citrus essential oil for boosted aromatherapy benefits

Combine all the ingredients in a mixing bowl and use right then and there or store in an airtight container. In the shower, apply the scrub in a gentle, circular pattern to boost circulation and slough away dead skin cells. Rinse and pat dry to let any oils stay on your skin for hydration.

RELAXING AROMATHERAPY FOOT SOAK

½ cup granulated sugar
½ cup olive oil
3 to 5 drops lavender or peppermint essential oil

EQUIPMENT

1 plastic or metal basin
Marbles for the bottom of the basin (optional)

This is best to do before bed or when you can put your feet up for a bit. In a bowl, combine the sugar, olive oil, and essential oil and thoroughly massage and scrub your feet, working deep into the pressure points at the ball and heel, and squeezing the tops of and in between each toe. This mixture will help to erase rough patches by removing dead skin and replenishing moisture. Place your feet in a basin of warm water and soak them. If you can, add marbles to the basin and roll your feet over them to give yourself a nice foot massage. Rinse well with clean water when you're finished soaking. Slather a rich cream over your feet and put on a clean pair of white cotton socks to allow cream to penetrate—this is great to do overnight! And especially nice to wake up to soft, soothed toes.

PRETTY MAKEUP

I remember watching my mother put her makeup on when I was young. What I learned from her is that makeup isn't about changing the way you look but about emphasizing those parts of you that are already gorgeous; it's less about the conceal and more about the reveal. Makeup application is truly an art and a creative way to have some fun, add some sparkle, and highlight your best features. When I'm on set at *The Chew,* makeup becomes a full-service affair. My makeup artist, Gaby, is a star! I simplify her expert tricks for when I'm doing it on my own at home—here are the basics!

Tinted moisturizer. All good things start with the right foundation, which means color as well as texture. Moisturize, then choose a base that matches your skin perfectly, even if it means taking a trip to the makeup counter for some expert advice. Back at home, you'll want to make sure you apply evenly, so invest in disposable makeup sponges to blend coverage for a flawless finish, and don't forget to work up into the hairline and down the neck onto the décolletage so all the skin that's showing matches. (The closer a match to your skin tone, the less necessary it becomes to blend all the way down—which will save your clothing necklines from unwanted makeup advances!)

Blush and bronzer. If you're adding some bronzer, apply it with a loose brush that won't leave streaks and blend it onto the high points of your face, where the sun would naturally hit: the cheek and brow bones, along your hair- and jawline, and over the bridge of your nose. Then lightly shade the deepest part of your cheeks for extra contouring. Apply cream blush with fingertips to the apple of your cheeks—the plumpest part when you smile. Cream beats powder if you're going for the natural flushed looked. If you're going for dramatic impact, brush a little powder blush with some iridescence over the cream blush—but remember, this double whammy tends to photograph better than it looks in life.

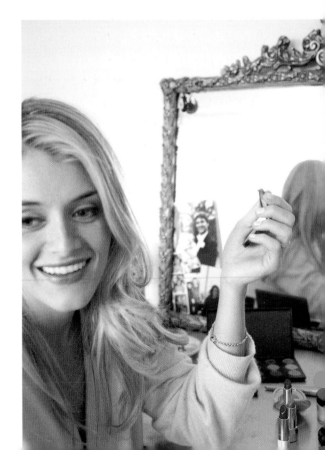

Highlighter. You're an angel, so shine like one. Apply to the high points on your face—cheekbones and brow bones—and the inside corners of your eyes for a celestial glow.

Eyeliner and shadow. On my days off from work, I'm usually good with just a simple warm brown or black line along the lash line, smudged out with a cotton swab or brush so the line is not so perfect and precise. This helps make your eyelashes look more thick and lush while giving your eyes a sultry shape. You can use a Q-tip to clean up any mess.

At the studio, my standard eye routine is to start with a neutral eye shadow over my lid, then gently blend a warm brown under the brow bone to create soft contour around the eye socket. I add some highlighter to the brow bone itself and at the center of my lid to open my eyes up, then a smudged swipe of liner and on to mascara. At night, I might add richer or darker colors, but I'm more a fan of dramatic shaping and contouring than bright rainbow hues. The most important thing is just to blend, blend, blend, so the colors seamlessly merge with one another.

Brows. Dramatic brows take a look to a whole new level—simply choose a pencil in a color one shade lighter than your natural brow color and delicately place little diagonal hash marks in between hairs to fill in and define those arches. Tweeze away any unwanted strays. To help give brows shape, raise your forehead and see the arch form your brows naturally take, then delicately work along those lines. I'm a fan of full brows, but you ideally want them to begin tapering just over the widest part of your eye. Typically, you want the outer corner of your brow to end at the tip of an imaginary line you draw at a forty-five-degree angle from the outer corner of your eye. Be careful not to overpluck—brows can be a brat to grow back.

If you find yours are too bushy for your liking, try brushing the hairs upward with a clean toothbrush and trimming the lengths with nail scissors to remove some of the density. If this sounds like a lot of work, it's because it is: I find it much easier to have my brows shaped once every six months and then maintain on my own once the professional has set the standard!

Volumizing curling mascara. Cheap is good when it comes to mascara, because you can replace it every month to keep it from drying out. If there's one beauty product I can't live without, this is it. Wiggle a well-coated wand at the base of each lash before drawing it up and over each one. Do on the other eye and then come back to the first for a second coat, this time leaving eyes closed and using the wand to scoop lashes up and out for a doe-eyed curl and lengthening effect. If you want to add another coat after lashes have dried, simply rewet with a little warm water on your fingertips. This helps prevent flaking and clumping.

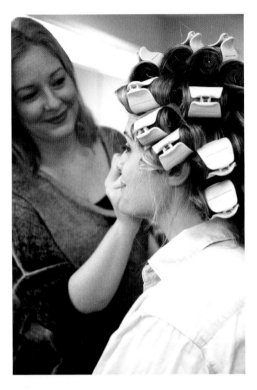

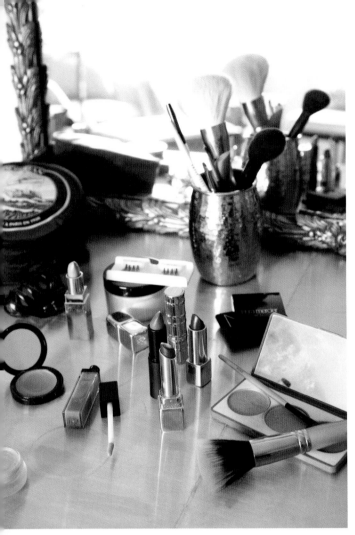

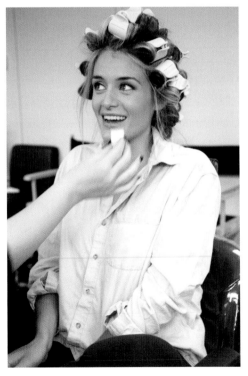

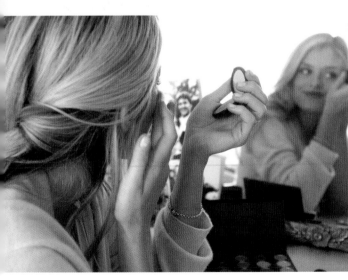

LOOKING DONE ON THE RUN

A makeup artist once gave me some great tips for streamlining makeup routines for busy mornings, which I now share with you. If you're pressed for time, use a swipe of eyeliner to bring the corners of your eyes up, because droopy eyes make us look tired. A swipe of thickening/curling mascara, a dash of blush on the apples of your cheeks, and a slick of bright lipstick (don't forget to blot with tissue paper!), and you're out the door.

Slept though your alarm? Just use cream blush (or pinch your cheeks!) and tinted lip balm for a "dewy angel" look. It's all in the sell, ladies!

Lipstick or gloss. Bite your lips. The flush that results is a good indication of the color family you want your lipsticks and glosses to be in. You may choose something with more or less pigment for more or less impact, but don't go too far off the bitten trail! A good rule of thumb is to choose either strong eye or strong lip, not both.

Bonus: DIY (sort of) manicure. I get my nails done every two weeks. At the salon, I like to get a bright or dark color since they're much harder to do yourself (though a cotton swab or tooth-pick rolled in cotton and dipped in nail polish remover works great to get rid of any coloring outside the line). I make sure to moisturize whenever I wash my hands to keep the cuticles soft and smooth. Three days in, I apply a top coat to prevent chipping and cracking and keep my digits glossy. Five days in, I remove the polish and let my nails breathe over the weekend to keep them from splitting and chipping. Then Sunday night, I file or buff and apply a base coat, nude polish, and top coat myself. I apply top coat again three days in and take it all off five days in. Then I get a manicure again on Sunday. This way, I get ten workdays of beautiful nails for around ten dollars—bargain!

Take It All Off

I always use coconut oil to remove my makeup, because it's all natural and works in seconds. It's antimicrobial and antifungal, so it blocks bacteria growth, keeping acne at bay. Plus it's incredibly moisturizing. And it doesn't need to be refrigerated, so you can keep that extra jar in the bathroom for maximum reachability. I just get a new jar each month.

1. Splash your face with warm water, and use your fingertips to loosen any kind of strong mascara or eye makeup. If you look like a raccoon, you're doing it right.

2. Turn the water off. Don't waste water.

3. Scoop out a teaspoon or so of coconut oil, and rub it between your fingers to melt it. Then rub it all over your face: your eyelids, your lashes, your forehead, everywhere.

4. Use a warm, wet washcloth to wipe it off, and then splash warm water on your face a few times.

5. If you were wearing a lot of makeup, repeat. If you feel you must, you may follow with a cleanser, but you don't have to. Then use your basic toner—I like witch hazel with lavender—and moisturizer, and you're done!

PRETTY CHIC

Now that what's underneath is primed and ready to go, time to get dressed.

Clothes exist to make you look good, and that means that they need to fit you just right. Even if it's on the cover of *Vogue*, if it doesn't suit you, do *not* buy that suit. When clothing is right for us, we feel confident because it accentuates our assets, holding in certain areas but also leaving some room for the imagination. Don't give everything away! It's great to show off delicate décolletage or toned gams or buff arms, but pick one and stay classy.

We've all seen how fashion advice changes by the hour, so don't fall prey to the idea that you can just follow along with what you see on catwalks and in magazines and be guaranteed of looking good. If only it were that easy! Figuring out how to dress best for yourself is a factor of your age, body type, coloring, personal preferences, and just the right amount of staying tuned in to the times—and of knowing when to skip a certain item's moment in the sun.

Trend Carefully

Every season, new looks hit the stores. Some are so flattering they become instant classics. Others should be avoided like a zombie bite. So know yourself! Don't be shy to experiment and change your style. Our bodies are changing all the time, so we have to keep trying new things to figure out what looks best.

When in doubt, ask a buddy who has good taste and fashion sense for her advice. That's the beauty of having a camera built into your phone: you never have an excuse to go it alone. If your friends agree that you can't pull it off, please, do yourself a favor and don't go there. If you're still not sure, tweet it to me and I'll give you the straight truth—@daphneoz.

EASY TO WEAR BEAUTIFULLY	TOUGH TO PULL OFF GRACEFULLY
Jeans and a blazer	Jeggings and a cropped jacket
Little black dress	Tiny black patent-leather dress
Pencil skirt	Short shorts
Trench coat	Studded leather coat
Kitten heels	Thigh-high boots

Creating the Perfect Wardrobe from the Ground Up

Here are my shopping rules of thumb: Listen to your gut before you show it off, play around with small things that are on trend but don't cost a fortune, invest in quality pieces you'll always want to wear, and have fun—since the rules are always changing, you get to play the game the way that makes you feel best!

1. Begin with good underwear. Whether or not you're into it, a *good thong* is a must if you're wearing clingy fabrics, and breathable cotton is best—no need for toxic, synthetic fabrics or polyesters that restrict blood or airflow. If you just can't handle the thong, then choose a more comfortable style (like a cute boy short), but make sure you're wearing clothing that hides any lines. Nothing ruins a great outfit like a full visual of your granny panties. Whatever your undies style, choose a shade that matches your skin tone for maximum invisibility.

2. No matter what, you need a few *well-fitting bras.* Not every bra has to lock and load the ladies, but make sure you have one that comfortably fits your rib cage (no back cleavage, please), gives breasts a good shape without squashing or smushing them, and has straps that aren't constantly falling off your shoulders. It should be made of a soft, washable material. While I don't usually discuss my décolletage with my colleagues, I made a note when Clinton Kelly, my cohost on *The Chew* and style expert of TLC's *What Not to Wear*, explained that "breasts should rest halfway between your shoulders and elbows," so try before you buy. Better yet, shop at a store where a bossy lady will tell you exactly what size you are, because most of us are walking around with a wrong number in our heads and on our boobs.

3. Then there are the better basics. First things first: *white cotton T-shirts* and a *crisp white button-down* in breathable fabric that still has shape to it. A clean, white top makes everyone look bright and put-together, and it goes with anything from pants to skirts to shorts. (Professionally pressed will get you the best results—unless you're an ironing champ!—but

an iron or steamer works well in a pinch.) Paired with a sharp jacket for luncheons or a comfy sweater on the weekends, your *best-ever jeans* (ones that fit you at the waist—low-rise and boyfriend jeans look good only on waifs—shape your butt and thighs, and are in a flattering wash) can be worn everywhere. If you haven't jumped on the *little black dress* bandwagon, do. It is absolutely necessary, and a great one is an equal star at the office, a meeting, drinks, dinner, or after party. Go for one that's not overly embellished, falls somewhere between the midthigh and knee, and is in a flattering fabric that doesn't show wear and tear too easily, because yes, you will be wearing it often. It's the perfect backdrop for fun accessories, and throwing on a chunky necklace and bangles, swapping them out for pretty pearls, or pairing the dress with a great scarf or jacket will get you fifteen outfits in one.

4. **This goes for all your basics:** Don't be afraid to *buy more than one* if you find a style or fit that matches your body like a glove. Nothing's worse than seeing your favorite sweater dress reduced to a pile of pills because you wear it every day without a buddy to rotate in.

5. **Now for the** *expensive essentials.* Pieces like cashmere cardigans, riding boots, a splendid little tweed jacket like the ones Chanel made famous, and a fab trench coat have been around forever because they make us look great with minimal effort. That's what you should strive for throughout your wardrobe: items that require little assembly for maximum effect. At the very least, invest in "lifetime" pieces that meet these standards. These are the places where you should (or at least justifiably could) spend a pretty penny to get really solid quality that will last. I live in my flat leather knee-high boots fall, winter, and spring—they're equally excellent for padding around town in jeans or with a cute dress. And yes, I shelled out a couple hundred bucks to procure them. But you know what? The money I've saved in Band-Aids, chiropractic appointments, and orthotic inserts, not to mention the years and years of excellent wear (and compliments!) I've gotten out of them, make it all worth it. This old Italian saying pairs perfectly with my policy on these things: "Buy less, buy better—cheap is expensive."

Shop Smart

If you want to be a savvy consumer, you'll need to let shopping be about the connection you feel to particular garments and not just the rush you get when you swipe your credit card. You can only wear one dress at a time, and a closet that is too full can be as stressful as one that is too bare.

We have a wonderful stylist, Fran, at *The Chew,* and she's been shopping without me now for over a year, always managing to find some choice outfits I will love. She does it by taking inventory of my body—an honest appraisal of my assets and cover-up zones!—and then looking for shapes similar to what she's bought before that I've liked.

So before you head out to go shopping, be your own stylist! Take a cue from your closet: Which are the things you wear most and that are most flattering? In the era of online shopping—especially when many of the best deals available are waiting at your fingertips!—taking clues from what's already in your closet and treating yourself like a client (meaning you take a real look at what your wardrobe needs and what suits your body best) will make you a much savvier shopper.

Other good things to keep in mind:

Bring your heels. If you're dress or trouser shopping, having the right shoes with you can make a huge difference when you're deciding if you should or shouldn't make a purchase. Instead of imagining how a garment will fall with your favorite party heels, bring them along so you'll know for sure. And having the shoes with you means that you can take the garment directly to the tailor if any alterations are needed to the hem or elsewhere, or take advantage of the shop's in-house tailoring service. You want your great new purchase to be ready the moment you need it!

Become an expert in asset management. When you're selecting garments to take up to the register, make sure you're being an expert in asset management, not just the latest trends. Perhaps you have slender, delicate ankles or a waist shaped like a corset, toned arms or a beautiful collarbone. Before you go into the laundry list of everything that is wrong with your appearance, consider what's right, and play those things up. Gorgeous eyes should wear colors that draw attention to those baby blues, glamorous greens, buttery browns and enchanting ebonies. Shapely figures should wear cuts that highlight tiny waists; the long-legged should let those gams peek out under shorter hems. Shopping is much more fun and efficient if you know to look for only what works on you.

Read the labels. Do your homework. Paying attention to what clothes are made of and the care they'll require over the long term will help you make smarter decisions. If you're a wash-and-wear kind of girl, leave the silk on the rack and opt for cotton instead. If your dry cleaner knows your name and also your Shih Tzu's, go ahead and put it on your AmEx.

Try it on. Sometimes items that appear draggy and unappealing on the store racks are exactly what you're looking for, but you have to get it off the hanger and onto your body in order to tell. And sometimes items that look perfect on the hangar don't suit your frame at all.

Remember that fit comes first, and you can only gauge fit if you try it on. Then be *honest* with yourself. The only person you hurt when you walk out of the store with clothes that are too small, too big, or just downright ugly is yourself, so make sure you really love something before you buy it! Even better, make sure each new item you buy goes with a few other items you already have in your closet or is so completely different from what you already own that it has no redundancies.

But remember, if you don't already own something similar, chances are there's a reason—make sure you're getting something that really is special and not just of the moment.

Make friends. Find a boutique you really like and shop there when you aren't under pressure to make a purchase. You'll be more likely to buy smart, and you'll have the chance to befriend the manager or salesclerk. Over time, she'll get a good idea of what you like and what suits you and can give you a tour of the store when you pop in that highlights all the items that she thinks will appeal. And once you're besties, you can prevail on her to set things aside in your size that will fit you to a tee—and give you a call when all the good sales are coming up!

Store/Closet Smart: Spring (Winter, Summer, and Fall) Cleaning

Part of keeping your wardrobe working for you is making sure you're holding on to only choice items and that you can actually see what you're working with (meaning no heaps of clothing, hangers stuck with fifteen pieces on them, stacks shoved in the back corner, and other fashion disasters).

At *The Chew*, Fran makes sure we have our foundations of closet essentials, and then she rotates in a few new choices each week so we have things to mix and match with but not so much stuff that we forget what was there in the first place. Here are some tips I've learned over the years for how to get the same benefits at home by curating your closet:

1. Once a year, try on every single piece of clothing in your closet to see how each actually sits on you (don't rely on how it used to fit or how you thought it would look on). See if it flatters your body, and if not, add it to the giveaway pile! If you have too many clothes to go through, no more shopping until you can get through it all.

Jeans that haven't fit for a decade need to go. That hideous dress your mother gave you when it didn't fit her anymore needs to go. Anything you haven't put on in months for reasons that are not seasonal needs to go. If you want to keep it: Use it. If you wouldn't buy it today: Lose it.

2. Another piece of Clinton Kelly wisdom that I've found totally indispensable: If you're at capacity, every piece of clothing coming in has to be able to be paired with at least two other items in your closet, and for each new thing coming in, something has to go out—either to storage or giveaway. Keeping your closet at a reasonable capacity means you won't get bogged down in sorting through the mess and forget about all your favorite pieces languishing in the back corner.

3. While you're trying everything on, check for any holes or spots you might not notice when clothes are folded in your closet; there's nothing worse than ending up on vacation with a pair of inadvertently crotchless pants.

4. Sentimental clothing items should be limited to either a half foot of closet space or one shelf, or whatever other metric works, depending on the size of your closet. This way, you can rein in the nostalgia and help yourself make the tough decision to let go of that unflattering camp sweatshirt you've had for twenty years. Reclaim your closet space!

5. Once a season, go through and organize your clothes into new purchases and favorites, old standbys, functional business wear, dressy formalwear, statement pieces, and accessories. You can certainly color-code within these categories, but this way your closet is already broken down into much more manageable subsections so you don't have to scour the whole place every time you're looking for a particular outfit.

THE PLEASURES OF DRESSING WELL

For too many of us, getting dressed is a hassle instead of a joy. We've all been there. A date coming in ten. A meeting starting in an hour. Or a husband already in the driveway leaning on the horn. And there we are, with *no idea* what to wear: everything looks terrible, or it's in the hamper, or we forgot to take it to the dry cleaner, or it no longer fits quite right . . . Sound familiar? So let's change all of that. Getting dressed doesn't have to be an anxiety-ridden affair. Like eating well, dressing well just takes a little bit of preparation and planning. Putting some thought and well-placed effort into your closet will shift your dressing rituals from stressful to streamlined, and from confused to confident.

It's easy to feel overwhelmed and underinspired when your closet is too full, especially if it's loaded up with pieces that don't fit properly, no longer appeal to you, don't go with other items, and don't help you create a wardrobe/outfits. And a closet that's too full of the wrong stuff doesn't leave you with any space to bring the right stuff in! By showing your closet some affection in advance, you'll never get caught with your pants wrinkled on the morning of.

So pledge to make getting dressed a pleasure instead of a chore. Remember that dressing up is part of what makes casual drinks into an event to be remembered, but having the outfit spring fully-formed from your closet without stress or numerous changes—now that's something to be excited about!

Dress Smart

Keep your ready-to-wear ready to wear. Nobody wants to get through two morning meetings before noticing her blouse has a mai tai stain on the front or that the zipper on her dress is busted and hanging halfway open. That's amateur hour! Be a smart girl: Learn to keep your closet in perfect array, your clothes clean and pressed, and your tailor on speed-dial. And don't forget to give yourself a good once-over before you step out the door! Check that your clothes are right side out and your tags are tucked in, and for new purchases,

---

PANTS ON, PANTS OFF

Yes, it's tempting to leave those jeans on the floor once you wiggle your way out of them, but instead, make the effort to put them away—in your closet, not in your drawers. Pants that are folded into deep drawers can be difficult to survey when you're not sure what you want to wear and tough to find even when you know exactly what you're looking for. Better: Stack your bottoms on shelves or hang them for easy viewing and selection.

make sure any sewn vents and pockets are opened and tags and outside labels trimmed off. It's the little things!

Protect your investments. Remember that pretty cashmere sweater you got at that sample sale last winter? How sad will you be next fall when you pull it out of your drawer, only to discover that the moths loved it as much as you did? Acquiring clothing you'll want to wear from season to season means caring for clothes so that they'll be ready to wear when you need them. Dry-clean coats before tucking them away for the season so they'll be crisp and not wrinkled when you suddenly realize it's fall again. Put your favorite clean and dry woolen sweaters into plastic bags for the spring and summer seasons to protect them from winged critters. Keep your cottons smelling fresh with lavender-scented sachets and cedar blocks.

Dress for fun—and function. Make sure you consult your calendar and the weather report as well as your style sense when you're making your sartorial choices. I don't care how much you want to wear that silk print number—it just won't work if you're going to be hiking up to Machu Picchu or stepping out in the rain. Rules of thumb: Avoid heels for a garden party where you're likely to be on the grass unless they're paying you to aerate their field. Go with flats or wedges instead. Don't wear a too-short skirt if you're at an interview or doing anything besides sitting pretty. And if you're expecting to make use of your umbrella, steer clear of white, unless you're hoping to win a wet T-shirt contest. But other fashion rules? Forget them! Years ago, jeans weren't appropriate for a night out and navy blue was a no-no with black. Now, that's all changed. If you want to mix and match, go ahead.

Hold a dress rehearsal. When you're going on vacation, you spend time thinking about what you'll wear for every occasion, and looking great becomes a breeze. You can use that same policy when at home. On the weekend, check your calendar so that you'll have a good overview of your clothing needs for the week ahead, then plan out a few mix-and-match outfits, leaving room for swap-outs if there's a change of heart, mood, or weather. This will save you from having to rush and compromise on a subpar outfit and probably earn you a few extra hits on the alarm's snooze buttons.

In general, you'll want to make sure always to have an outfit on hand and ready to go for the following occasions: a business meeting, a job interview, a date, a cocktail party, and a funeral. Even if you aren't looking for a job and you're already married, you never know when a work opportunity might arise or your husband might score a reservation to that awesome new restaurant downtown.

CARING FOR CLOTHES

Now that your closet is curated to perfection so that only your most eminently wearable pieces remain, time to uncover a few tricks for keeping these favorite pieces fresh so getting dressed continues to be a joy for as long as you want to wear them!

Tinker, Tailor: How to Sew a Button

So you've lost the button off your favorite skirt, or you notice your boyfriend heading off to work in a shirt sans closure. Avoid unwanted games of peeka-boo (and impress your dude) with your super sewing savvy. You'll need the following items:

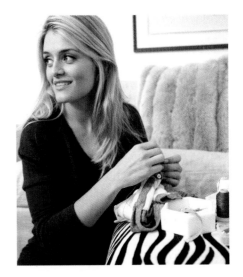

Needle
Matching or contrasting thread
A button
Chalk (maybe)
Thimble (maybe)
Scissors

1. Observe how the buttons are sewn onto the shirt. Are they using contrasting or matching thread? If the buttons have four holes, is the thread sewn in two parallel rows or two rows that cross? You'll want to sew to match the style of the rest of the buttons.

2. Use matching thread, contrasting thread, or whatever emergency thread you have on hand. Cut off an appropriate amount (about twelve inches should do the trick). Thread the needle, doubling up the thread and knotting it at the bottom.

3. Place your button exactly where it should be. If there's a pucker mark from the lost button, bully for you. If not, button up the shirt and make a tiny chalk mark or pencil mark where it belongs. Slip a thimble on the pointer finger of the hand that is not sewing if you're worried about sticking yourself or need a little extra support to push the needle through thicker fabrics.

4. Starting from the back, slip the needle in the fabric, sliding it through one of the button-holes. Pull the thread through all the way, so that the knot is sitting on the fabric. Slip the needle back through the buttonhole directly above or beside it. Repeat. Repeat. Repeat. Don't

go too tight or too loose—check to match the other buttons. You want just enough space for the material to fit smoothly when the garment is buttoned.

5. When the button seems nice and secure, finish your last stitch with the needle on the inside of the fabric (where people won't be able to see it). Sew a mini-stitch, but don't pull the thread through all the way. When you're left with a small loop of thread, put the needle through the loop and then pull it snug. Repeat once or twice to make sure the button is secure, then trim off the thread, leaving a half inch or so of thread next to the knot.

6. *Extra credit: Dress up a boring cardigan.* Why wait until the Case of the Missing Button to hone your needling abilities? Sharpen up a bland twinset with your new skill set by purchasing some awesome fascinator buttons (antique coins, rhinestones, mismatching), and replace the existing boring closures with something a little more sparkly and special. Just make sure that your exciting new buttons will fit through the buttonholes before you buy them!

Laundry List

If you don't have a washing machine, perhaps you send the laundry out, in which case it will always come back properly cleaned and folded. If you're lucky enough to have your own, or you don't mind hanging out at the local Laundromat with a pocket full of quarters, you'll need to have the know-how. And with this handy information, you'll always know how to get the job done well so you can put your best foot forward in a tidy outfit.

How to Get the Stains Out

I've learned a lot working on *The Chew*—and I've occasionally had to embarrass myself to gain that knowledge. During a special segment on getting rid of stains, I had to wear a sweater with very obvious artificial (!) armpit stains—exactly what you don't want to wear in public, let alone in front of millions of viewers on television. Yet there I was, taking one for the team. So if my shame helps you avoid a similar circumstance, then it was well worth it. Note that these are pretreatments, so you should wash as usual afterward. And read the labels! Pouring liquid on dry-clean-only silks is always a no-no!

Greased lightning. For grease stains, use Dawn or other grease-fighting dish soap.

Bottoms up. For red wine, pour salt or baking soda on the stain to soak up the damage, then blot with cool water.

Inked. For pen ink stains, blot with alcohol.

Cuppa joe. For coffee stains, mix 1 teaspoon white vinegar in 1 quart cold water, then blot onto the stain and wipe clean. Baking soda also works: Just mix with water until you have a toothpaste consistency.

Home sweat home. For sweat stains on a white sweater, prepare a 1:1:1 solution of water, hydrogen peroxide, and baking soda. Scrub the mixture into the stains with a hard toothbrush and let it sit for a half hour before washing as usual. Remember: Though it may be tempting, at no point should you give in to the urge to use bleach! It will just darken the stain, exactly the opposite of what you're trying to accomplish.

My accidental silk/chiffon discovery! Don't quote me on this because I have absolutely no idea why it works, but I once accidentally reached for a Lysol wipe when I thought I was getting a baby wipe to clear some makeup off a silk blouse. Not only did the Lysol wipe take the stain completely out, it left no watermark stain! I've since tried it on all kinds of silk/chiffon-type delicate fabrics and had incredible results. It's my secret weapon!

How to Keep It Clean

1. Always read the labels. Silks and other delicate fabrics should go straight to the dry cleaner, no matter how tempting it may be to just do it yourself. Unless you want to give my little Lysol trick a try—it's worked for me!

2. Lingerie, tights, stockings, and bathing suits should be washed by hand and air-dried. Yes, it will make your bathroom look like you live in a sorority. Do it anyway.

3. For cottons and other basic washables, split the laundry into two groups: white and colors. If you've got heaps and heaps of laundry to do, you can even separate into three groups: whites; dark colors; and light colors, like pastels.

4. White towels and sheets can be bleached and washed in higher temperatures, depending on how delicate and soiled they are. To bleach in top loading washers, turn on the water, and add bleach along with detergent *before* you put the clothes in. Once the bleach is diluted, add whatever needs a good whitening. Make sure to choose a non-chlorine bleach alternative—these are meant to be less toxic than the conventional. If you have a side-loading washer, put your whites in, turn the cycle on, and add the bleach and detergent to the running water (most washers will mark which section of the loading tray is for bleach versus detergent versus fabric softener). For towels, skip the fabric softeners since they actually reduce absorbency. Never use bleach on colored clothing unless you're a fan of the tie-dyed look.

5. In general, you want to do all your laundry on the coldest possible setting with the least amount of detergent—totally counterintuitive!—to help fabric fibers maintain their flexibility and shape. I stick with warm water for lights and whites, cold water for darks. I skip the hot water unless something needs to be sanitized.

How to Get the Wrinkles Out (Iron Not Required)

My husband's mother ironed his socks until he was twelve. I love them both, but you won't catch me doing that anytime soon. I throw his shirts in the dryer for a few minutes to get the wrinkles out and then hang them up. For my dresses, I just hang them and let them dewrinkle from the steam of the shower while I'm sudsing up. If you do need to use an iron, here's what you need to know:

1. Read the labels and follow the instructions on your iron for your fabric type. Generally, cotton and linen get a high setting, cotton blends and wool get a medium setting, and silk and nylon get a low setting.

2. Preheat your iron. Make sure to use distilled water in the iron—water from the tap, depending on its mineral content, could actually stain your clothes over time.

3. Stretch your garment flat across the ironing board to avoid adding wrinkles while ironing.

4. Iron with long, smooth movements, and don't let the iron rest on your garment.

Okay, so now you have bright skin; soft hair; great makeup; pretty nails; clothes that fit you like a glove, and nary a stain, loose button, or wrinkle in sight! So why not call your friends over for an impromptu cocktail party—all the recipes you need are coming up!

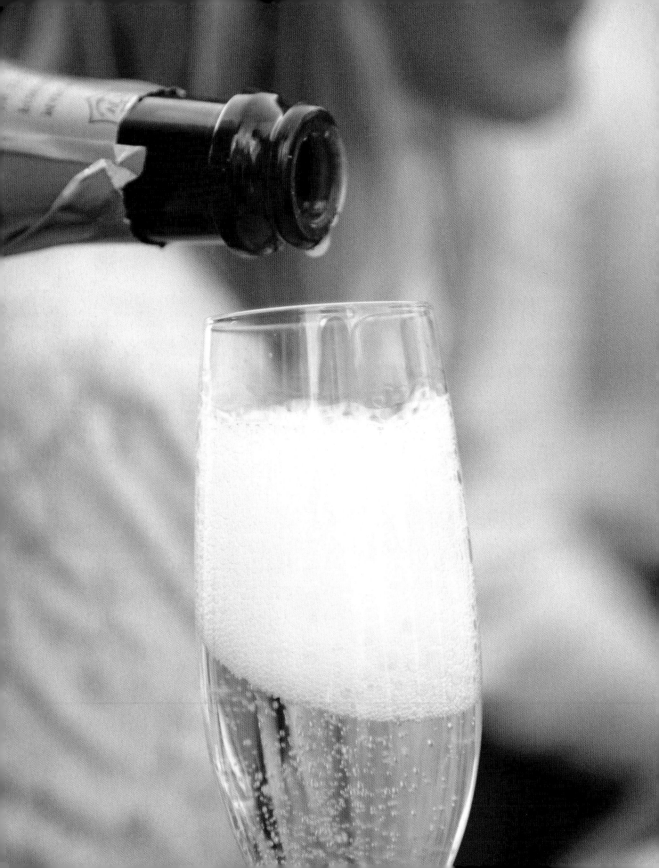

SEVEN

TIME FOR A DRINK

cocktails

One martini is all right. Two are too many, and three are not enough.
—JAMES THURBER

I'VE GOT TO BE HONEST: I'M NOT USUALLY A MARTINI DRINKER, and you won't find a recipe for old-timer drinks in this chapter. Though I love the classics, I suppose I like my cocktails a little more quixotic. But before I get too far ahead of myself, let's be clear that no matter your preference, drinks are meant to be relished responsibly.

There's nothing wrong with cracking a few bottles of beer or opening a merlot when friends come over. But imagine their amazement when you roll out the bar cart or whisk away to your alcohol cabinet—a stylish and sophisticated touch in any home!—to whip up your signature cocktail. My, my—you are the well-rounded hostess! So leave the jet fuel behind in favor of some more thoughtful party beverages, like a creamy milk punch, a classic Champagne cocktail, or a steamy mulled cider. And say hello to my personal favorite, Sombrero Aloha—a bewitching elixir of tequila, pineapple, lime, and a splash of seltzer for days when Mexico is a little farther than you'd like, but a home-thrown fiesta is just the ticket.

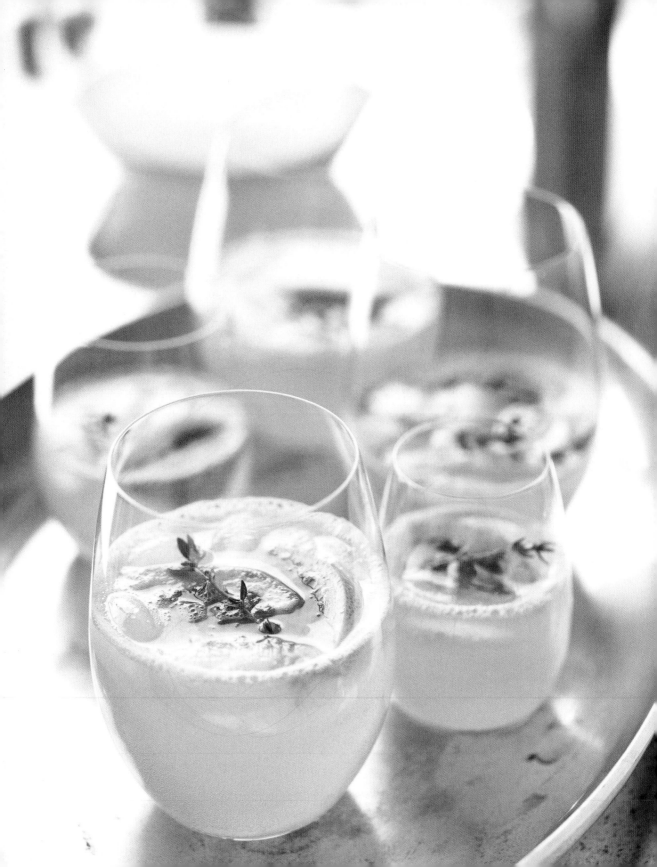

GRAPEFRUIT THYME SPRITZ

serves 4

THIS DRINK IS RIPE for the riffing—feel free to nix the vodka if you prefer a virgin version. You could also swap the seltzer for something with a little more party in it—like a cheap and cheerful cava! You might not think of fruit and herbs going together, but thyme (and mint, too) lend a delicate aromatic boost to help make this drink sophisticated and refreshing.

½ cup sugar

½ cup water

10 fresh thyme sprigs

¼ cup fresh lemon juice
(from about 2 lemons)

1 cup grapefruit juice, strained
(about 3 grapefruit)

8 ounces (1 cup) vodka

20 ounces (2½ cups) seltzer

Fresh grapefruit slices
for garnish

1. To make a thyme simple syrup, in a small saucepan over low heat, combine the sugar and water. Bring the mixture to a boil, stirring gently, until the sugar is dissolved. Gently bruise 6 thyme sprigs by banging them with the back edge of a knife or the heel of your palm and add them to the simple syrup. Remove the mixture from the heat and set aside for at least 2 hours. Strain the liquid just before using to remove thyme; reserve the syrup and discard the thyme.

2. Combine the lemon juice and grapefruit juice in a pitcher and add simple syrup to taste (about 1 tablespoon per serving); stir to combine. Store remaining simple syrup in a sterilized glass jar in the refrigerator for up to 1 week.

3. To each glass, add ice, 2 ounces of vodka, and a quarter of the grapefruit mixture. Top with seltzer. Garnish with a few fresh grapefruit slices and one of the remaining thyme sprigs.

GINGER MINT JULEP

serves 4

½ cup sugar

½ cup water

One 2-inch piece peeled fresh ginger, cut into thick slices

1 bunch fresh mint, leaves coursely chopped (about ½ cup) 4 mint sprigs reserved for garnish

8 ounces (1 cup) bourbon

28 ounces (3½ cups) seltzer or ginger beer

I NORMALLY TRY TO CONTAIN MYSELF when it comes to purchasing ultraspecialized kitchen items, but mint julep cups are worth it, especially since you can invest in silver-plated ones bearing your initials for under twenty dollars—totally fetch! Toss them in the freezer to frost for a few minutes and you'll be using them to serve perfectly icy derby drinks to dazzled guests in ginormous hats for years to come! And if monogrammed cups are not in the cards just yet, this drink is equally classy in a pretty glass (or a plastic one if you're outdoors at the races).

To make a ginger-mint simple syrup, in a small saucepan over low heat, combine the sugar and water. Bring the mixture to a boil, stirring gently, until the sugar is dissolved. Add the ginger and mint leaves, remove from the heat, and let stand for at least 2 hours. Strain out the ginger and mint and add 2 tablespoons of the simple syrup to the bottom of each glass. Add 2 ounces of the bourbon to each glass and stir to combine. Fill each glass with ice (preferably crushed) and top with seltzer. Garnish each with a sprig of fresh mint.

DASH

To make crushed ice, you can buy an expensive ice crusher—or your refrigerator might have a "crushed" setting—or you could try this blender trick! Add ice by the handful to a blender with just enough cold water to blend on "ice crush" setting. Crush until desired consistency is reached.

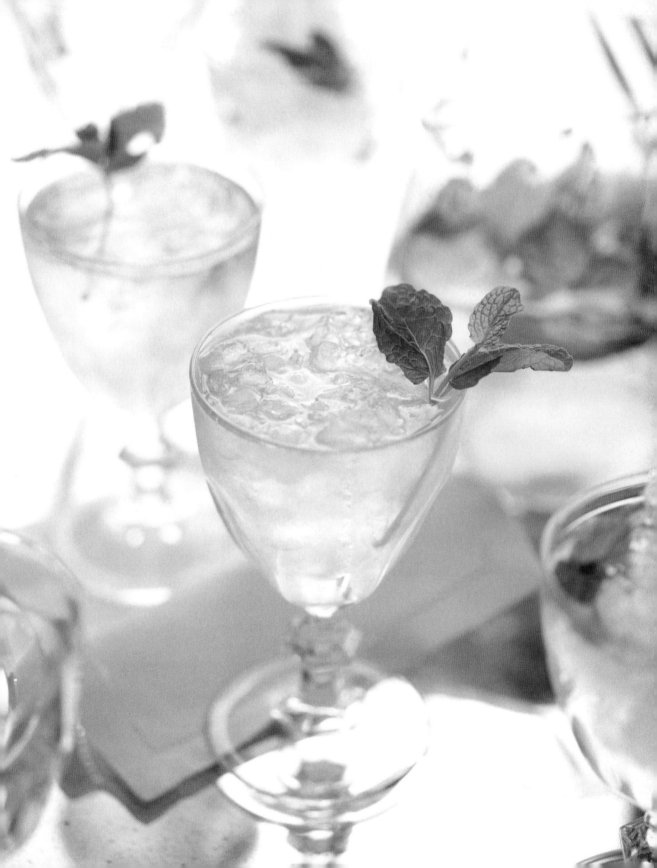

LAVENDER CUCUMBER LEMONADE

serves 4

½ cup sugar

5 ½ cups water

1 teaspoon dried food-grade lavender (check your grocery store's spice section)

1 medium seedless cucumber, peeled

1 cup fresh lemon juice (from about 8 lemons) plus 4 lemon wheels for garnish

8 ounces (1 cup) gin

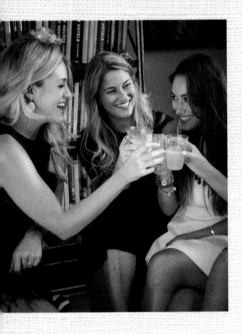

THIS DRINK FEELS like the South of France in a glass. Crisp, cool cucumber plus fragrant lavender, and there you are in St. Tropez by way of Provence. To bring it a little closer to home, I like to serve this in a handled mason jar—the perfect picnic drink! But like any well-rounded lady worth her salt, this drink is as lovely in delicate stemware and a summer dress as she is in a glass jar and overalls.

1. To make a lavender simple syrup, in a small saucepan over low heat, combine the sugar and ½ cup of the water. Bring the mixture to a boil, stirring gently, until the sugar is dissolved. Gently bruise the lavender by banging with the back edge of a knife or the heel of your palm and add it to the simple syrup. Remove from the heat and let sit for at least 2 hours. Just before using the simple syrup, strain out and discard the lavender.

2. Puree the cucumber in a blender until smooth (hold back 4 slices of cucumber for garnish if desired).

3. In a large pitcher, combine the lemon juice, 5 cups water, and the cucumber puree. Add simple syrup to taste and stir to combine. Fill each of 4 glasses with ice and add 2 ounces (¼ cup) of gin. Top with the lemonade mixture. Garnish with wheels of lemon or cucumber, and get the country jams going.

If I'm not feeling up to hand-juicing eight lemons, I'll peel them with a paring knife and blend on high in a blender until pureed, then strain the liquid through a fine-mesh strainer. The result is basically lemon juice (you might even end up with a little more than you need, since no juice is wasted)—plus you preserve some of the bioflavonoids—immune-boosting, anti-inflammatory antioxidants your body loves, found in citrus's white pith!

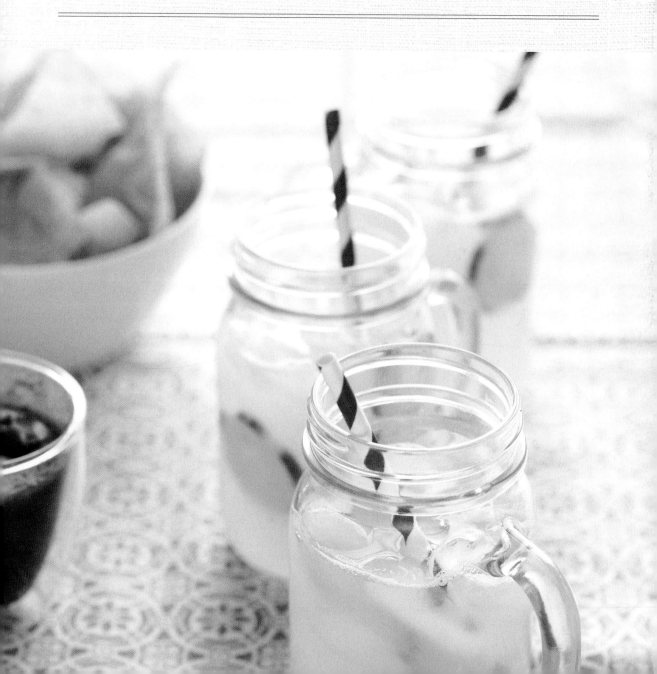

SOMBRERO ALOHA

serves 4

8 fresh mint sprigs

¼ cup fresh lime juice
(from about 3 limes)

8 ounces (1 cup) tequila

8 ounces (1 cup) pineapple
juice

16 ounces (4 cups) seltzer

AHH, MY FAVORITE. This is my signature drink because (1) it tastes so good—refreshingly light and not too sweet; (2) it's equally good for day or night; and (3) it comes together in a flash with plenty of flavor. If I'm having a party, I make the base of pineapple and lime juice with mint ahead of time and leave it out with ice, tequila, seltzer, and glasses for guests to help themselves as they filter in. Best part: I never have to worry whether people are having a good time!

In a large pitcher, muddle the leaves from 4 of the mint sprigs (or leave the sprigs whole, if desired) and lime juice with the bottom of a wooden spoon. Add the tequila and pineapple juice. Add ice to each of 4 glasses and fill the glasses halfway with the pineapple mixture. Top with seltzer and garnish each serving with a fresh mint sprig.

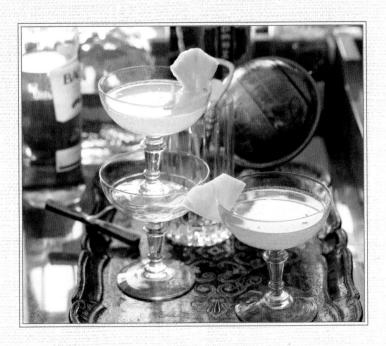

STRAIGHT OUT OF A BOTTLE

WINE is not as fancy and foreboding as you might think. Unless you're a connoisseur, don't get caught up on the price tag or the points—the best rule of thumb is just to drink what you like! Good palates come from trying lots of different wines, so pay attention to regions or varieties you like and then try various bottles in those categories. Here are some of my favorite wines by region:

Sauvignon Blanc from New Zealand
Pinot Noir from Oregon
Chardonnay from California
Cabernet Franc from France
Nebbiolo from Italy

BEER isn't just for the Super Bowl. Artisanal beers are as elegant as a long-necked bottle of wine (and sometimes just as expensive). Instead of Budweiser, look for microbrews or seasonal beers or the very delicious Framboise, which has the fresh bite of raspberries mixed right in. And just because you're serving beer, don't assume you need to go straight for the burgers or pretzels. Like wines, different beers have their own tastes and characteristics, and pair delightfully with cheese.

IPAs with cheddar
Hefeweissen with chèvre
Stout with Brie
Porter with Gouda
Amber ale with pecorino

CIDER Apple juice isn't just boxes with straws anymore. When it's been fermented, the juice of the apple exchanges its child-friendly ways for a grown-up take that makes me very, very happy. Hard cider has an alcoholic content of 2 percent to 8.5 percent, and offers a creamy, earthy bite with a faint hint of its former sweetness that's a pleasure to drink whenever you'd have a beer. Though it's a pub favorite in London, it's still slightly unexpected in the United States, which of course makes it all the more alluring. I love it paired with a fancy grilled cheese in any of these delicious flavor combinations:

Sweet cider with blue cheese and pear
Dry cider with chèvre and caramelized onion
Norman cider (from the Normandy region of France) with Brie and apricot jam

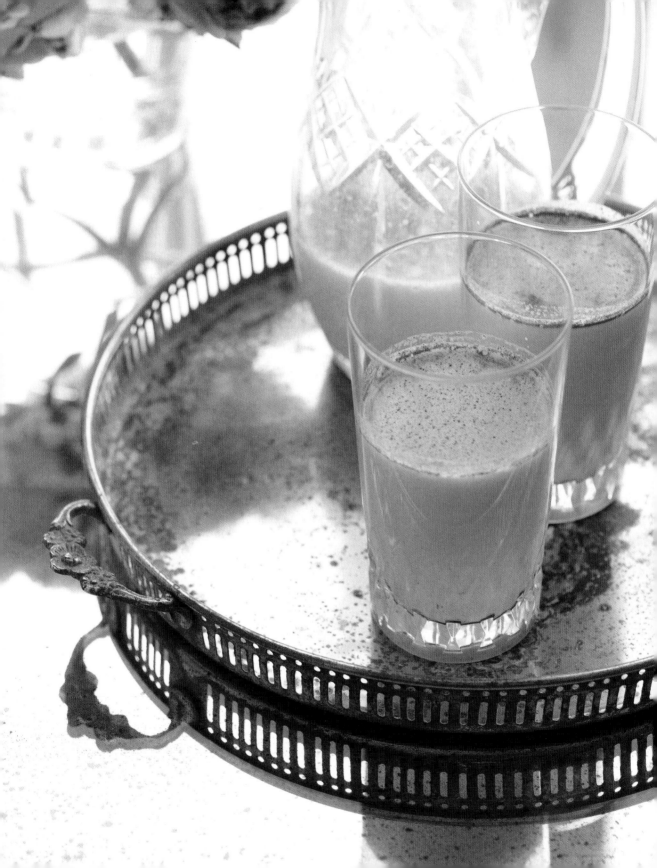

MILK PUNCH

serves 4

THE BEAUTY OF THIS COCKTAIL is it can be served warm or cold. I love it served tall over ice, or warm in a mug, while I'm curled up on the couch in a cozy sweater with an old movie playing; I'm happy—and a little sleepy—just thinking about it. If you had a different sort of evening planned, add brewed coffee in place of some of the milk and you have a delicious pick-me-up that's pure winter fun. Hello, après-ski!

3 cups whole milk

2 tablespoons pure vanilla extract

2 tablespoons sugar

¼ teaspoon freshly grated nutmeg plus more for serving

¼ teaspoon ground cinnamon plus more for serving

8 ounces (1 cup) light rum

1. In a medium saucepan, combine the milk, vanilla, sugar, nutmeg, and cinnamon over medium-low heat, stirring constantly to dissolve the sugar and being careful not to burn the milk. When the milk is scalded (there will be a thin skin on the sides of the pan), after about 5 minutes, remove from the heat and allow to cool to drinking temperature.

2. To drink warm, divide the milk mixture into 4 heat-proof mugs and add 2 ounces (¼ cup) of the rum to each. To serve cold, fill 4 tall glasses with ice, add the rum, and top with the milk mixture, swirling to combine. Serve with freshly grated nutmeg and a dash of cinnamon.

WHITE WINE SPRITZER

serves about 6

18 green or red grapes

One 750 ml bottle white wine, chilled (I like dry Spanish Verdejo or Italian Verdicchio varieties, or a floral Napa Sauvignon Blanc)

18 ounces (2¼ cups) seltzer, chilled

6 ounces (¾ cup) 100% white grape juice, chilled

THIS IS WHAT I'M DRINKING in the bewitching hour between a long day at the pool or beach and the arrival of dinner guests for our weekend summer barbecues. But it's perfect for anytime (post-12 p.m. local), really! I like to add a drop of white grape juice to blow up the fruity flavor of the wine and add a fancy touch with frozen grapes— they help keep my drink icy cool without diluting and are quite delicious on their own as a hot-weather snack.

If you're looking to make an individual glass, the ratio is 4 parts wine to 3 parts seltzer to 1 part grape juice. Happy sipping!

THE GLASS MENAGERIE

Why are there so many different shapes of glasses? Stemware is designed to keep warm fingers from heating up the bowl of the glass. The wider the mouth of the glass, the more oxygen hits the liquid, which influences its taste. Champagne glasses with their narrow nozzles keep bubbly bubbly. And the cone shape of a martini glass keeps the ingredients from separating—genius!

But that's not to say you can't use whatever glasses you feel like—see my white wine spritzer in cognac glasses!

1. Rinse the grapes, pat them dry, place them on a baking sheet, and freeze them for at least 2 hours.

2. To make the spritzer, add the wine, seltzer, and grape juice to a large pitcher and gently stir to combine. Place ice cubes and 3 frozen grapes into each wineglass. Top with the spritzer.

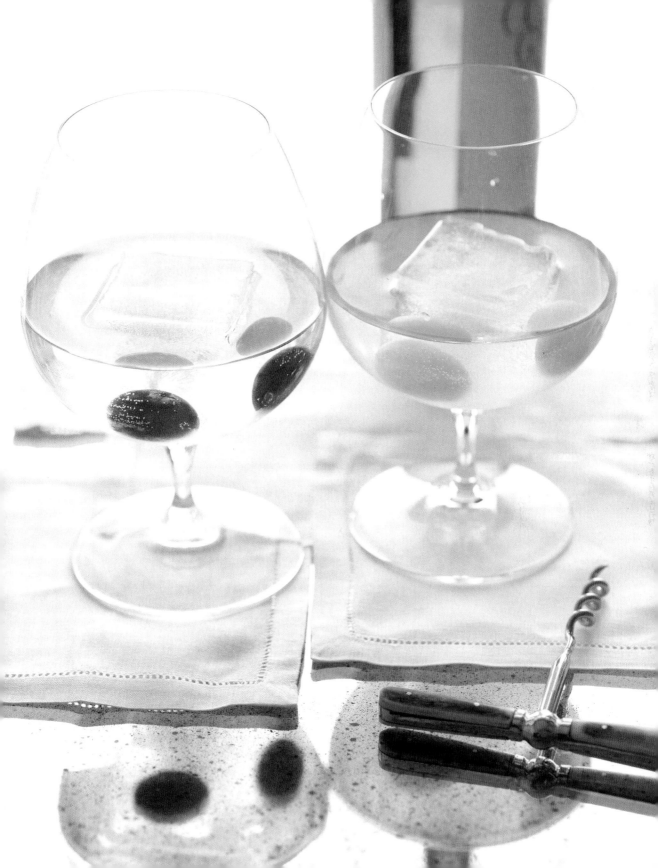

WINE AND CHEESE

The best way to enjoy wine is of course . . . with cheese! When you're shopping for your wines and cheeses, there are a few ways to go to make sure that you're going to love what you bring home.

Do your homework. There are myriad magazines, books, and blogs that focus on wine and cheese selections, so read up before you hit the shop.

Try before you buy. Many wine and cheese shops have organized tastings or let you taste as you go, so don't be shy about asking.

Trust yourself. Don't be afraid to like what you like and dislike what you don't! People will tell you tobacco or wood or earth flavors are desirable, but if you hate them, that's your palate. Buy what you like, not what you're supposed to like.

Ask the experts. Boutique wine and cheese shops employ individuals who know what they're talking about, so let them know what you like, and ask them what they like. They may be able to steer you to special selections you'd never think of on your own.

Take notes. If you find yourself in a restaurant eating a particularly delectable morsel of goat cheese, or sipping on a marvelous bottle of Sancerre, make note of it so you can look for it later. No pen and paper? Use your smartphone to snap a photo of the menu, the cocktail list, or the bottle you're finding so compelling. I keep a whole digital album with photos of food, drink, and other special finds I want to try again.

Here are some pairings to consider:

If you like apples and figs, try Chardonnay. Pair with Camembert.

If you like herbal flavors, you'll like Sauvignon Blanc. Pair with Gruyère.

If you like citrus, try Grüner Veltliner. Pair with Gouda.

If you like pepper, try Zinfandel. Pair with Parmesan.

If you like plum and black cherry, go for Cabernet Sauvignon. Pair with aged Cheddar.

If you like cherry and spice, try Pinot Noir. Pair with Asiago.

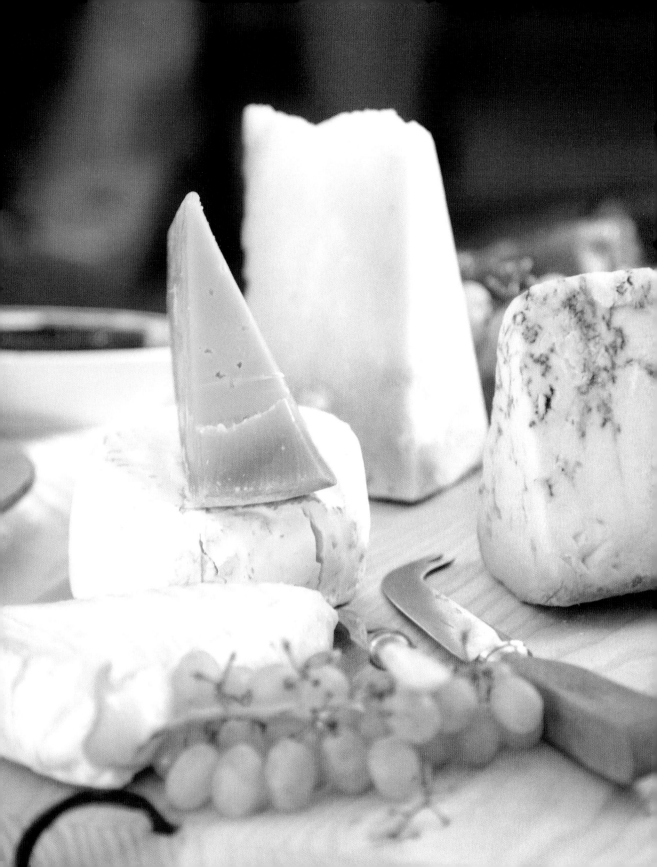

SPICED WINTER WINE

serves 6

¼ cup pure maple syrup

8 cinnamon sticks

One 1-inch piece fresh peeled ginger, sliced into 4 rounds

6 cloves

¼ teaspoon ground nutmeg

10 cardamom pods

1 vanilla bean, halved lengthwise and scraped

Zest and juice from 1 orange

1 lemon, sliced into rounds

Two 750 ml bottles red wine (Cabernet Sauvignon, Malbec, or Chianti work well) or apple cider

IN THE WINTER, I crave spice, sweetness, and the warmth of mulled red wine or cider. I love heading to winter festivals where you can smell this stuff brewing a mile away, and nothing says housewarming party like the apple-pie aroma of spiced winter wine simmering on the stove. For those of you looking to skip the alcohol, apple cider works great in place of wine in this recipe!

If you use cider and want to put the alcohol back in, serve the mugs with a shot of bourbon!

1. In a large saucepan, combine the syrup, 2 of the cinnamon sticks, ginger, cloves, nutmeg, cardamom pods, vanilla bean, and orange zest and juice. Heat over medium heat to boiling, then immediately turn off the heat, cover, and set aside 10 minutes to steep. Add the lemon rounds and steep 2 minutes more. Add the wine and heat over medium-low heat until simmering, taking care not to boil.

2. Strain and divide among 6 heat-proof mugs and garnish each with a cinnamon stick.

===== DASH =====

I love to serve these on a tray decorated with a sprinkling of cardamom pods—the aroma is intoxicating!

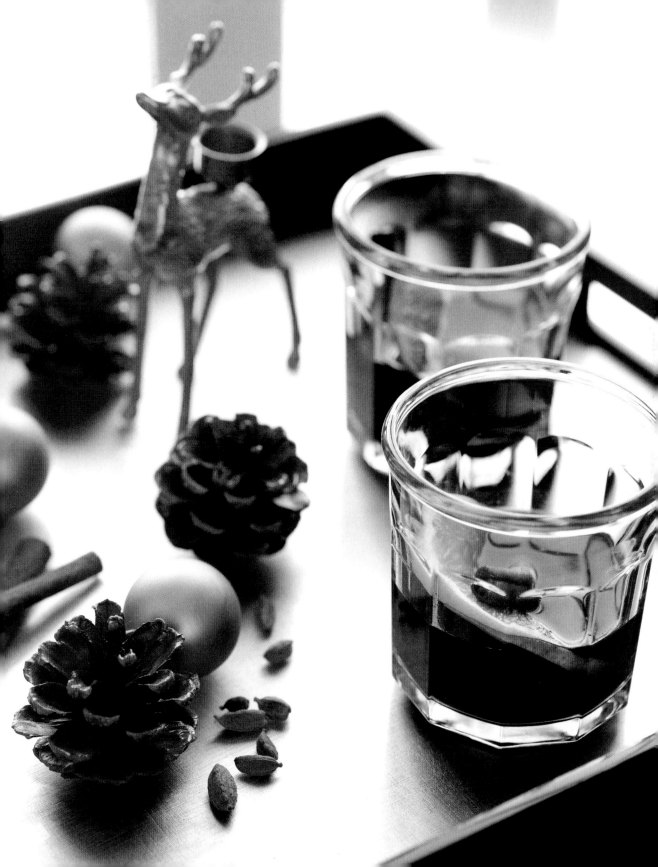

(ALMOST) CLASSIC CHAMPAGNE COCKTAIL

serves 4

4 white sugar cubes
(see DASH)

8 dashes of bitters

4 ounces (½ cup) Cognac
or other brandy

Enough Champagne to fill each
flute, about 16 ounces (2 cups)
total

Juice of ½ lemon

Juice of ½ orange

4 thin orange slices for garnish

FOR THE CLASSICISTS who may have been thrown by all this talk of herbs in drinks and spins on the originals, this one is for you.

The best way to drink Champagne is straight out of the bottle—ahem, I mean leave it alone, silly! It's perfect the way it is and simply the best. If you want a little pink in your drink, a gorgeous Kir Royale is decadent but understated—a drop of crème de cassis liqueur floating in a heavenly bed of bubbles. If you want to go cheap and cheerful, substitute Champagne's Spanish compadre, *cava, or Italian Prosecco. But if you absolutely must get fancy on us, there's the Champagne cocktail, a rich, earthy drink tinged with your grandpa's Cognac and a sugar cube for good luck. And though I promised you no old-timer drinks, this one is a worthy exception to the rule. I leave off the dreaded maraschino cherry because I hate them, and add a little lemon because I like its brightness, but play with this recipe to fit your taste!*

Place 1 sugar cube at the bottom of each of 4 Champagne flutes and add 2 dashes of bitters to each cube to start to dissolve the sugar. Add 1 ounce (2 tablespoons) of Cognac to each flute and swirl. Top the glass with Champagne and finish with ¼ teaspoon of fresh lemon juice and 1 teaspoon fresh orange juice. Garnish with an orange slice.

===== DASH =====

Cava and Prosecco make the perfect wallet-friendly base if you're serving mimosas (bubbly plus orange juice) or bellinis (bubbly plus peach puree), since money spent on champagne quality is wasted when the fresh fruit flavor takes over.

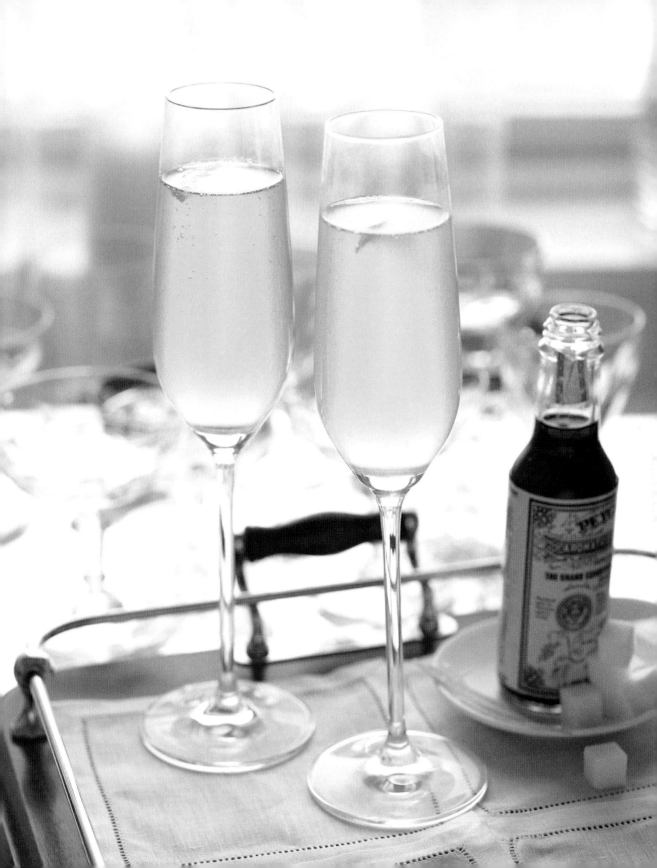

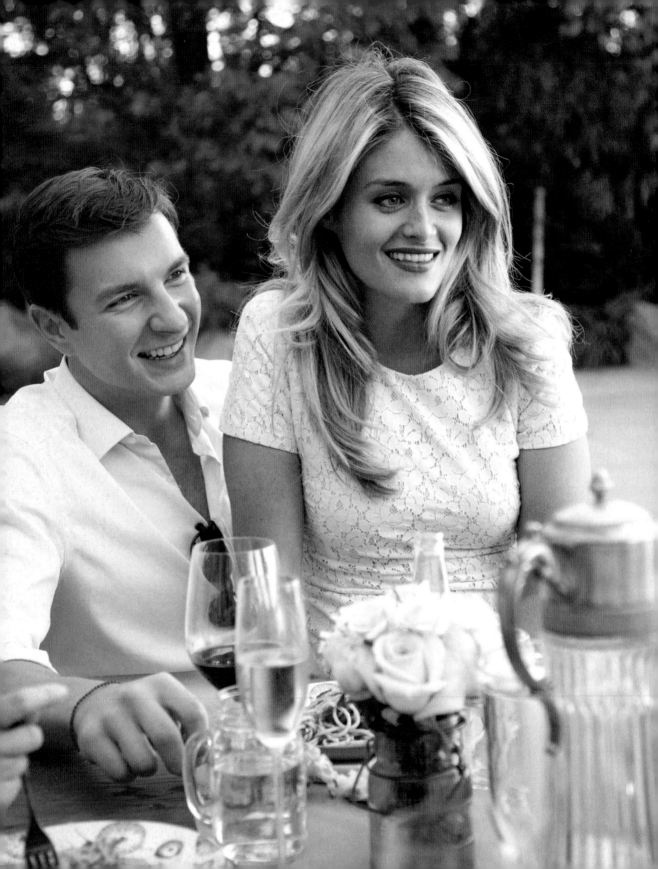

EIGHT

THE HIP HOMEMAKER

creating a home that's your own

Luxury must be comfortable, otherwise it is not luxury.
—COCO CHANEL

WHAT MAKES A HOME A SWEET HOME? I'VE BEEN IN HOMES that are lavishly appointed and visually perfect, but the couches are too stiff and the fabric is itchy and there isn't anywhere to put your glass. That's one end of the spectrum. Then there are the homes that are organized around family and comfort and maximum livability, and whether the chairs are imported from Italy or IKEA they are a joy to curl up in with a mug of cocoa and a favorite old book.

These are the types of homes I grew up in: the ones that are always loaded with aunts, uncles, cousins, grandparents, staged for family game nights and giant feasts and quiet time. Friends were always welcome around the table—and for those who showed up before the meal or stuck around after, the more the merrier for Oz family Olympics! (We hold epic football/basketball/any-sport-at-all challenges whenever we reach a certain threshold of people in the house. Stop by sometime! Bring Band-Aids.)

There were rooms that were set up for "company," and they were luscious and elegant, but the rooms I spent the most time in are the ones with worn-in, comfy couches, threadbare carpets worn from years of trampling, and a stack of cards ready for battle. And of course, our family always manages to convene in the kitchen, the place where hundreds of thousands of meals have been prepared, enjoyed, and lingered over. These rooms embodied my family's personality and contained most of our memories, and they were the ones we wanted to live in.

We all love beautiful things. But what makes something truly beautiful, truly luxurious? Like Coco says, if it isn't comfortable, it isn't luxury. What makes a homemaker a savvy homemaker? She understands that a luxurious home is one that is driven by comfort as well as aesthetics, where you feel relaxed and replenished, where you can get creative and get cozy. The goal is not to copy someone else's taste but to cultivate your own, creating a space that complements your needs and your lifestyle, raises you up, and brings you back to center.

THERE'S NO PLACE LIKE HOME

My very first home was a one-bedroom apartment that I shared with my parents and my little sister until I turned five. With a limited floor plan, we made use of every square inch of space, and the kitchen became our de facto hang zone. I remember "helping" my mom make dinner, standing on tiptoes or sitting on the counter so I could see every step of the process, stealing tastes and whining when I eventually got tasked with washing lettuce (the worst!) to keep my hands busy and me out of the way. That kitchen was where I first fell in love with cooking, despite all the lettuce washing.

When we moved into a new, bigger apartment, my mom started to experiment with her interior design style and let her WASP-plus–Staten Island roots show. (Think wooden antiques bought at auction, satin sofas with velvet pillows, and lots of animal prints!) With four kids running around, she often had to choose comfort and durability over her ideal style, but she still managed to put her own spin on each room, giving our home personality while taking into account all the people who lived there. She was also conscientious about including my dad's Turkish heritage, so there was a real mix of influences at our house. There was plenty of decoration, but it was a lived-in fullness rather than embellishment for its own

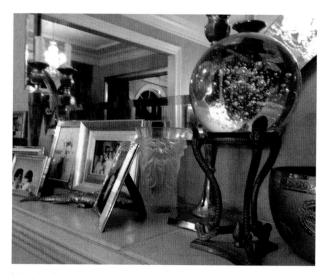

Here's the crystal ball my parents brought back from China—glued together and good as new!

sake—every item had a reason for being there.

Every time my parents took a trip, they brought home special trinkets that would be displayed in cool areas around the house. Take the huge, brass soup samovar from the Turkish bazaar that my sister and I used to brew "magic" potions in (which magically ruined the samovar). Or the giant ten-pound crystal ball that my dad lugged home from China, which now stands on the living-room mantel. It broke in half during a particularly wild fight among my two sisters and me over whose turn it was to "read fortunes" from the orb's depths, but my dad gamely superglued the two halves back together, and on it lives in our home.

As we moved into different homes, we would jettison old junk and bring with us those things that we loved, and the new places would feel just like home with a slightly different layout. Logistics might be different in the newer spaces—location, architecture, the height of the ceilings—but there was a constant quality to our home life that came from us and from our belongings. The wooden armoire my parents got from my aunt Carole for their wedding. The grand piano and treasured family pictures that adorn it. The sofa that never dies and just keeps getting reupholstered to match changing environs. Those objects created a visual consistency that bridged the gaps and created an environment that always felt like ours. But I only realized the importance of these components once I was trying to create a space of my own.

After college, I moved into an apartment with a roommate and the two of us went to IKEA and selected furniture essentials like bookshelves, a TV console, a little dining table, headboards, and bedside tables. But these things didn't make the apartment feel like a home. Not until I went to my parents' and retrieved my favorite bedding, borrowed a rug, and installed my great-grandmother's shell mirror and my favorite pictures did it start to feel like a place that was specifically mine and not anyone else's.

I'm not a control freak or a perfectionist. Working within a budget and on a quick timeline often means using what you can get. But I know from experience that it's totally possible to dress up generic pieces and make them play a solid backdrop to the special items that make a space mine. I believe in smart, practical luxury, and I don't need a decorator's degree to know what I like—and neither do you! Be patient; be proactive. Even if it comes together slowly, if it looks and feels like you and not just a page out of *Architectural Digest* or a home-goods catalog, then you've succeeded in creating a space you can call your own.

Ultimately, I want to feel good when I walk in the door. I want everything I need within reach. I want my history represented, I want to feel like my personal taste is reflected, and I want others to feel welcome and taken care of.

Finding your decorating identity is like finding the right haircut: Lasses who don't want to visit the salon every five weeks may not opt for edgy cuts that need upkeep. Likewise, if you've got five dogs who don't respond to the command "Sit!," you probably don't want a white sofa. But if you've got a cleaning staff of seven, by all means, white silk it is! Know yourself. Know what works for your life. And then build your taste into that reality so you can enjoy it and make having a beautiful home a practical luxury.

MAKING A HOME

In the old days, private and public life were kept carefully apart. Hosts entertained in designated spaces like parlors; kitchens were hidden at the back of the house and areas reserved for family were tucked away and not open to guests (think: *Downton Abbey*!). Nowadays, life is a lot more casual (thank goodness!), and especially in apartments and smaller houses, you can expect guests to visit all parts of your home. In our first apartment, my parents' bed was in the "living room" and became the de facto couch, coffee table, and coat check. You may have a bit more room, but when you consider your home design, keep in mind that you'll likely be sharing your personal space now and again. All the more reason to make all the component parts a beautiful part of the whole.

For every room in a home, my decorating keywords are *tasteful*, *practical*, and *comfortable*. A well-appointed room is like a well-dressed woman: every piece in place, every piece on purpose, every piece a necessary and delightful part of the whole.

Tasteful: Does My Home Feel Like Me?

First things first: Taste is inherently personal, and there's no right answer. Think of all the different interior designers and the millions of different ways they could conceive of a space, and that's just the tip of the iceberg. I'm a die-hard fan of Mary McDonald's designs (all rich wood, plush, oversize couches, and soft fabrics), but I also love Kelly Wearstler, with her affection for harsher elements of bright colors, stone, leather and metal—less for everyday space, more for statement areas. I like to blend the two, so I took a huge wooden-framed mirror and added it to my entry hall along with a cast-iron candelabra that would have looked crazy anywhere else. Then I added a plush velvet-covered bench to soften up the look. I put stacks of books on either side—more an act of desperation, since I didn't have room for bookshelves—and voilà, decor that has pieces of me, is functional for my things and for what I needed to do with precious space in my apartment, and creates a statement out of an area that could have been just a boring white hallway.

You can cull inspiration from all different sorts of aesthetics, and there's no rule that says you have to stick to one specific look. It's about finding what makes sense in a particular space and what makes you comfortable. All you have to do is play!

Living with taste is much more about having there be some story you are telling through design and the way you live your life, some continuity and clarity. Even then, the story you're telling could be totally random and a hodgepodge of everything; I wouldn't be comfortable living in a room packed with a rainbow of colors, prints, patterns, and textures, but hey, you haven't asked me to live with you, so have at it!

Even if you've never thought about defining your taste, chances are your brain pretty well already knows what you like. To help suss it out, head over to a magazine stand and see what you gravitate to in the home-decor section. Are you more of a sleek, modern kinda gal, or do you like lots of patterns and objects to draw your eye? If you're looking at a fashion magazine, do you like to see monotone colors or contrast?

Take clues from the kind of homes you've been in that you like best; the way your wardrobe (or dream outfit) looks (is it all structural angles and shiny embellishments, or is it draping chiffon in a simple silhouette?); the way you feel in different spaces (do you feel strangled in cozy places or anxious in wide-open ones?). Think about the decor in the house you grew up in—did you love it or hate it?

Honing taste is about trial and error, letting yourself be inspired by what's around you, and paying attention to how you instinctively respond to certain looks. It's also about working within your budget and getting creative to maximize its potential; decorating and keeping a home were never meant to be elite activities! They're just about taking care of what's yours and making the most of what you have. If you haven't got your taste totally pinned down yet, don't fret—it's the work of a lifetime. You've got plenty of places (start with your desk at work and go from there!) and time to play around, change your mind, and try something new.

Practical: Do I Have the Things I Need?

Practicality is creating a home that works for you, and sometimes that means taste takes a backseat to livability. If you have a million messy kids, it's probably not a genius move to cover your home in delicate brocade and porcelain. If you're an avid outdoorswoman, maybe skip the fancy foyer in favor of a tricked-out mudroom with places for all your hiking boots and a basin to wash up in when you come through the door.

Understanding your own specific needs is crucial. A magazine can show you cool color schemes and layouts you might not have thought of, but it can't tell you what makes you *you*. Some of us need lavish kitchens; others would rather cook in a Crock-Pot and have a backyard, if that was on the table. Walk-in closet versus cupboard space; guest room versus room with a view; space for a bookshelf or space for an armchair?

Once you understand your basic taste and practical needs, you can start allocating those most precious of decorating resources: funds and imagination! If you're the kind of girl who can't sleep without the coziest bed ever, then budget for an expensive mattress instead of a fancy couch. If you can't afford a luxe headboard, scour online for budget options with a similar look, or get creative and make your own!

Comfortable: How Do I Want to Feel When I Look Around?

Comfort is more than just a physical feeling: It is also an emotional sensation. What makes you feel at home, taken care of, relaxed? When we decorate, we are doing more than deciding how a room will look. We are establishing an aesthetic and creating an atmosphere. Walking into a stylish, well-appointed home that truly reflects what you think is beautiful is a joy! When we can find the things we need easily and walk into a room knowing that everything's in its place, we feel that we belong in the space, too.

Whether the style is streamlined modern or decorative antique or casual vintage or a blend of all the above (though this certainly takes more practice to master than any of the more basic looks), everything in the room needs to make sense. A well-thought-out room is not too adorned or too bare, not too stuffed with furniture or too empty; it's not a storage locker, but you have all the things you need; it invites you in to sit, to talk, to linger.

Once you've reflected on what makes you comfortable and made sure to include those elements—a cozy place to read or channel surf, a brightly lit kitchen—then you tackle atmosphere, choosing new colors that make you feel vibrant and alive, displaying heirlooms and souvenirs, and finding a dining table and a new couch—or reupholstering an old one.

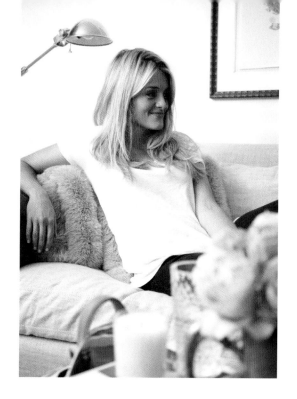

At the end of the day, putting your home together should be simple—figure out ways to make use of what you already have and get rid of stuff you hate. Get the essentials, and then recognize that a beautiful home comes together with time! Don't rush to buy random junk you don't need just to fill a space out. Let these things find you, whether they jump out at you at a vintage store, leap into your hands at a market, are gifted to you by a friend or family member, or call to you from a magazine ad.

And remember: More stuff isn't always better, especially if it feels generic. No one wants to live in a furniture showroom. More stuff that's all you is what you're looking for.

PROJECT INSPIRATION

If you're not sure of your style, the best way to help crystallize it is to buy a few decor magazines or spend some time scavenging around on the web—there are so many incredible interior design mashups and blogs these days that you can get all your inspiration for free!—and tear out or bookmark those rooms that really appeal to you. Some of my favorites include the Improvised Life, Design Sponge, Apartment Therapy, A Cup of Jo, and StyleMePretty, and Tumblrs like Wit & Delight and I Wanna Be Gwyneth, and of course, the Pinterest boards I follow give me tons of amazing interior design inspiration.

Keep a physical or online filing system for your inspirational images, sorted either by room type or aesthetic. My mom has drawers full of these things, so she was able to pull from years of brainstorming and honing her vision when it finally came time to design her own home from scratch. I'm not doing that just yet, but you better believe I kept my choice of magazine clippings close at hand whether perusing online or in stores when I was picking out furniture for John's and my apartment, and it made narrowing the options and staying within my vision much easier because I already knew the types of spaces I wanted to create. Plus, because I knew some of the specific items I wanted ahead of time (like particular light fixtures I'd found in a magazine spread)—and how much they were going to cost—I was able to build the rest of the room around them so I could figure out where to spend and where to save to create the room I wanted without going over budget.

I also keep tearsheets for everything from makeup and hairstyles to clothing looks to vacation escapes I'd like to take—everything goes in a labeled folder in a filing box specifically reserved for inspirational images. I call it my "dream box." Every year, usually around the holidays when I have some free time and am planning for the new year, I filter through all the various images and articles I'm holding on to, weed out the ones that I don't love anymore (tastes change as we do!), and remind myself what I want to see more of in my life. It's a good idea to keep the things that inspire you close at hand and fresh in your mind so you can look for ways to bring more and more of them into your everyday living.

MAXIMIZE YOUR SPACE

Whether you're working with a studio apartment or have a guesthouse out back, there are a few things we all do at home—*eat, sleep, relax, store up, create.* We need to make room for all these needs, even if our floor plan does not, by maximizing every inch.

In the next few pages, we'll first consider how to give your home bones—the essential structure that holds it all together—and ways to organize and prioritize space to get the most out of it. Then we'll determine how to flesh out your home with all the personality, style, and history that make sure each room serves its function and its fun. Along the way, you're going to get a little dirty playing handywoman around the house. And then we'll look at the best ways to get and keep your space clean with products you likely already have in your pantry.

START WITH THE BASICS

Basic does not mean boring. It means essential. What are the basic needs of a home? You need a place to eat (your kitchen or maybe a dining room); a place to sleep (your bedroom or a dedicated corner of space with a place to rest your head); a place to relax and entertain (your living room); a place to store up and keep safe (shelves and storage space); and a place to work and create (this can be anywhere you can get productive and creative, whether it's a proper home office or a lap desk). Let's lay the foundation for a home that takes care of you by making sure each room covers the basics and then some.

Every room has a different purpose and should be organized around its main functions, based on who will be using the room and what they'll be doing there. Once you've covered the basics, you can design, decorate, and accessorize to your heart's content. Below, I've included my top recommendations for *basic* essentials, *better* improvements, and the *best* finishing touches to help you create the perfect balance of form, function, and fun in every room in your house.

An Excellent Entry

An entryway is the *aperitivo* to your home's main meal—it's there to whet the appetite! A welcoming entryway makes you comfortable the moment you walk in the door—and doesn't require a great deal of space. Whatever your floorplan, the entryway should be designed to make life easier and ground the home. It will be the first and last thing you see, so it's important not to miss an opportunity to make an impact.

BASIC

Somewhere to hang your coat. Whether it's a coat stand or a closet, make sure you have somewhere to leave your outerwear as soon as you walk through the door so you're not tempted to leave it in a heap on the floor or sling it over furniture.

Somewhere to leave your keys and sundries. Nothing is more frustrating than spending twenty minutes hunting for your keys morning after morning, so take the guesswork out by designating somewhere specific to leave the essentials. I prefer to have a narrow table with a pretty bowl to toss these items into, but a hook on the wall works just as well.

A mirror and some light. You want to be able to snag a last look before you run out the door but don't have time to run back to the bathroom, so put a mirror near the door—the bigger the better, since mirrors also help to create the illusion of more space. Make sure it's well lit so that you can see if you have spinach in your teeth and are left with a glowing impression, not a bunch of shadows.

BETTER

Drawers or extra shelves. Give yourself a little extra storage space near the front door. Extra shelves give you a place to leave incoming and outgoing mail so you can keep track; storage bins give you a way to organize different types of shoes, umbrellas, and other things that don't have a place farther inside the home.

A bench or chair. This is a very useful thing to have as you try to pull heavy boots on or off.

BEST

Fresh scent. Give your home its own signature scent by greeting yourself or visitors with a scented candle or fresh flowers in a vase as soon as they come through the front door.

Photographic memory. So many great pictures we take get buried in photo albums or digital archives and never get seen. Give yourself something fun, happy, beautiful, or meaningful to look at every time you come and go. I stick snapshots of my hubby, family, friends, pets, vacations, or anything else I want to look at over and over again in the corners of the mirror in my entryway or in their own frames. Guests especially love to see the goofy one of me as a kid in a pink snowsuit looking beyond put out. Seeing all these memories as I come or go always puts a smile on my face.

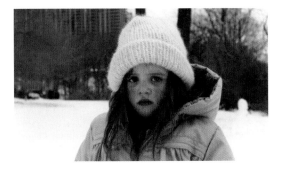

If you're stuck in a New Jersey snowstorm, you might as well be decked out in head-to-toe pink—even if it does restrict your movement to waddling only.

Curios. Use your entryway as a place to display some of your greatest finds, whether it's an architectural piece you picked up at the flea market or a ceramic bowl you threw at pottery class that's perfect for holding loose change and gum.

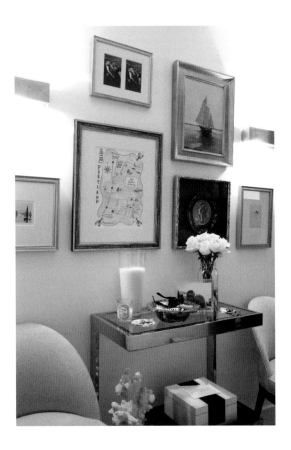

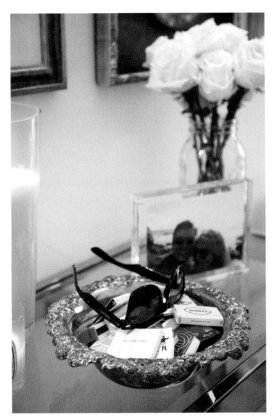

A Tricked-Out Kitchen

I could sleep in a cubby as long as my apartment has three things: good lighting, fresh air, and a great kitchen. A studio apartment with a chef's kitchen appeals to me much more than a one bedroom with a palatial closet and a hot plate. Maybe you feel differently, and you should pay attention to the space you care about most when you're creating your home. In order for me to be comfortable at home, and to feel inspired to prepare the foods that will keep me and mine feeling happy and energized all week long, I must, must, must have an easy-to-work-in kitchen. I need room to make a mess! And I need my kitchen necessities (and maybe a few extravagances, too). Hey, if you love it, it's worth it.

BASIC

A quality chef's knife and paring knife. Your chef's knife should be sharp and rest comfortably in your hand, because you'll use it to do everything from slicing to dicing. Make sure you test it in the store to see if you like the way the handle feels, how heavy the knife is, and how long the blade is. And your paring knife—a slightly smaller knife that gives you more precision and control—will come in handy for smaller vegetables or peeling duties.

A cutting board. Invest in a good-quality wood cutting board, and a couple of plastic or silicone ones that are easy to throw in the dishwasher to sanitize after cutting fish, meat, and poultry. Chopping on a board not only protects your knives from getting dull, but it also protects you by preventing the blade or whatever you're cutting from slipping.

An open space to chop. It's equally important to have an open place to do your chopping—if you're hunched over under a cabinet and uncomfortable, there's no way you'll love to cook. The only thing I care about in your kitchen is that you feel comfortable and happy in it. Because as Carla Hall, my cohost on *The Chew*, likes to say, if you're not happy, the only thing you should make is a reservation. A backache does not a happy cook make.

An eight-inch skillet. This is your all-purpose utility cooking instrument. If you get nonstick, it's best to look for a coating that has been tested for off-gassing. Otherwise, stainless steel is a good basic and just needs a little bit of fat in the pan to prevent sticking.

BETTER

A cast-iron pan. This is a totally worthwhile investment, and if you take care of this thing, you'll have it for at least twenty-five years. Skip your manicure this week, or say no to that expensive drink, because you need to have a cast-iron pan. It does everything. Go for an eight- to ten-inch skillet. You want it to be large enough to hold two steaks or fish fillets, and you can also use it to make pancakes, corn bread, hash browns, a frittata . . . anything! It's a really good conductor of heat, and it creates a wonderful crust on whatever you're making. (Just remember to keep it away from soapy water—no soaking! Clean it up by letting it cool slightly, then rubbing it with coarse salt to soak up any cooking oil and remove debris. Wipe it out with a clean cloth and season it by rubbing with a little olive or canola oil.) To sanitize, you can heat a clean cast-iron pan in a 350°F oven for 20 minutes. Remove and allow to cool, then season the pan with oil.

A high-powered blender. I got a Vitamix for my birthday a few years ago, and it has completely changed my life. I use it to make smoothies every week (it makes short work of frozen fruit and ice) and to make dressings or creamy soups (hot or cold!), and it's a must-have when margaritas are on the menu.

A food processor. I have a small one that I use for any kind of mincing work—throw a few peeled garlic cloves in, press a button, and presto! It's also great for emulsifying salad dressings. Larger ones have different attachments and are perfect for everything from throwing together a quick dough to chopping/dicing/slicing vegetables.

BEST

A Le Creuset enameled cast-iron Dutch oven. I live in my Dutch oven. I use it to make soup, for braising, baking, roasting. Because it's enameled, you don't have to care for it as carefully as you would cast-iron—just wash with soap and water, and it's done. Plus it comes with a lid and goes safely into the oven or fridge. Brilliant!

A standing mixer. I wouldn't go so far as to say this is essential, but it does look gorgeous on a kitchen counter and makes putting together all sort of doughs a snap. Plus, the myriad attachments you can purchase—for everything from meat grinding to pasta making—mean this is an appliance that will grow with you as your culinary skills increase.

DON'T BE A BAG LADY

I am fanatical about keeping reusable bags with me all the time (hate to waste all that plastic and paper!), but I never put bags on the counters. Or on the bed. Or the couch. It's a simple rule, and one that keeps a lot of gross germs off the surfaces I use all of the time. When I ride the subway and put my bag on the floor, or drop my purse next to my chair at a sidewalk café, or bring home bags from the grocery store, I just know that the bottoms of those bags, are covered with leftover germs from the people who walked there, who walked their dogs there, who did who-knows-what there.

So if you wouldn't invite everyone in the neighborhood to come in and walk all over your counters before you chop a salad, keep the bags on the floor.

Dining in Style

Now that you've cooked a meal, you need somewhere to eat it!

Before moving from one apartment to the next, my husband and I held off on getting a new dining table because I wasn't sure which kind I would need. We got rid of our old one—a junky thing I'd bought online and never thought I'd hold on to as long as I did, but lots of great meals were shared at that dinkey piece of plywood!—thinking it wouldn't be a good fit for the new place and sure we would find an alternative pronto. (Lesson 1: out with the old only *after* the new is in!) For two months, hubby and I ate cross-legged on the floor, and though this seemed romantic and "picnic-y" at first, it quickly got tired.

Relationships happen around the table—it's where families commune, where partners discuss, where roommates find out about each other's weird habits. Eating on the floor is all well and good for those moments of rustic inspiration, but find a way to give a table space in your home, even if it has to work triple duty as a coffee table, desk, and lamp stand, too. When everyone knows where they're meant to gather at mealtime, it adds a homey rhythm to life.

Given my love of food and cooking, not having a dining-room table felt like someone took the anchor off my ship, and the whole apartment was out of whack as a result. Waiting to find our "perfect" table meant that we wound up hovering in the kitchen, snacking out of containers, or eating out rather than lingering over romantic dinners together at home. Meals were rushed, uncomfortable, insignificant—and I probably put on five pounds, to boot. When you aren't paying attention to what you're eating because it doesn't feel like a meal, chances are you're not going to be easily satisfied. Tables are what help make food feel like meals; all we were doing was snacking.

We should have been relishing our time together, not scavenging uncomfortably on the floor. Not having a proper place designated for eating won't (and shouldn't) ruin a relationship, but it won't give you the benefit even a simple forty-dollar collapsible version could provide: a place to share, to make moments out of meals. To enjoy one another.

Learn from my mistake. I don't care if you have to make it yourself: Get a table or, at the very least, designate a real space for sharing meals. It may be at the kitchen counter with stools pulled up, in a breakfast nook, at a foldout table, or in a proper dining room. Whatever space you're working with, here are the things you'll need to make sure you and your guests can enjoy your meal properly.

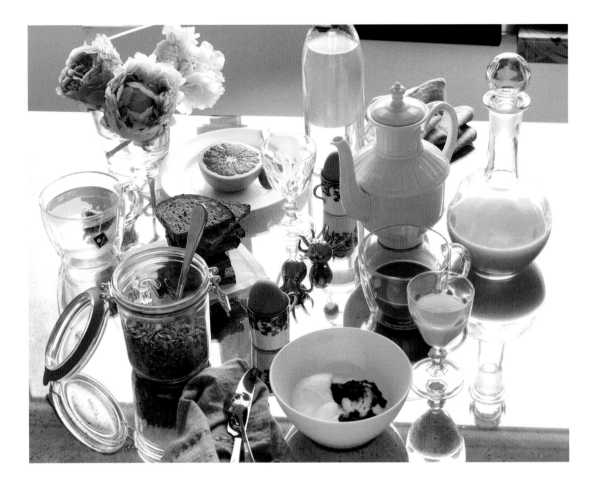

BASIC

A table that fits. My preference is for a rectangular table that allows you to face people directly, converse and share food easily, and maximize the number of people that can sit along its sides. If you don't have space for a large table, or you like to be able to bring it out only when needed (or, if you want to be prepared in case you need more seating than your current table has), keep a folding table in the closet. A lovely tablecloth fixes up even the least fancy of card tables. Whatever table you choose should fit in the allotted space so that it feels proportional and should be as large as possible, while leaving room for everyone to get in and out of their chairs comfortably.

Comfy chairs. If you or your guests are going to want to linger over sumptuous meals, you can't have bad seating. Choose chairs with back support and a slightly padded cushion. Armrests are a nice touch for extra support and comfort, but they do take up space.

Good lighting. People want to see what they're eating, so don't set your table up in the darkest corner of your home—if you do, you'll need to supplement with lots of artificial light.

Simple cutlery, plates, and glassware. It may not be the fanciest collection out there, but basic stainless cutlery, simply decorated white or cream plates, and clean, clear glassware will help you put together beautiful tablescapes without the worry that your most precious items will be damaged every time someone proposes a toast. Plus, they're generally pretty easy and inexpensive to replace when someone does accidentally clink too hard. Having a neutral canvas also gives you more room to play and add fanciful fun with candles, flowers, napkin rings, or other trinkets, if you want to doll the presentation up.

BETTER

Candles. Adding candlelight to the table is a wonderful, simple way to add grace and atmosphere to any gathering. I collect interesting candelabras. I know, it sounds fancy (and perhaps a little unnecessary—but isn't that half the joy of collecting?), but there are cool ones out there made from everything from ceramics to nuts and bolts. Sterling silver is all well and good, but that's a lot of polishing I don't have time for, and I'm just as happy to have a few pretty crystal pieces or to buy interesting wooden ones and spray-paint them in the hues I need. The most important thing is that candlelight casts beautiful uplighting, which will give all your guests a generous glow that overhead lighting cannot.

Cloth napkins. Linen or cotton napkins nicely bridge the gap between über-traditional and über-modern, and they add a touch of class to any affair, even if you're standing over the counter and eating leftovers by yourself. They dress up a table and they're good for the environment. My go-to is white cotton napkins, which always match and are easy to bleach when I want to sanitize and remove stains. If you have more than one set of napkins, get a bright color or seasonally appropriate pattern. A little bit of embroidery or a pretty hem is also a nice touch, but make sure they're not totally irreplaceable—people will be wiping food on them, after all. And the fancier the napkins, the more special care has to be paid whenever you want to wash them—so think of how much hand-washing you're up for before you commit to the lace!

BEST

Mix-and-match china. In addition to my basic whites, I have plates in varying shades and patterns of blue, crimson, and gold that can be combined in any number of ways, as needed—for anything from a spring lunch to a fall dinner (that's the beauty of having both cool and warm tones to play with). Even better: If one breaks, it's not the end of the world, because it's not part of a perfect set.

Specialty items. I have a reserve selection of unique glassware and decorative items that I like to scavenge for in different little markets and vintage stores. Breaking out some funky salt cellars or colored wine goblets makes the setting extra special without needing to pay particular attention or spend a ton of money getting a full matching set of something.

The Best-Ever Bedroom

Your bedroom should be a place where you can really kick back and be yourself; where you can feel cozy and cosseted, warm and protected; and where, of course, you can entertain admirers. But the most important thing to do in your bedroom, aside from romantic interludes, is sleep.

Think of the biology behind sleep—generally, we're most comfortable when we re-create the way we felt in our mother's wombs, so the perfect sleeping quarters must include darkness, white noise, warmth. Solid shut-eye for most of us depends on re-creating these environs. And it's important that you do, because sleep is an active and necessary state of being for humans.

Sleep allows our minds and bodies to recharge so that we can face the next day renewed and invigorated, and it's the time when your body does all its basic household chores to make sure you're in tip-top shape. Plenty of sleep means you're better able to deal with stress and be creative. And because sleep gives your body time to shed toxins and replenish healthy cells, you can also think of it as essential to aging gracefully. So creating a space that is conducive to maximum rest is a must.

BASIC

Supportive mattress. If you can't even remember when you got your current bed, it's time for a new one. Turn your mattress (so your head is where your toes were) once every six months, and flip the mattress over (so the top becomes the bottom) once a year to prevent odd lumps and divots from forming. And invest in a mattress cover! Basic ones will prolong the life of your mattress by protecting it from bedbugs, stains, and the like. Pillowtop covers will upgrade your mattress tenfold and make you feel like a princess on a cloud.

Cozy pillows and comforter. I'm a pillow fiend—and I opt for at least a 90 percent down fill and then encase my pillows in pillow protectors to keep the feathers in and any bacteria, mold, and mites out. Good pillows cost forty dollars of more, and the protectors help them last longer, so protect your investment in a great night's sleep! (Same goes for my down comforter, a medium fill that's good for summer and winter and everywhere in between.) Get some firm pillows that can be arranged for comfortable reading, thinking, and journal keeping with proper back and lumbar support, and a few plush ones to sink your head onto at night.

THE DOS AND DON'TS OF LIGHTING

Beautiful lighting is one of the most important ways to create a luscious home environment. It refracts against objects and changes the color of the walls. It keeps us from bumping into the furniture. And it can make the difference between looking like a rosy young beauty and an ancient, sallow crone. (Score!)

Know your lighting. There are three kinds of basic lighting: task lighting, ambient lighting, and accent lighting. The lamps that you read by are task lighting, as are the lights that help you see when you're chopping salads in the kitchen. Ambient lighting is light that comes from all directions, spilling over an entire room to illuminate when sunlight is not available. Accent lighting highlights a particular part of a room, such as a painting you want to show off.

Instant facelift. Uplighting sends light bouncing upward, creating highlights as opposed to shadows the way overhead lights do. This helps faces shed fifteen years, and the under-eye bags to prove it. You can achieve this effect by having light at different levels in your home—a variety of floor lamps, table lamps, wall sconces, and recessed lighting, for instance—since the rays will bounce and play off each other. You can also try lamps with diffusers that do not cast downward rays because the light is being bounced off of a surface to create a more uniform, surrounding glow. If that's not an option, best to provide lots of candlelight to help balance out the harsher brightness of artificial lighting.

Brighter is not always better. You don't necessarily want every corner of your home flooded with blinding light at all times. In fact, you need variation and some shaded areas to create atmosphere—think mood lighting. Without having to invest in dimmers for the whole house (although these are awesome if you can swing it! Like having multiple light fixtures in one), try using spot lighting to draw attention to a particular feature in a room—since your eye is drawn to light, this is a great way to make small spaces feel larger.

Use a bold fixture to anchor your dining room table. If you have a chandelier or other dramatic lighting fixture, position it just above the dining-room table. Like a headboard over your bed, it creates the idea that the table absolutely belongs where you've placed it, even if it isn't in the middle of the room.

Pay attention to ceilings. A too-long fixture hanging in an area where people pass is a bruise waiting to happen. Dangling lights are fine over a table, because it's not a walk-through zone, but shorter fixtures are more appropriate in areas like hallways or the parts of a room that are high-traffic zones. If you are doomed to overhead lighting that came with a home and you can't—or don't want to—invest in changing it (though I will tell you that an electrician can often do it in about an hour and you may want to consider!), you have two options: (1) Crowd out the bad lighting effects by filling your home with other light sources—pretty standing and table lamps, candles, even string lights throughout your home to diffuse light and make it more forgiving; or (2) Move.

Count your threads. When it comes to sheets, spend the extra forty bucks to choose the ones that feel the softest to you with the highest thread count you can afford—try to go somewhere in the 300 to 600 thread count range. Generally, the higher the thread count, the softer and more durable sheets will be—so you won't be finding holes in your sheets in a few months' time. You sleep on your sheets every night, so do your own nails this month and spend those dollars on counting sheep.

HEADBOARDS

The purpose of a headboard is not just support while you're reading juicy novels late into the night. If you want to anchor the bed and make it look like it belongs exactly where it is, invest in a headboard. Or make one yourself! I love crafts, but I—like most people these days—never have the time to perfect my skills or project and am often left with little more than a jumbled heap of glitter, glue, and pipe cleaners to show for my efforts. This is the type of DIY that I adore because it's actually possible to accomplish in a reasonable time frame without an art school degree.

WONDERFUL MAKESHIFT HEADBOARDS:

Vintage finds: A beautiful old door or screen can be reclaimed and mounted over your bed. Same goes for metal grating, colored-glass windows, or any antique find that is a likely shape. (Note that items painted before 1977 probably contain lead paint, so take care that the paint isn't flaking, and a coat of sealant is probably a good idea. When in doubt, check with an expert to be sure.)

Fine fabrics: A favorite piece of fabric can be mounted over a painting canvas or framed and hung up over your bed to create a decorative backdrop.

Paint a canvas: Simply paint a blank canvas your favorite tone—the bolder the better!—and hang. This is your chance to try a shade you might not use to cover the entire wall.

Paint the wall: You can also use painter's tape to mark off the section where the headboard would be, and paint it any color that strikes your eye, using color and shape to create definition and frame your bed beautifully.

Frame a gorgeous piece of wallpaper: If you love the look of designer wallpaper, get the whimsy of your favorite design without all of the fuss. Simply purchase a small roll, cut out the desired amount, and frame the desired section. Voilà! Charming.

I generally opt for white or light colored sheets because they're easiest to clean, and the lighter the dye color, the softer the sheets. Make sure they're freshly washed—at least once a week to keep them clean and smelling fresh—and store them in a cupboard with dryer sheets in between the layers to help remove static and keep them freshly scented. You should have two sets of sheets per bed: one in use and one being washed or in the closet. Using different light colors for each bed will make it easier to sort them and find what you're looking for.

Mood lighting. You want to limit bright lights before bed of any kind, so either dim the over-head lights or nix them and opt for candlelight or a bedside lamp if you're going to read your-self to sleep.

Hydration. Set a pretty, covered water jug and glass by the bed. Drinking water before bed helps the body excrete salt, wastes, and toxins so you don't wake up puffy in the morning.

BETTER

Bedside table and lamp. This is a good place to keep your light reading, a candle for mood lighting, and the water and cream you want to have near you before bed and when you wake up in the morning. From a feng shui energy perspective, you should try to have matching side tables on either side of the bed for balance.

Creams and balms. Keep lips, hands, and feet moisturized by stashing your favorite products at your bedside for easy application before tucking in.

Curtains. We all sleep better in darker environments. Blackout curtains are awesome, but sometimes it's just a matter of angling your bed so light doesn't shine toward your pillow.

If you go for sheer window coverings, you can keep prying eyes out but let morning light filter in—natural wake-up calls are good for the brain and the soul. Plus, sunlight helps set your internal clock—which is why most of us need darkness to fall into deep slumber, and why sunlight helps us feel energized and alert in the morning. If you can manage it, a double layer curtain—sheers to close for light coverage and a second layer of more opaque curtains to shut when you want to sleep in—is the best of both worlds.

BEST

Dress up your bed. Little bursts of color define a room and make a bed look more impressive and put-together. Even if you want to keep most of the room a neutral palate, you can have some fun choosing accent pieces like throw pillows, blankets, dust ruffles, or a duvet cover. I try to stick with colors I might find at the spa: relaxing, uplifting shades of deep blue, soft lavender, or creamy coffee, but burnt orange or zebra-patterned can be luscious, too.

Boot the TV. The best thing I ever did was throw the TV out of our bedroom, opting instead for a stack of relaxing reads (try short stories—for ultimate relaxation, it's nice to be able to shut your eyes at the end of a story or chapter rather than leave your mind racing on the edge of a cliffhanger).

Perfume dreams. Essential oils like lavender and mint (again, think spa!) are a great addition to any bedtime ritual. They help all your senses relax and can be mixed into cream or a carrier oil like coconut or jojoba, or used in a diffuser. Candles with the scent of lavender or vanilla help you feel relaxed, and the warm glow sets a romantic tone. I like to go for soy-based candles because they're clean burning and don't release as much smoke into the air. But any one with a scent you love that isn't cloying or overpowering is perfect.

Pad and pen. I always keep a pad and paper by my bed because I inevitably end the night with ideas floating through my head as I drift off to dreamland, and I'm afraid I won't remember my subconscious inspiration if I don't write them down then and there, which of course keeps me wide awake! Jot yourself a note and you'll be counting sheep in no time. Even better, writing down the thoughts and inspirations that float through your head as you drift off to sleep will let you harness the genius of your subconscious! I've retrieved some of my best ideas from my bedside notepad . . .

A Wonderful Washroom

The bathroom is a room that isn't often discussed but gets a lot of traffic, from bubble baths to quick morning showers, exfoliating, mud masks, and removing those eyebrow stragglers, so it should be set up to be as pleasant as possible. Some bathrooms are blessed with gorgeous tiling and fixtures, some have skylights and steam showers, and others are dank, windowless, cramped affairs with plastic shower curtains and a prefab cabinet—but they all can be made better!

BASIC

Medicine cabinet. Keep all the essentials—toothbrush, toothpaste, floss, deodorant, face wash and cream, and so on—somewhere clean and easily accessible. It's also a good idea to keep a reserve supply of first-aid bandages, antibiotic cream, ibuprofen, acetaminophen, aspirin, and anything you might need for that time of the month always in stock.

Mirror, mirror. A clean, well-lit mirror is a must for makeup application and pore inspection, so if your mirror doesn't pass muster, this is a good place to begin for initial improvement. Get one that has a magnification option but also a regular surface so you can get up close but also see the full picture. If you don't have great lighting elsewhere in your rub-a-dub room, opt for a mirror with a lit rim you can turn on when you need to feel the spotlight.

Extra TP. Keep extra toilet paper on hand in an easy-to-reach location. There's nothing as frustrating as reaching for the roll and discovering at an inconvenient time that it needs replacing—even if you're the one who forgot! And there's something comforting about that row of clean, white rolls arranged tidily on a shelf or in a pretty basket.

Fresh towels. Leave the brightly colored towels at the beach and stick with light colored, white, or cream towels in the bathroom. This makes it easier to keep towels in neat matching sets, since colored alternatives will fade at different rates if they're not always laundered together. And promise yourself you'll get rid of any towels as soon as they're frayed or full of holes. Old towels can be used for cleaning rags; just cut them to the right size and scrub away. I like to keep at least two fresh, dry towels in the bathroom at all times so I never get stuck reaching for a cold, wet one. You can roll them in a basket or fold them neatly on a shelf, so you're never caught out in the rain.

BETTER

Wash and dry. Hand towels in pretty pastels, jewel tones, or bright whites are an inexpensive and easy upgrade. I'm a big fan of whites and creams, because they can be easily cleaned and sanitized regularly without risking color loss, but if you love color, go for it! Shy away from patterns that can look dated or be hard to match, and skip the scratchy embellishments.

Pamper your toes. There's something horrible about stepping out of a warm shower onto cold tile, so put a cozy bath mat between your piggies and that ground. It also helps to keep dripping and slipping to a minimum. Just make sure you get one that can be easily washed and dried since you'll want to do that at least once a week.

Don't skimp on hand soap. Even if you haven't gotten that promotion yet, spending a bit more for a luxurious hand soap and softening cream in a scent you love adds a touch of luxury (and hygiene) for a relatively small investment.

BEST

Space savers. For smaller bathrooms, hanging shelves and hooks adds valuable real estate to tiny quarters. In larger bathrooms, a vintage wooden chair or detailed bench or minimalist stool adds visual interest and is a great way to display and store a stack of clean and neatly folded towels. If you don't have enough cabinet space or you hate the one that's currently hanging, check out local markets and vintage shops for an antique that looks cool and is equally adept at housing your aspirin, Band-Aids, and nail polish. I'm a big fan of the antiqued mirror look, but find one that doesn't look out of place in the rest of the bathroom.

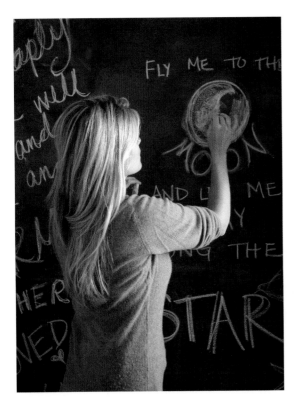

Eye candy. Something to look at, like a sharp little piece of art, can create an entire space or feeling of a room—yes, even a bathroom!—with minimal effort. Hey, if you have to spend time in here, why not make it beautiful? Frame a postcard, or a sophisticated black-and-white photograph, or a little painting that just wouldn't fit anywhere else. A bathroom wall is also a wonderful place to use some splashy paint you might not use elsewhere in your home, like hot pink or canary yellow or the prettiest cobalt blue you ever did see. If you're into modern art, try bold stripes, different colored walls, a painted mural . . . Let the rainbow be your guide! (Just don't forget to put a tarp or plastic sheet over the toilet, sink, and any other surfaces you don't want to add color to). And if you just want to maintain a calm vibe, opt for pretty pastels. I actually decided to paint my bathroom wall in chalkboard paint and have invited everyone who visits me to give it a little TLC, so it becomes a mural created by the people in my life. Every couple months we wipe it down and start from scratch . . . and it makes for a great babysitting tool whenever my little cousins come to play.

Flower power. If you've got windows or a skylight, include a plant on a shelf. If you don't have enough natural light to keep a plant alive, one beautiful bloom with its stem clipped can be floated in a stem vase or glass bowl of water for an elegant touch.

The Loveliest Living Room

An ideal living space is equally well suited to give you space to lounge about in your pajamas on a lazy Sunday morning as to host an impromptu Saturday night soiree. Setting your space up to host the kinds of gatherings you're partial to will make impromptu fests (virtually) effortless and encourage planning if you're the type who likes to pencil it in well in advance.

When John and I were dating, I traded apartments with a friend and had only three months left on the lease. And so I thought, logically, *Why should we bother spending time making this apartment nice? We're gonna be moving out in five seconds.* I didn't really have the furniture to fill

SMELL FRESH

Smells can impact us emotionally, triggering memories, feelings, and responses that go well beyond "good" and "bad." The nose, it turns out, leads directly to the brain. And the brain might not look as pretty as a heart on a Valentine's Day card, but it's still where our emotions live. When you take a whiff, your olfactory receptors deliver the information to the limbic system, the most ancient part of your brain and the part where your feelings are housed. And the information travels quickly. By the time you guess that what you're sniffing is basil, you've already had an internal reaction to the scent.

Aromatherapists use specific smells to make us feel relaxed, energized, aroused, less stressed, and more focused. You don't have to be an aromatherapist to know that the reek of garbage makes us cringe and leave the room, while orange flowers, eucalyptus, and vanilla make us breathe in deeply and say, *Ahhhhhhh . . .*

Light a match. Banish any stale odors instantly by lighting a match. The quick flare will release sulfur dioxide into the air, which will quickly take care of any offensive smells.

Light a scented candle. Scented candles are wonderful, but it helps to tailor them to the environment. The best part is that having individual scents for different rooms gives people a whole different sensory experience in each area, making your home feel more personal and larger because each space is identifiable. Here are some of my favorite scents for different rooms:

Kitchen: clean scents that don't overpower the food, such as lemon verbena and mandarin

Living and dining room: fragrant florals that give the impression there must be giant bouquets all around, like jasmine and gardenia

Bedroom: warming scents that create comfort, like vanilla, amber, and musk

Light a diffuser. Essential oils not only smell great but can enhance feelings of relaxation and energy, and adding a few drops to a diffuser over a heat source helps to quickly perfume a room naturally and therapeutically.

If you want to *relax*, try lavender or vetiver.
If you want to *energize*, try lemon or neroli.
If you're *stressed*, try chamomile.
If you need *clarity*, try clary sage.
If you *feel queasy*, try grapefruit or peppermint.
If you want to *feel calm*, try rose or sandalwood.
If you're cooking or serving dinner, try lemon verbena.

up the space properly. I had one giant chaise longue that was plopped in the middle of the room. There was a random console against one wall. I stuffed an odd leopard-patterned chair into a corner and then decided to spend money to have my television professionally mounted onto the wall. It was a completely bizarre layout, a total nightmare, and exactly how *not* to think about putting an apartment together. Only when John and I went to watch TV from the only sitting spots in the room—the aforementioned floating chaise longue and nonmatching leopard chair—did we realize that the TV was at the wrong height for viewing comfort, and our individual seating islands made for intensely awkward hang-out time.

What I learned from that experience was that by not paying attention to how I might want to use a room, I wound up wasting space and spending money on the wrong things rather than making them count. Rather than relishing the opportunity to host amazing gatherings and hang out comfortably on our own, the space became a lobby, somewhere to drop our things and watch the news on our way to other rooms. Our current living room has been organized in a completely different fashion: by maximizing comfort and functionality instead of simply using what we happen to have around. We learned our lesson from that ill-advised living-room setup and did the work to create an intimate space this time around—a real couch, a comfortable chair, a beautiful ottoman, and a TV at a height we can watch without booster seats. And now that we've created comfortable personal space, we're happy to welcome others in, too.

BASIC

Chat fest. The living room is where you'll likely be doing the most entertaining, so consider the flow of conversation when you plan your layout. Think about organizing the seating arrangement(s) in a way that maximizes seats while minimizing wide-open space that can feel empty when it's just you sprawling on the couch. If you have the space for it, opt for a few smaller seating areas branching off the main seating area so that people have space for deeper conversation without having to bellow over the group, even if it's just two chairs in a corner with a small table and lamp, or a La-Z-Boy and a bunch of throw pillows for floor seating. Think in terms of conversation—you want maximum interaction, so give people ways to face each other comfortably. If you're tight on space, opt for a sofa with no arms—presto, two more seats on either end!

Sit tall. If you do have a television in your living room and are planning to either hang it on the wall or store it in a TV console, make sure you first take a seat on the couch or chair where you'll be watching from so you can gauge the right height for your viewing comfort.

Be versatile. Especially in tighter spaces, having multifunctional pieces is crucial. One of my favorite double-duty pieces is a medium or large ottoman—you can set a few trays on top as a coffee table for daily use and remove the trays if you need extra seating. Ceramic drums, blocks, or tufted cushions that can be both side tables and stools also come in handy.

BETTER

Downsize. It's always tempting (and often economical) to hang on to available couches and chairs, but consider balancing your budget so that you can replace the giant hand-me-down couch that takes up the whole room in favor of a love seat that's more your scale and style.

Customizable coffee table. I have always loved really structural coffee tables—ones made from salvaged wood or architectural metal. They're an easy way to add lots of visual interest to a room that otherwise plays it safe, but they are extravagantly pricey, which is why I still don't own one. Instead, I've opted for simple glass ones that can be spiced up with candles, trinkets, pictures, and reading materials. Another great technique I've used is to push stacks of books into the middle of the room to create the grounding element of a table without having to invest in another piece of furniture. I leave the stacks at different heights (all decently low to the ground so they aren't at risk of toppling over) so there are different layers to the "table"—and it's a great way to store heavy books and show off your literary stores! If you can make all the stacks an even height or create four stable corners for the foundation, you could consider putting a sheet of glass or marble on top.

Homework. Whether or not you actually work from home, work always seems to follow you there. Even if you don't have room for a desk complete with assorted pens, stapler, and hole-punch, create a corner of space in your home where you can be productive, write your emails, and make your plans and keep them. Especially when you set your own schedule, valuing your time as if you were truly on the clock is essential to getting work done, meaning you can't schedule random coffee breaks or shopping dates with friends if you're meant to be putting in some solid time. So put your phone on silent, cut the distractions, and get down to it. Creating an environment that lets you work efficiently means more time to sit back and relax later.

BEST

Reading rainbow. I love to be surrounded by books—old favorites and new recommendations—magazines, coffee table reads, and paper goods in general. I keep most of my collection in the living room so that guests can peruse, and so that I'm reminded of the options on hand when I have a moment of downtime. If you have tons of bookshelf space, more power to you, but books are equally great stacked by theme or color against a wall (spine facing out for easy selection). But avoid being buried under books—and make room for new ones!—by lending out or donating copies you don't feel the need to keep on hand.

Paint job. While I was away on a business trip one weekend, John asked if he could paint our living room and I came home to mint-green walls. More appropriate, perhaps, to an island escape than a New York apartment, but it was incredible to see how radically different the room looked in this color—and oh, my handyman husband! A fresh coat of paint (in the right shade) can add tremendously to a room's look—think of how dramatic a warm brown or slate blue wall behind a collection of metallic frames would look compared with whitewash. If you're thinking of making the jump to boldly colored walls, test out a painted section for a week or so and see how you like it, how the light in your apartment plays with it, and how it meshes with the furniture you already have.

Create. Whatever you love to do in your spare time for fun, make sure there's either room for it at home or that your tools can be safely stored for easy access. Create the space for creativity and it will flow more freely. Removing the blockades—physical or otherwise—that make it difficult for you to find time to have these rejuvenating moments of personal growth, advancement, and *fun* is the first step to making it a regular experience rather than an occasional luxury.

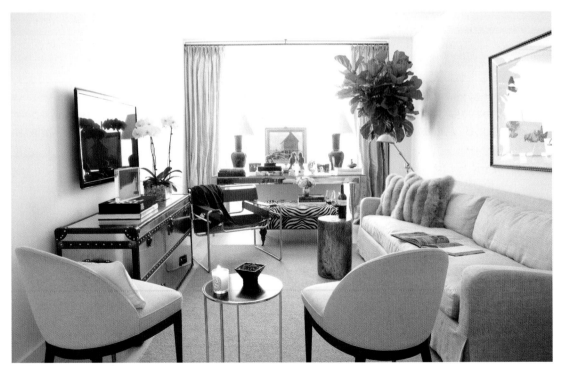

Here's a snapshot of my apartment living room, set up to maximize comfort and conversation.

GET PERSONAL (STATIONERY)

Generally, I don't stand on tradition. Traditions can be wonderful, but they can also be totally tiresome, irrelevant, stuffy, and old-fashioned (in the worst way), and I often find it's better just to make our own. But one old-fashioned thing I absolutely believe in is the value of the handwritten thank-you note. Email suffices for most things, but the surprise of getting a handwritten note to "just say hello" is bound to score you major brownie points with your mother-in-law, grandmother, colleague, and best friend. No one can resist its charm!

One of the many things my great-grandmother did well was write letters—not too effusive, just the right amount of appreciation or gratitude or sincere apologies and condolences so that the recipient felt every bit of her sincerity and class.

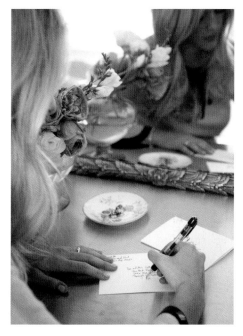

It takes a little bit of practice—and in the meantime, always better to err on the side of being too thankful than too cavalier—but crafting the perfect missive is an art that does not get overlooked.

In the end, it doesn't matter if your stationery is elaborate or simple. One of my favorites was a cutout piece of watercolor paper my aunt painted a few clouds on in fanciful colors—so definitely feel free to make your own! If you're not so crafty and can't afford professionally done stationery, just get some nice cards at a stationery store, write your name on it—and it's yours.

And it tells whomever you choose to write to that you are theirs, too.

Shelve It

Organization is always stylish, and it helps you maximize the space you have. I'm a firm believer that order around you helps breed order inside you, so make sure you're creating a home environment that feels purposeful and stable.

Everything you own should have a designated place to go in your space, from shoes to spices, guest towels to that thing you use to scrub the toilet. Spare yourself the headache of

THE PAPER CHASE

I love my e-reader, but I still get my paper delivered and invest in bound books and beautiful paper magazines. Your bookshelf paints a picture of who you are—what you're interested in, who you learn from, the type of prose or poetry you like to read, the magazines you subscribe to. Make sure you're presenting who you are and who you want to be. Get rid of books you'll never read again and ditch multiple copies (unless they're first editions!). Your personal space is precious, so don't waste an inch on material things you can afford to live without. Plus, the more open bookshelf space you have, the better—more room for newly scavenged books!

How to manage your library:

Color-code. Organize your books by shade to create fun blocks of color on the shelves that add a whole new dimension to home decor without costing a penny.

Be a librarian. Organize your library by theme: poetry, fiction, history, cookbooks, travel. Thematic is easier and more fun than alphabetizing, and it's a simpler task to glance through one shelf than twenty when you're looking for something specific to read, reread, or loan to a friend.

Be ruthless. Curate your perfect library by getting rid of the books you don't absolutely love. If space is limited, try the one-for-one technique: For every new book you bring home, one must be gifted or donated.

Get in line. Make sure that books line up with the edge of shelves. Pushing them back to create space for knickknacks gives rooms a messy, crowded feel, while keeping them flush to the edge gives a neat line, no matter how they're sized. Then again, a few curios or pretty bookends on the shelf can be lovely—just don't overdo it.

Tear and toss. If you tend to save all your magazines, as I do, make it a project every so often to leaf through them, rip out and file the articles and inspirational images you'll really want to refer to again (put them in your dream box—see page 180), and get rid of those piles!

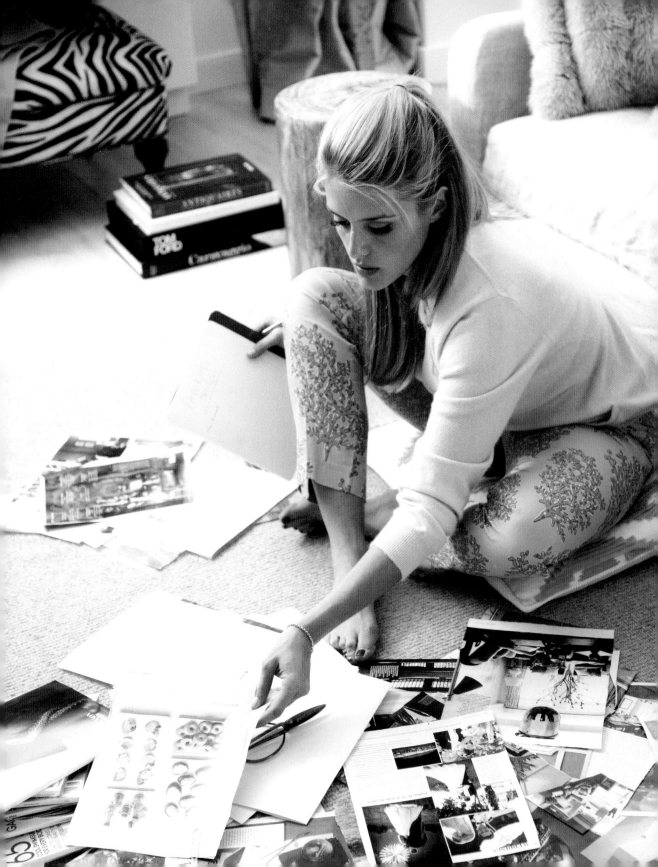

never knowing where anything is and invest a little time in cataloging, stacking, alphabetizing, storing, vacuum sealing, or whatever else you might think necessary.

Let your inner OCD roar! It might not sound fun, but it really is—especially when it's over. Do it when you can—even if it's just while you're chatting on the phone or in between appointments—a little bit of work each day is just as good as an all-out weekend clean fest.

And you don't have to do it alone: Invite friends over to help you sort through things, make executive decisions about what stays and what goes (they'll probably help you part with your favorite and totally moth-eaten college sweater), and then you'll have a few hands to help carry out the garbage—or turn one woman's trash into another woman's treasure!

BASIC

Hang a shelf or two. Adequate closet space and shelving is integral to not feeling overrun. Invest in a couple shelves you can install yourself, or a few rolling racks that can quadruple your closet space with minimal assembly or investment needed.

Keep like things together. If you can, create a special linen closet for your sheets, towels, cloth napkins, and tablecloths. Keep like-size and interchangeable items together. If there's no room for this kind of closet allocation, store items near where you use them—bedroom stuff in your closet; kitchen stuff in the pantry; cleaning stuff under the sink; bathroom stuff on a shelf or in a cupboard nearby. Items you use all the time go at eye level and within arm's reach; things you use rarely go on higher shelves or at the back of the closet. Don't cram, or everything will get wrinkled.

BETTER

See-through storage. Those flat plastic bins they sell at Bed, Bath & Beyond and The Container Store are a godsend when it comes to making use of the storage space under your bed, on top of shelves, and in the backs of closets for summer clothes in winter and vice versa. Anything you don't need to use for the next couple months, box it up and put it safely away. The best part of clear packaging is that you'll know exactly which box to head for when you need to retrieve something.

Label it. Oh, if you only knew my pathetic love of automatic labelers. I label my computer cords, my closet shelves, and my spices. Anything that could possibly be confused for someone else's, or any space that could potentially be cluttered with junk that doesn't belong gets a label. It prevents confusion, and it also helps make sense of why condiments go on one shelf while spices go on another.

BEST

Private eyes. We all have so many user names and passwords in our lives that we're sure to forget the combinations now and then. Keep a few super-top-secret lists of categories of user names and passwords that only you know how to find, whether it's password-protected on your phone or filed away in a safe if you prefer. Break down the lists by finances, news accounts, social media, online shopping, and so on, so they're easy to find. Add new user names and passwords to the list as you get them so you're never scrambling to remember whether it was your mother's maiden name or the name of your first cat that will unlock whatever you're trying to get at. And try to steer clear of storing your passwords for frequently used websites if you can—if it's worth putting a password on, it's worth keeping that password private!

Standing order. Instead of struggling to remember things one by one, or having to dash to the store every ten minutes, dedicate one shopping trip a month to filling up your supply cupboard, or set up a running order online. Keeping enough supplies around creates a feeling of abundance and preparedness, like your home is really taking care of you.

DETAILS, DETAILS, DETAILS

Now that you have what your home *needs* in place, it's time to deal with what your house *wants*! What you're looking for are ways to fill your home with the things you love. Some of my favorite things are chalkboards, the color hunter green, vanilla fragrance, fresh flowers, and linen. A chalkboard in the kitchen gives me space to jot notes, to-dos, and recipes I might

A GREAT GUEST ROOM

If you have one of these, you're a lucky girl. Capitalize on the opportunity to host friends and family by creating a space where guests can relax and feel at home. Guest rooms should be kept spotless, just in case you get a last-minute visitor in town. When not in use, keep a sheet over the bed and furniture to avoid spending hours shooing away dust bunnies.

If you're going the extra mile, one of the simplest yet fanciest amenities I've had while staying at a friend's house for the weekend was access to monogrammed drink coasters and paper napkins: Your initials aren't changing anytime soon, so go ahead and invest in a bunch. They'll help protect your furniture from water rings and spills, while making your guest feel extra cared for.

Other wonderful additions to a perfect guest room:

- A bottle of water on the nightstand

- Hand lotion—consider picking a signature scent for your house or each room for a double dose of luxury at minimum cost

- Tissues—hide the ugly cardboard box under a decorative overlay

- A local guidebook—or even a self-printed booklet of your favorite local spots and adventures, especially if you live somewhere out of the way or in a big city where guests might be expected to fend for themselves and will want to feel like insiders

- A stack of current magazines

- An extra toothbrush, toothpaste, and a razor, just in case

want to try—and are a fun way for guests or regulars to leave little messages. I have a hunter-green cushioned bench in my bedroom. I mixed my own blend of essential oils into a perfume that smells like vanilla and coconuts. Gardenias are my favorite flower, and when they're in season, I like to have one or two floating in a bowl on the kitchen table—or a lush bouquet of my second favorite, pink peonies, in my bedroom. And linen is flowy and breezy, perfect for curtains that keep prying eyes out while letting the sunshine filter in, and it reminds me of vacations on the Mediterranean where linen shirts are the status quo. Since vacations are another favorite thing (duh), it's a two-for-one deal.

Make a love list of pretty, fun, or whimsical *objets* that give you little bursts of joy in life and try to find ways to adapt them for your home. Whether it's a color, a texture, a scent, or a flower, take note of the stuff that fills your heart with pleasure, and plot a way to bring them into your home.

INSTANT UPGRADES

You're a grown-up, so your apartment should look like a grown-up lives there. We've all lived in dorm rooms and inexpensive digs that felt as temporary as they looked, but now we're trying to settle down, not just settle. Growing up means giving up "just for now" style and adopting a more sophisticated approach. So let your apartment know that it's time to move up in the world with a few simple upgrades:

Replace the futon with a couch. Yes, I know it turns into a bed for guests with ease, but it's more suited to freshman year than your fresh start. So get a couch. It doesn't have to be expensive, and it doesn't have to be the couch you have for the next ten years, but it should be something that makes the room look a little bit sophisticated instead of a lot sophomoric.

Frame those posters. Movie posters, concert posters, that amazing French advertisement from the fifties that you scored at a flea market in Paris—put them behind glass instead of reaching for the thumbtacks, and presto! Artifacts become art, instantly.

Be a matchmaker. The stacks of towels you "borrowed" from your mother's linen closet ten years ago have become, frankly, gross. I'm not suggesting that you need to invest in mono-grammed linens, unless you have a penchant for that kind of thing, but a new set of match-ing towels in the bathroom and in the kitchen are a simple and inexpensive way to make the details count.

Vive le vase. Recycling is a wonderful thing, but find something else to do with those wine bottles. If a date or a dinner guest goes to the trouble of bringing you a luscious bouquet, shouldn't you have somewhere equally luscious to place it? A pretty vase makes a nice objet d'art even when the flowers (or the relationship) have lost their bloom. Keep a couple low square or rectangular clear glass vases, plus a few taller, more decorative ones so you have all your mod, clean, classic, and fancy vase bases covered. When you don't have flowers, you can arrange empty vases in a collection and make them a centerpiece of their own.

Get the hang of it. It's easy to dump your coat on a chair or hang it on a hook, but nothing says "mature" like using proper hangers and keeping coats in the closet. I still haven't fully mastered this, but I'm working on it! Being conscious of the problem is the first step to remedying it. Not only does it look messy to have outerwear all over your apartment, but hooks can ruin the shape of finer garments (which I am now meticulous about hanging up after an unfortunate incident with a spiteful family cat and my favorite vintage blouse), while wooden hangers help them maintain their drape, which means that you'll look neater when you leave the house, too.

MAKE IT YOURS

Sometimes our homes are furnished quickly, with everything picked up from IKEA or Pottery Barn in one fell swoop. The issue? A bland look that says hotel more than personal retreat. The quick fix? Adding individual touches that turn those factory settings into something fabulous.

Personality plus. Don't just move a bunch of furniture in and call it home. Add a pillow embroidered with your favorite phrase, a blanket from your mother, a slipcover you sewed by hand. Paint one wall a funky color and then live with it for a month! It may not be all you thought vermilion would be—or it may! Give a room personality with pops of color, a fresh scent, and beautifully textured textiles. Even if you can't afford to get your whole couch reupholstered in your favorite Liberty of London fabric, try buying a swatch and making it into throw pillows, curtains, or a little satchel to keep potpourri in.

Show off. Curate a collection; highlight a hobby. World travelers can gather curios from travels abroad on shelves or in hanging boxes for a 3-D scrapbook. Thoughtful displays personalize your space, remind you of what you love, and give visitors a glimpse of your passions. Interesting hobbies make you more interesting.

Picture imperfect. And what about that hysterical photo of you with braces and frizzy hair from the eighth grade, or the romantic snapshot that your cousin took of you and your sweetie over Labor Day weekend? Adding personal photographs and snapshots allows you to create your own gallery of memories. Think about all the photos we never get to enjoy because they're buried in boxes or even albums that don't get thumbed through nearly often enough. Dig through the mess of albums and scour your hard drive and iPhoto and get some photos framed. Keeping them in view is the best way to make sure that you get to enjoy them.

Go green. Another way to improve the view, instantly, is to get yourself some potted plants (remember to water them). There are so many good reasons to create an indoor garden that it would take an entire book to list them all. For instance, cut flowers need to be replaced often, whereas plants last for years if you treat them right. And they're useful! Your windowsill herb garden lets you add basil to salads at will while making your kitchen look homey and loved. Even nonedible plants such as money plants aren't just pretty to look at: They're hard workers, filtering the air you breathe. Feng shui, the ancient art of directing energy through home design, encourages the use of plants to represent creativity and spring—think renewal and new energy in your home. Busy girls need plenty of energy . . .

Fire it up. If you don't have a fireplace, opt for something more portable. Invest in three hurricane lamps or cylindrical vases that can hold pillar candles and arrange them in a row under a makeshift mantel or against a wall to create a pretend hearth. Even if you do have a fireplace, the hurricanes can be placed within for a mess-free, ash-free glow. And everyone looks better in candlelight!

LITTLE MISS FIX IT

Part of keeping house is knowing how to fix little things when they break. No, I'm not going to teach you how to plumb a pipe—call in the professionals!—but you should know how to do everything from hanging a picture to filling in holes in the wall with a bit of spackle. And for the inevitable mini-crises that crop up—a broken fridge handle, loose shelf, or the child's toy that needs its battery replaced—always be prepared by keeping these tools within reach.

HANDYWOMAN'S RECIPE FOR A STARTER TOOLBOX

1 hammer and a handful of nails in different sizes

1 flat-head screwdriver and a handful of screws

1 Phillips screwdriver and a handful of screws

Pliers

Wire cutters

Measuring tape

Extra credit: A girl with her own drill sets a mighty fine example and can hang pictures, hooks, and shelves with ease. Consider going down to your local hardware store and investing in a drill with a keyless chuck, which means that you'll be able to change the drill bit without needing an extra piece. (But don't worry. Just ask for it at the shop. They'll appreciate your savvy.)

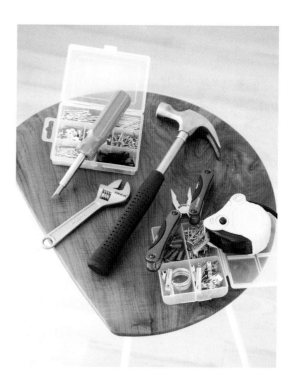

How to Hang a Picture

Play hangman! Gone are the days of hanging your pictures on the wall with thumbtacks or Scotch tape or, even better, that tacky goo that you rolled into a ball and that took off half the wall with it when you had to take it down; gone, too, are the days of using a plain old nail and hoping it hangs on to the drywall. Now graduate to the easy-to-use picture hook.

INGREDIENTS

Picture
Picture hook
Nail
Hammer

1. Decide where you want your picture to hang. A wall of photos should grow organically over time or be laid out on the ground in a measurable grid before you attempt to hang in a pattern on the wall.

Individual pieces of art should be centered on empty walls, used to anchor a space in a loft apartment, or hung evenly over the nearest large piece of furniture, be it the sofa, the dining room table, or a desk. Many people hang art too high. The focal point of the artwork should be at eye level, ideally. When in doubt, put the center of the painting at eye level, making sure that the top and bottom of the piece are well out of the way of furniture and anything else that could bump or scratch your art.

Test to make sure the place you want to hammer is made from sheetrock or another material that is easy to hammer into (not brick or cement!).

2. When it comes to showing off a collection of artwork, I find that both minimalism and over-crowding can look very chic, if done correctly. I tend to like symmetry, especially in places like bedrooms where you want a very calming atmosphere. But I also love the look of a wall hung with tons of different styles of paintings, sketches, photographs, notes, and memorabilia, all of different sizes and styles, framed in wood or metal of the same color family so there is some uniformity and a clear indication that you didn't just throw a bunch of stuff up haphazardly. Plus it lets you put all your goods up on display so nothing is languishing in the back closet!

If you have a particular piece you want to highlight—maybe it's a favorite picture of you with friends or family, or a painting your kid made you—let it stand alone with plenty of space and good lighting. An inexpensive picture light can be bought for about twenty-five dollars online and takes your homemade art to gallery glory.

3. Once you're set on the location and the space, get precise. Make a tiny pencil mark on the wall, exactly where you'd like the center of the top of the piece to rest. Measure the distance between the hook or wire on the back of the frame and the top of the frame: We'll call this the "hanging distance." Measure the "hanging distance" from the pencil mark and make another tiny pencil mark. That's where your picture hook and nail will go.

4. Hold the picture hook up to the pencil mark with your left hand, holes at the top. Now slip the nail in the holes with your right hand, hold it delicately against the wall with your left hand, and hammer the nail into the drywall with the hammer in your right hand. Try a few light taps to get you started and position the nail in the wall, and then it's best to go for a few strong blows to make sure the nail stays straight—just watch those fingers! (Heavier items need special attention—think mirrors and things more than twenty-five pounds. Often you'll need to purchase anchors or studs for added support. Best to check with your local hardware store first.)

5. Hang your picture. Pat yourself on the back.

A Guide to the Simple Spackle

If the measuring didn't go exactly as planned, or you've got ghostly holes haunting your living room from paintings past, fear not. A bit of spackle and a swipe of paint and your landlord will be none the wiser—I actually used toothpaste in the days when they would charge you an arm and a leg for leaving a dorm room pockmarked where the Audrey Hepburn photograph once hung. Obviously, this is no longer my preferred method, and with this easy spackle tutorial, you'll never need to resort to such devious tactics again!

> Hole
> Lightweight spackling compound
> Putty knife
> Sandpaper

If this list is already confusing, don't sweat it. The nice people at the hardware store are well acquainted with the need to fix scrapes, holes, and bumps in drywall, so don't be afraid to march on in and explain what the situation is and ask what they've got to help you remedy it.

Knights in shining armor are still around; they're just waiting for you at the local paint and keys emporium. Ask them for help and they will eagerly comply—or at least educate you and sell you the tools you need to get on with it yourself.

1. Gather your supplies.

2. Use the knife to schmear (that's the technical term) some of the spackling stuff over the hole, filling it in.

3. You may have to repeat step 2 to get the hole really filled in so that it is flush with the wall.

4. When it's filled, leave it be. Don't touch it, sand it, or poke it, no matter how tempting that might be. Let it dry fully (a few hours at least; overnight if you're practicing your patience).

5. Sand the area if necessary to smooth it out, then paint to match the wall. Depending on how long the wall color has been up, you may need to paint the whole wall, as color fades with time, especially if it's constantly exposed to light. But that's for the perfectionists among us . . .

CINDERELLA, CINDERELLA

In the sixteenth century, a rich Roman banker named Agostino Chigi lived in a villa that overlooked the Tiber River. He was well known as an incredible host, a man whose al fresco dinner parties were the hot invitation in town. After each course had been consumed and praised, he would encourage his guests to toss their soiled plates and forks into the river. Impressive! But Chigi was no fool. As soon as all of his guests were gone, his servants would go down to the river and pull in the nets they had installed beneath the water's surface, thereby saving the tableware for the next party.

The moral of the story? Dishes always have to be done.

Even though we have dishwashers and laundry machines and vacuum cleaners to make life easier, and just because we have careers and social lives and interests that make life busier, we still need to embrace our inner Cinderellas and scrub those floors if we want our homes to be neat and clean. But don't fret. The key to keeping house is to keep it simple. Getting too complicated undermines what you're trying to do, because a goal you'll never stick to is useless. So don't swear to alphabetize the spices if you've got a hundred; do promise to put your socks in the hamper when you pull them off.

And remember: The health and psychological impact of getting organized is as powerful as the time-saving, fiscally responsible benefits. A study at the University College London found that even just twenty minutes of housekeeping a week lessened feelings of psychological distress. That's twenty minutes well spent!

My technique is to do ten minutes a few mornings a week (every morning, ideally, but sometimes "snooze" gets the best of me). A quick scrub of the bathroom with disinfecting wipes, sweeping the kitchen, clearing out a cabinet of old toiletries, emptying the trash, or folding the laundry gets my blood pumping and wakes me up, so that by the time I hop in the shower, I'm ready to start the day alert and energized. And by keeping up with the cleaning regularly, I don't (usually) end up spending my Sunday nights doing chores, which is far less enjoyable than game night with hubby and friends or curling up with a glass of wine and *Game of Thrones*.

CLEAN GREEN

When I can, I skip the conventional cleaners and turn to my kitchen cupboards for cleaning supplies. I prefer to clean more often with more natural stuff so I can rest easy knowing I don't have toxic chemical residue all over my home.

Vinegar and baking soda, always useful in the kitchen, can be used to freshen counters, toilets, and your breath (seriously). Those common ingredients are happy to do double duty and have the added value of being good for you and the environment as well as already being close by, readily available, and affordable.

White Vinegar

Counters and windows. Vinegar can be used as a counter spray by mixing with water in a 1:1 ratio and storing in a spray bottle. The same mixture can be used to clean your windows. Steeping hardy herbs like rosemary or lavender in with your vinegar solution may help to limit the strong acid smell, but be careful to test this solution on any porous surfaces like marble.

Bathroom. Toilets benefit from a cup of straight white vinegar poured into the bowl and left to stand for twenty or thirty minutes before you scrub.

Baking soda

Kitchen odors. Place an open container in the fridge and freezer to soak up smells.

Stinky clothes. Sprinkle directly on gym clothes that are waiting to be washed (especially boy socks!).

Carpets. Baking soda also makes an effective carpet odor neutralizer when sprinkled on a rug and left for fifteen minutes before you vacuum.

Kitchen counters. If your kitchen counters need more than a quick wipe with a cloth and a spritz of your homemade vinegar/water cleaner, turn to baking soda's natural grittiness. Sprinkle the baking soda on a damp cloth and you'll have an instant wholesome counter scrub.

Teeth. Since it's nontoxic, you can use the same counter measures for a gleaming smile: A little bit of baking soda on your toothbrush can kill bad breath, stop bacteria growth, and whiten teeth! Great in a pinch for when you run out of toothpaste, too.

REMEMBER: If you're using conventional cleaners, never mix ammonia-based products (like Windex) and bleach-cleaning products (like Clorox spray) together because a toxic gas results. And all we're trying to get rid of is the dirt, not you.

STAY COOL

The point of keeping house is not to stress you out . . . It's to create an environment where you can feel relaxed precisely because you are organized, clean, and prepared, so your impeccable style won't be hidden under layers of spiderwebs and dust. Housekeeping is really just about picking and choosing your battles. I'm not going to detail the stove with a toothbrush every time something falls between the grates. And I'm not about to stainless-steel polish everything. But I will give it a once-over with a disinfecting cloth after cooking a messy meal, and I'll take a Swiffer to the floor two or three times a week because I don't like having dust fly up into my face when I open the door, and I'd rather my feet didn't stick to the floor after a spill.

So, roll your sleeves up and play Cinderella. But don't forget to take a break when it's time to go to the ball!

Now, mistakes happen. Messes happen. People forget to take out the garbage. Managing your house is as much about managing expectations as it is managing people and chaos—especially if you're living with roommates or squatters. So keep your wits about you, and even when someone loses the screwdriver, try not to lose your cool.

Wipe spills when they happen. Little fixes prevent big cleanups. So put things away after you use them. Sweeping up? Put the broom away the moment you're done. Coming in from the cold? After you take off your boots, put them in the closet. Finished with yoga? Roll the mat up and put it back where it belongs. Little efforts rather than massive marathons go a long way in making house management feel manageable.

Spring clean in spring, winter, summer, and autumn. Simply wiping down counters is not going to keep your whole house looking spiffy and neat. So don't save the spring cleaning for spring! Every change of season is another excuse to roll up your sleeves, get the chairs off the floor, and get down to business. A good scrubbing now and again is key if you want your home to look tidy, smell fresh, and have floors that are *almost* clean enough to eat off of. Better yet, give your closets, cabinets, and cupboards a good cleaning each season, too—out with old food, old makeup, old clothes, old anything you don't want anymore. In with organized, clean, beautiful, simplified living! Put on the Billie Holiday or the pop stars or the techno, and have at it.

Run a democracy, not a dictatorship. Everybody who lives in your home needs to pitch in to keep things running smoothly. And since it's not your job to boss everyone else around, take a cue from our Founding Fathers and go with a democratic system. Instead of telling each member of your household what their responsibilities are, call a meeting and let them figure it out themselves.

And remember: Dishes left in the sink is not a conspiracy. Socks left on the floor is not a major crime. The key to staying cool while keeping clean is to be on top of things without making too much of them. So when there are other looming priorities, dusting can take a backseat, no problem.

WHISTLE WHILE YOU WORK

It's really not all bad—I kind of love cleaning: In some weird way, it calms me. Or maybe I'm just choosing to enjoy it. Either way, it's got to be done. There's company coming!

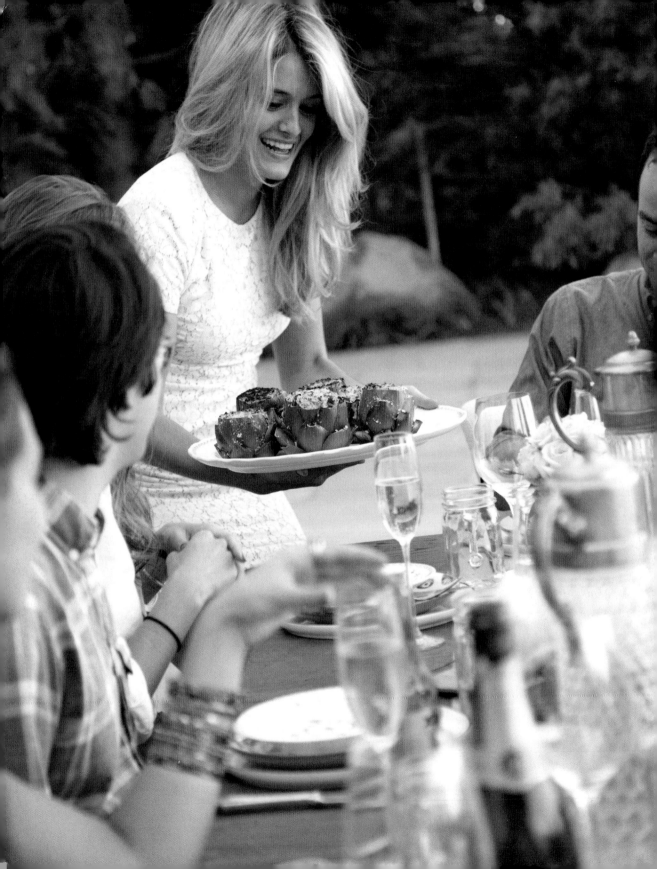

NINE

THE STRESS-FREE HOSTESS

throwing a party like you mean it

"And now," cried Max, "let the wild rumpus start!"
—*WHERE THE WILD THINGS ARE*, MAURICE SENDAK

ENTERTAINING SHOULDN'T BE STRESSFUL. IN FACT, IT SHOULD be—dare I say it?—entertaining! And not just for your guests—for you, too. Whether you're hosting a sit-down dinner for twelve or a casual backyard barbecue, whether you're marking a particular event or celebrating just because it's Monday, it's your party and you should enjoy it! The trick is to plan for perfection, cross your t's and dot your i's ahead of time, and then, once the doorbell starts ringing, put your party dress on and never look back. Even if trouble arises or guests drop in unannounced, with a good head on your shoulders and a few tricks up your sleeve—and sometimes, just enough courage and panache to turn mayhem into magic—you can manage it like a pro and make your party even better.

Case in point: When I was younger, I had this amazing cat that we rescued from a shelter. He was four when he joined our family, and we quickly discovered that he had a crazy personality. He was called Batman, but he probably should have been named Houdini, because he could open locked doors, unhinge birdcages, and escape any scenario—all without opposable thumbs.

We were living on the ground floor of a building in New Jersey that had a patio overlooking the Palisades, an overgrown, rocky area. Batman would go hunting and, of course, bring us "gifts." One evening, as a dinner party got under way, Batman came home with a writhing snake held delicately in his mouth. Our guests were (understandably) horrified. My mother, with a twisted sense of humor, decided that because Batman was clearly so proud of his capture, she would just make the snake the evening's centerpiece. She gathered some twigs and rocks and put them and the snake in a huge glass vase in the center of the dinner table. There he sat contentedly until the end of the night, when we released him back into the wild.

The guests were bewildered, then intrigued, then positively enthusiastic about this recent addition to the decor. Not only was this snake the talking point of the evening, its presence set the tone for what became an even crazier night.

A couple of hours into the party, one of our guests stood up to tell a story that apparently required a lot of wild gesticulation. As he flung his arm back during a particularly dramatic part of his tale, he knocked over an iron candelabra (which I still have in my apartment, a tribute to this ever-so-interesting evening—and believe you me, it has proved a great conversation starter itself over the years), right into the curtains. Moments later, as we all hurled water at the corner of the room to extinguish the flames, and the snake sat peacefully in his vase observing the whole scene, my mom just kept rolling with the punches.

Imagine if she'd lost her cool? Freaked over the snake on her doorstep or her clumsy guest? Decompensated into a heap of tears? Instead, she jumped into action and set the tone for how her guests would react by treating the whole thing as an adventure. In my experience, the evening becomes infinitely more memorable the moment a reptile is made the guest of honor or anything is set ablaze (not that these are the only or preferred ways to make an event exciting!). And aren't brilliant memories the whole point of entertaining?

So before you obsess over how the roast turned out or why you never seem to have enough bowls, remember: Snakes are appropriate centerpieces, fires can be put out, and without your cleverness, your wit, your style, and your social know-how, this event would never have happened. Thus, the most essential element to successful entertaining, my dear hostess, is *you*. You keeping calm. You carrying on. And *you* having fun!

THE ELEMENTS OF A GREAT PARTY

First things first, let's get the basics sorted. There are certain things every great party needs: a reason for being (the standards are pretty loose on this one!), people to celebrate with (I trust your friends are up to the task), divine food and drink (plenty of *Relish* recipes in your arsenal), an inviting ambience (now that your home is your haven, this should be a snap), and a hostess who knows what she's doing (or will very shortly!). We'll get to making you the stress-free hostess supreme in just a second, but lay the groundwork by making sure you cross the following items off your list as you plan your next fete:

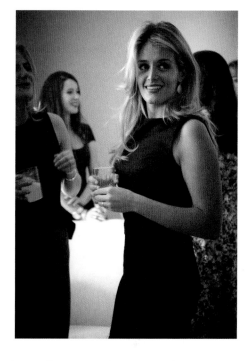

The occasion. Some parties are in honor of occasions; others are "just because." So whether you're having a brunch, a dinner party, or a how-many-people-can-we-cram-into-the-living-room bash, the purpose will inform your guest list, menu, and decor. Choose the date, select the hour, determine the dress code or theme, and then (if it's the type of event that calls for such things) send the save-the-dates or invitations, so everyone can get it on their calendars. Emails work just fine, but a paper invite is so lush! Impromptu gatherings can be just as fun as those planned far in advance, and a phone call to invite friends over for cocktails tonight or dinner Friday is just about as old-school fabulous as it gets—no one ever actually calls anymore, so make it your thing!

The guests. For an intimate dinner party, you'll want to carefully calibrate who you invite. If everybody on your list is best friends with one another, you may not want to invite someone who will be an odd man—or woman—out. Unless the point is to introduce the newcomer around, he or she will likely be bored by the memory sharing that often arises among groups who know each other very well. If everyone is a stranger to each other, consider their interests and proclivities and invite folks who will mesh well with others and can offer some scintillating conversation over the meal. If you're throwing a blowout bash, invite anyone and everyone. Between the cocktails, the crowds, and the dance music, it'll be less about the intimate chats and more about throwing down, so the more the merrier.

LESSONS FROM GATSBY

I love the illusion of control. In theory, I know it cannot be real, but time and time again I hope that if I organize and map out and double-check, things will go according to plan. Of course, the universe has a funny (and often sadistic) way of proving just how foolish we are when we expect the expected.

A few summers ago I decided to throw my mother a birthday party. I set the date, invited her friends, and then got right down to business planning the menu.

Our mouths would travel all over Italy, Lebanon, and Turkey as we savored creamy mozzarella with vine-ripe tomatoes and arugula salad, tabbouleh, hummus and baba ghanoush on pita crisps, couscous with currants and pinenuts, rosemary-roasted sea bass and a spicy lentil stew. Dessert would find us back in America with a vanilla chiffon cake decorated with my mother's favorite gardenia buds. I created a specialty drink in her honor, "Lisa's Lemon Elixir"—a Meyer lemon lemonade infused with basil that we topped with a little Hendrick's gin for the adults at the party. It's just as enjoyable without the alcohol if you have guests who'd rather pass—always good to have a virgin option on hand!

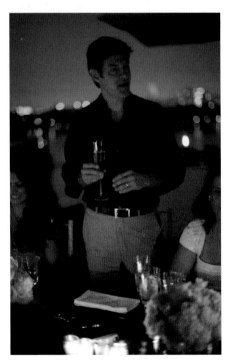

My dad making a birthday toast to my mom.

As the day approached, everything was coming together nicely. I decided to set the tables in a "nautical chic" theme with navy blue and white linens, stainless-steel and white ceramic service, and loads of star paper lanterns and candles. For the flowers, I bulk-ordered white roses, hydrangea, and freesia and arranged them in bunches in the glass cylinder vases I'd discovered at a floral supply shop near my apartment in Manhattan. Processing the flowers was a fun (and economical!) way to be creative and to have the final arrangements look exactly the way I wanted—totally worth the six hours I spent hunched over in the basement! Between the food and the decor, I hoped the party would be as close to a night on the Mediterranean as New Jersey could get!

My mother is a July baby, so contending with the heat is always something to be expected. This year, the thermometer read 100°F at six o'clock the night before the big day. Everyone tried to convince me to move the party indoors, where at least we would have the benefit of air-conditioning. Being the stubborn eldest child that I am, I refused. All of my decor had been planned to feature and accent the outdoor location, and I wasn't about to compromise the aesthetic experience and sacrifice all of that hard work just to spare guests a little sweat.

The day of the party, we began setting everything up outside as planned. The first couple hours went smoothly. We all hustled about, laying out the place settings, the many candles, the flower arrangements,

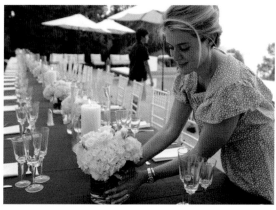

Putting the finishing touches on the table before guests arrived.

and so on. And then our entire county suffered a massive power outage. That's right. There were no lights, no refrigeration, no air-conditioning, no nothing.

The electricity stayed off through the entire party until 2:00 a.m., when suddenly every light in the house came on. And you know what? It was the most memorable birthday party my mother has ever had. She got to spend time with her very closest friends and family without the distraction of music (no electricity for our iPods), with no air-conditioned rooms to escape to, and no landline calls to receive (and most of our cell phones had died at this point, with no hope of being recharged). There was nothing to do but relish simply being with each other, and that's what we did.

The caterer cooked by candlelight, and we enjoyed a delicious meal prepared entirely on gas-top stoves. We sipped iced drinks (one more reason to always buy bagged ice for a party, just in case!), and mercifully there was a strong breeze blowing across our table, which would never have reached us if we'd been seated indoors (Ha! I was right about one thing). One of the guests remarked that the entire experience was very much like a scene out of *The Great Gatsby:* We had inadvertently been transported to a period dinner-party setting where we were without the many modern-day conveniences that make us comfortable but that also sometimes prevent us from living in the moment and enjoying real connection with each other, which is precisely the reason we go through all the trouble and expense to throw and show up at a party.

And so with all of my well-intentioned plans laid to waste, we were hot, but we were very, very happy.

The moral of the story: If you can go with the flow, realize that even the best plans sometimes run amok, improvise, and make the best of a situation, you'll be ready to tackle anything. And luckily for perpetual planners like me, sometimes things that don't happen according to plan turn out even better than we'd hoped for!

The menu. When I plan a menu, I think about food from the perspective of variety: of *taste*, *texture*, and *temperature*. When it comes to taste, you want to ensure your meal isn't all from one food group—fondue, followed by mac 'n' cheese, followed by bread pudding—or all in one taste category: sweet, salty/spicy, sour/tart, or bitter. It's also a good idea to get in a variety of textures. Are all your foods soft? Crunchy? Chewy? Smooth? And you can play with your color wheel as well, pairing bright orange, red, and yellow with crisp green or deep aubergine.

A very important consideration, especially when it comes to party planning, is what on your menu needs cooking and what can be served room temperature or made before and chilled. Your game plan should be to have all your cooking done an hour before guests arrive, with only a few things needing to be reheated right before eating. If you absolutely must put your cookie tray in as guests are walking in, don't leave its fate to chance: Set a timer for yourself so it doesn't go up in smoke.

A fail-proof plan is to have hors d'oeuvres that are either chilled or are good both hot and warm (if they start hot, they'll cool as they're passed around), such as mini-quiches and pizza pitas. If you're skipping passed food, or doubling up on pre–main meal eating, the appetizer is a good place to choose something to be served cold or at room temperature, such as salad or stuffed artichokes. Your main course should be served hot, since this is the anchor of the meal, meaning that you'll likely need to pop it back in the oven for a few minutes, so this is the place you need to budget time for yourself to be near the stove. And then dessert can be whatever you please, since people usually like a little time to digest between the main course and dessert, so you'll have time to scoop frozen ice cream or heat up warm cookies. Or, spare yourself the extra work and serve something that's easy to make ahead of time, like banana pudding or a cake!

Do make sure you've made all the dishes on your menu before the big event! If you want to try your hand at a soufflé, practice getting it right well *before* your party. Otherwise you may find yourself serving guests store-bought brownies instead. Not the worst thing, of course. But if it can be avoided by a practice session, get your practice on.

The decor. Decorating is not always about hanging a hundred paper lanterns from your ceiling or making everyone wear masks. It can be as complex as renting a visiting merengue band and as simple as arranging a beautiful bouquet of flowers, buying themed paper plates, or placing candles around the room.

Also part of planning decor that's both fun and functional is preparing for all the things your guests might need to feel comfortable. Consider the kind of food you're serving and what your guests will need to enjoy it. Are there messy items that will probably require extra napkins? It's probably best to stick with finger foods if you're not providing places to sit or sturdy knives to cut through larger items. Will you put out water for guests to help themselves to?

The idea is just to have your space reflect the kind of atmosphere you want your guests to enjoy. Are formal place settings in order, or a buffet? Are you drinking out of scavenged glass coupes or Solo cups? Give your guests clues about the kind of affair you're looking for—chances are they won't take up an impromptu game of beer pong if you've laid out your best china—by letting your table setting and decorations do the talking.

HOW TO BE A STRESS-FREE HOSTESS

There are three types of hostesses in my book: the do-nothings (they take casual to a new level of laziness), the do-too-muches (forget about getting your own drink or finishing your own sentence), and the just-rights (stress-free hostesses fall into this category!), who manage to make everyone feel warm and welcome while creating a magical affair that feels totally organic. If you try too hard, guests feel overwhelmed. If you don't try at all, guests feel lost and, frankly, a little bit duped—part of enjoying a party is the thrill of being taken care of, so they shouldn't have to track down their own ice or search the back cupboards for mixers.

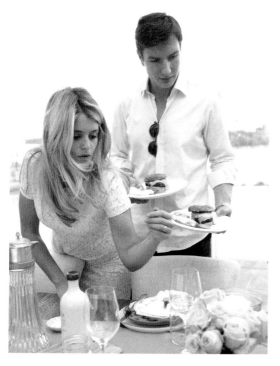

Balance is everything, and the first step to successful entertaining is to remember: It's a party, so have fun! But smart, stress-free hosts take care to plan ahead so they can relax once the guests arrive. Take, for example, my friend and cohost Mario Batali. He's the consummate host, always ready to enlighten those around him by sharing from his world of experience, whether it's business, happiness, philanthropy, music history, or food (obviously!). He gregariously makes sure all his guests are taken care of and entertained without leaving too much up to their decision making: Your drink is already fixed (you're having what he's having); your meal is already planned (and it's delicious); and your dinner companions are curated specifically for your enjoyment (so

FLOWER POWER

I planned my dream wedding with the expert help and guidance of my wonderful wedding planner, Kate Parker (otherwise known as KP) of Kate Parker Designs in New Hampshire. It was a totally collaborative process, and I learned a ton from her about how to give a party personality, focus on the aspects that matter to you, reach for perfection, make your guests feel wonderfully at home, and still be cool and calm enough at the end of it to let yourself enjoy the event like a guest, too!

Now that the wedding is over, I still think about these elements when putting together smaller soirees (even pizza parties for four deserve this love and attention). But of all the wisdom KP had to share, I am most grateful to have picked up some great tips for putting together a simple and elegant floral arrangement for everything from cocktail gatherings to special occasions to easy bouquets that brighten up my home.

Kate was kind enough to break down some of her best advice for everything from how to care for and preserve flowers the longest to how to style a floral design that gets you the professional florist look without the price tag for me to share with you here! Now you'll be able to do so much more than just stop and smell those roses.

Roses. Rose stems should be cut at a wide angle and placed under water as soon as they're cut. You have to remove the extra leaves and thorns before arranging them to prevent any injuries to yourself—you can do this by purchasing a six-dollar garden stripper that quickly cleans the whole stem—and while you're at it a pair of gardening gloves go a long way toward protecting yourself against nicks and scrapes. A rose needs quite a while to be rehydrated after being shipped from a wholesaler, so don't be alarmed if they're a bit droopy when you get them to your house. If freshly cut and given a few hours in water, they should perk right up. You can remove the first few petals around the outside of the rose, called the security petals, which will allow them to open quickly and more widely. If you want a more natural look, you can keep the security petals on. They tend to be a bit darker and more ruffled compared to the rest of the petals.

Peonies. Peonies are available for a very limited time in early to mid spring and are usually unavailable after the last week of June. Peonies start as hard balls and soften and spread out as they open. If you want to force a peony to open, you can cut the stem and put it in lukewarm water. Don't scald the flower. You can also speed up this process by completely submerging the head and stem in warm water for twenty minutes. Peonies are very fragrant and have a large scale, so they're perfect for entrance arrangements or even as just a single stem in a clear glass container—a great way to stretch your budget.

Tulips. Tulips have a tuberous, water-filled stem, so they don't need to sit in a large amount of water. In fact, if you put tulips in water too high up their stems, they actually absorb so much that they thin out and wilt prematurely. Place your tulips in just an inch or two of water. You can also drop a penny in the water to help keep the stems upright, making it much easier to arrange them with other flowers. Nifty!

Lilies. Lilies come in a number of different varieties and can range in fragrance. As a general rule, stick to Asiatic lilies for scale and scent—these are the huge white ones. The Stargazer lily variety can be extremely (read: overpoweringly) fragrant, and many people are actually allergic to them. They're also very large in scale, so they're a great flower for distance arrangements—such as in a foyer or as an entrance piece in your home or for an altar arrangement at a wedding.

Hydrangeas. Cut hydrangea stems with the widest angle possible, allowing the maximum amount of water to enter the stem. Like roses, make sure you put hydrangeas into water immediately after cutting the stems. The fewer air bubbles up the stem, the longer your hydrangea will last. If the hydrangea has started to wilt, recut the stem and fully submerge the head underwater to rehydrate for twenty minutes. You should get a good seven to ten days out of hydrangeas if they're cut properly and in plenty of water.

KP's Top Floral Designing Tips

Height. The best rule of thumb when arranging flowers is to keep them either low enough to talk over and enjoy or high enough that they're not in your sight line. If you're sitting at a table, place your elbow on the tabletop and make a fist. This height will be in the middle of your sight line, so your arrangement should be either significantly taller or shorter. There's nothing worse than not being able to see your invited guests across the table!

Flower variety. Limiting the number of different kinds of flowers in your arrangement allows guests to notice and enjoy the composition without overwhelming them. It also helps keep your budget in check because you don't have to overfill the container with tons of different flowers. Select no more than three to five types of flowers when arranging to keep things clean and simple.

Composition. Create a flower arrangement that suits your style and personality. For a classic design, consider a silver compote or glass vase filled with hydrangeas. Add peonies, freesia, or even gardenia blossoms, and keep the arrangement tight and compact.

For something more modern, consider a monochromatic arrangement using just one variety of flowers. A cluster of thirty canary yellow calla lilies in a sleek square vase really makes a wow factor statement with its architectural lines and simplicity. For a more relaxed look, consider wildflowers from your local farmers' market and place them in mason jars or old galvanized buckets. Queen Anne's lace, delphinium, and dahlias organically composed look like you just picked flowers in a wildflower field and placed them in a vase. In a pinch, float a single bud—or three—in a low dish or glass cylinder of water for a serenely simple and chic arrangement.

many fascinating people don't turn up by accident!). It's an absolute art form, and the best part is you'd think it all happened by serendipitous chance, to look at how relaxed he is.

What takes practice is making ultimate attention to detail look like an act of whimsy. Great entertainers make everything look effortless because they put the effort in ahead of time! And then they *relax* at their own parties and let the plan unfold. It takes a master . . . but we all have to be students someday, so start now.

Here are the things you can take care of ahead of time to lay the groundwork for an epic party and be ready to deal with any last-minute items that might crop up.

Setting the Table

In days of yore, homemakers fretted over the proper placement of an array of serving utensils, from salad forks to liqueur glasses. If you feel like it, you certainly may purchase and arrange the nearly thirty objects it takes to create a traditional table setting. Me? I go with the mood of the party at hand and the relatively minimal number of accoutrements needed to let my guests drink and dine comfortably.

If you're having a picnic-style meal or buffet, utensils and napkins can go into buckets, and plates can be stacked neatly for everyone to help themselves. Paper goods are fine, especially if you're heading outdoors. There are some excellent eco-friendly options available—I love the ones from Verterra.

Think about the things your guests might need if it's more than the traditional picnic fork, knife and napkin. Serving lobster? Make sure you include bibs, extra napkins, and nutcrackers or mallets. Soup? Include spoons. It may seem obvious, but it's your job to think preemptively about what your guests will need in order to enjoy their meal with minimal mess and maximum comfort.

For casual sit-down meals, perhaps family style or buffet, either put out stacks of plates, cutlery, and napkins near the food or lay them on the table informally with a plate at each seat and a napkin rolled around a cutlery set (fork, spoon, and knife) on each one.

For more formal seated affairs, I still opt to go with as few items as possible: dinner plate under salad plate at the center of each setting (or a place-holding charger that will be cleared away if plates are being brought out later); spoon protecting the knife on the right, knife blade facing the plate; cloth napkin to the left under a salad fork protecting the dinner fork; if you want to include it, the bread plate and knife go above the forks; glassware goes above the knife and spoon in this order, right to left: water glass, white wine, red wine. Two additional pieces are the dessert fork pointing right underneath the dessert spoon pointing left that go centered

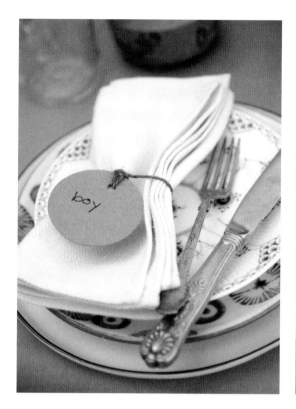
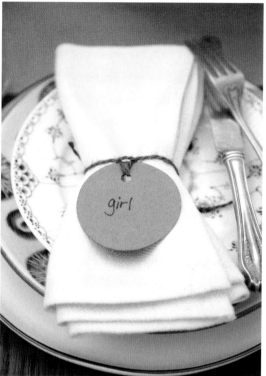

over the dinner plate, but my table doesn't always have space for these, so I bring them out with dessert most of the time.

If you have extra time on your hands, you might choose to fashion a napkin that looks like a sailboat or a swan or a star, and the Internet is full of such ideas. Be sure to send me a pic of the finished product: @daphneoz!

The Music

Music sets the tone for any evening, and even if you're not a DJ, you can still pull together an awesome soundtrack—or task one of your music-loving guests with getting a playlist together on his or her iPhone. I'm constantly scouring music websites like Hypem for new releases and asking my tapped-in little siblings and friends for their recommendations, and Shazam is one of the few apps I use on a daily basis: Whenever I don't recognize a song I love, Shazam to the rescue! Here are my guidelines for the perfect sound at each stage of the evening:

When guests arrive. The music should be upbeat to fill the space and get the mingling started but not so loud that they can't meet and greet. This is your chance to test out your new favorite artists but nothing too avant-garde. You want guests to feel comfortable in the space, and an easy way to do that is to have them listen to music they're already familiar with. Sometimes the easiest way to do this is to load a Pandora channel of one of your favorite artists so you know the genre without having to pick each song individually while you're running around welcoming everyone and making final preparations.

SIMPLE WAYS TO GO FANCY

Not all parties are planned well in advance, and one of the tricks to successful entertaining on any time line is knowing how to make the ordinary extraordinary with a few easy embellishments!

Cheese and crackers become an elegant cheese plate. On a regular Wednesday, you might serve yourself some cheese with crackers. At a Friday night party, add some fresh fruit, scented honey or spiced jam, and fancy biscuits, and it becomes extraordinary. Always good to have a reserve supply of these accoutrements on hand for when unexpected guests drop by!

Soup becomes an *amuse-bouche*. Soups served in a bowl are ordinary. Soups served in shot glasses with a dash of flavored chili or truffle oil as an *amuse-bouche* to excite and wake up the palate before the main course are extraordinary. Though homemade is preferred, this is also a great way to gussy up canned soup.

Champagne goes over the top. A glass of bubbly is an everyday luxury. A glass of bubbly with a few fresh raspberries dropped in and a splash of St. Germain or creme de cassis is extraordinary. This is also an easy way to make less expensive effervescent options like cava and Prosecco feel just as special as Champagne.

Cake gets dressed. A slice may be nice . . . but a slice topped with ice cream and chocolate sauce, or berries and homemade whipped cream, is extraordinary. Adding homemade topping, even if you had to buy your cake at the store, will lend your dessert plenty of homegrown goodness.

Coffee indulges. Coffee is always delicious. Coffee with condensed milk—hot or iced—is immediately, extraordinarily divine. In fact, that goes for almost anything with condensed milk.

When you sit down to dinner. The music should be soothing, so guests don't feel rushed through their meal and so conversation can flow freely without being interrupted with a thudding bass. When in doubt, go for subtle, not electrifying, with medium tempos or softer, soothing voices that will blend into the dinner conversation rather than super loud, staccato, or squeaky background distractors. If you're old school, think Ella Fitzgerald, Sarah Vaughan, or Bobby Darin—there are also more modern remixes of some of these favorites that are the perfect balance of fresh and familiar—or something classic like the Rolling Stones or Simon & Garfunkel for starters (you don't want one artist playing for the entire meal, though, so don't just put the Beatles' *Abbey Road* on and call it a day!). If you want something more present day but don't know what you feel like, try a Spotify search of your favorite new movie soundtrack to get a little inspiration.

As the meal is wrapping up. At this point in the evening, I usually go for lounge music, or what I call "boat music," because it's what I imagine is playing 24/7 on yachts in St. Tropez, like the compilations from Buddha Bar, Hôtel Costes, and Maison Kitsuné. It's good digestion music but interesting enough to keep revelers alert and engaged.

What happens next. Now is your time to determine whether the dance party is going to come next—in which case, I recommend high-energy techno, rock, and pop that people recognize— or whether you want to invite guests to linger over something more soothing or shut the music off altogether to signal the night is winding down.

Theme parties! All the rules go out the window when you're doing a theme party, because you'll be sticking to the music of a genre/age/region. Nothing gets a bunch of eighties-dressed partygoers going like nonstop Journey on the boom box!

Helping Hands

Now, the framework is in place and you're almost there. The party will be in full swing soon!

Though hopefully you'll have taken my advice and gotten everything done an hour before anyone is meant to arrive, even I am sometimes caught running around like mad right up until the last minute. And then guests who want to "help" start arriving—and all you really need them to do is get out of your way so you can finish up!

One thing I always do is put out a cheese plate with crackers or a few simple appetizers and alcohol, mixers, ice, and cups—and maybe a premixed specialty drink to make it easier—in an easy-access spot for guests to help themselves to as they filter in. This gives any early arrivals something to busy themselves with, helps them get comfortable, and buys me a little extra time before I run in to join the fun. You can also ask them to help greet new guests as they arrive and take over DJ responsibilities if you haven't fixed your playlist yet. Fingers crossed you like the same music!

If your significant other or best buds really do want to help, never say no to capable helping hands! You be the judge of whether they can be trusted in the kitchen or need a job elsewhere. If you're hosting as a couple, division of labor is a great thing and takes some of the pressure off you! If you're lucky, he'll be doing the heavy lifting and you can have the extra time you'd like to curl your lashes and add a swipe of lipstick. If not, let him do what he needs to do. Then, make sure he has a snack (and so do you! No hostess worth her salt starts her own party on an empty stomach), a shower, and a fresh shirt and let him get the merriment going with your guests—you'll be there to join in soon enough!

The Art of Great Conversation

Now that everything else is in place, time to mix and mingle! Your guests are there to fill the fun into your party—and you can help them by being the ringleader of top-notch chat. The art of great conversation is honed over a lifetime, but here are a few pointers to get it flowing that tried-and-true hostesses agree upon:

Make introductions. As your guests arrive, it falls to you to make sure they all feel welcomed and included, so make sure everybody has someone to talk to. If people aren't already acquainted, targeted introductions are a must. Don't just say, "Peaches, this is Georgia." Be specific to help get their conversation started. "Peaches, this is Georgia. She's an artist who creates sculptures out of cabbages. Georgia, Peaches just opened a charming gallery downtown." Now that Peaches and Georgia have instant topics to explore, you can continue to move around the room. Movement is important. As the hostess, you want to encourage people to get to know one another, but you're most certainly not a babysitter and should not ever feel as if you have to entertain one person in particular.

Play bellwether. At the table, and especially in smaller groups, the hostess sets the tone for the group, so make it enlightened and/or lighthearted, and remember that humor is always welcome. Be aware of how people are responding and reacting. Sometimes a topic is just too serious or too light for a given group, and it falls to you to be the bellwether and keep checking the collective atmosphere.

Listen closely. Since I started chatting on TV every day for a living, I'm often around people who are really good at talking. But the best among them are the ones who are truly great at listening. That's because they're better able to catch a topic that may have been casually mentioned, ask probing questions, and elevate a conversation to its most interesting level. They're the ones who look you in the eye instead of staring over your shoulder or down the table checking to see who just walked into the room.

If you're not a natural-born listener, think about it this way: Everyone has something to offer, so approach each conversation with the goal of plumbing the depths of that wisdom. The game is to figure out what makes each other tick. Chances are the more you learn about a person and understand where they're coming from, the more you'll like them! And studies show that the more questions you ask and interest you show, the more they'll like you. Win-win!

Hostess Survival Skills

Mishaps make memories, and you can always make the best of them. Here are the most common party fouls—and how to navigate the treacherous terrain like a champ:

Über-inebriation. Serving a delicious Grapefruit Thyme Spritzer (page 155) sometimes means that one of your guests may be compelled to overindulge. If that occurs, don't sweat it. Just calmly lead them away from your other guests and any breakable items with a cup of coffee and some bread. If they're too far gone for these efforts, offer them a place to lie down to sleep it off or get them home safely in a cab. Hopefully nothing more drastic is needed, but it's always a good idea to stay with your friend until you're sure all is well.

Menu emergency. Perhaps you didn't heed my advice and you tried that new soufflé recipe moments before your party began—and it fell. Or you made one of your most surefire recipes, but someone (thanks for your help, dear) left it under the broiler for a few minutes too long and your perfect lasagna got burned to a crisp. Don't freak out! Whatever the reason, skip the blame game and spring into action. If your fancy feast fails, just remember: Everyone loves comfort food. So open up another bottle of wine and whip up some grilled cheese sandwiches or order a pizza. I promise, your guests are there for you, not for your homegrown five-star restaurant (unless you really run a five-star restaurant, in which case, get back in the kitchen).

ICE BREAKER: PARTY CONVERSATION FOR THE ADVENTUROUS TYPE

Occasionally, the best way to break the ice is to just smash right through it. In an effort to crack the code of the individual seated next to me at a dinner party, I have been known to, let's say, ask questions of a less than delicate nature. Like, Why did you get a divorce? Are you still in love with your wife? Do you think you are emotionally withholding? You catch my drift. Perhaps not what you immediately think of as polite dinner conversation, but life is too short for boring conversations.

Still, there is tact involved. When it comes to posing questions of this ilk, it's about how you ask, and your emotional motivation, that signals your dinner companion to see you as charming—or at least cheeky—rather than a meddlesome, prying jerk. I'm not digging for dirt; I'm just curious to learn more about people, to see how we can connect and relate. Being honest, attentive, and reflective when they do answer your questions is also a must—no one likes to bare their soul, much less to a total stranger, and feel as if that person isn't even listening.

In these conversations, most people are generally willing to speak candidly, or at least they haven't proved so mortally offended that they turned on their heel and never spoke to me again. Many people actually seem thrilled to engage in conversation that goes a little deeper than the traditional cocktail party chatter we're all used to. For my part, hearing about how others think through their own lives helps me better understand and consider my own.

Then again, you have to use your best judgment before really grilling your hapless seatmate: It's not always appropriate to jump into the deep end of the conversation pool until you know someone a little bit better.

In the interest of self-preservation, and to give myself some boundaries that still allow for riveting, eye-opening, joyful conversations to take place, I've taken the liberty of rewriting some of the rules of polite dinner conversation (contract negotiations and hostile takeover proceedings excluded) so that nothing is really off limits, though it falls to you to determine whether your party companions are the sort who will enjoy certain topics or not. You may have spent the last three weeks studying intellectual property law in the digital age, but it won't be everyone's cup of tea. Who knows, though—maybe you can teach them something! It's generally best to keep to a subject everyone can contribute to.

With that in mind, I offer you my "How Not to Look Like a Jerk at a Party and Otherwise Be Totally and Magnificently Scintillating" guide to party conversations:

Experts only. This category covers politics, religion, and money. These are always going to be touchy categories where emotional attachment runs high—but hey, sometimes that's just the sort of rowdy chemistry you're hoping for. At the very least, go in with an open mind, not just to hear yourself speak.

Proceed with caution. Sex and relationships. Not everyone is interested in hearing you air your dirty laundry, but if you choose to and you trust your dinner companions, then this can be a great opportunity for free therapy—though be aware that you'll likely have to relive any accusations after you and your paramour have made up or be haunted by that *Fifty Shades of Grey*–inspired interlude you'd rather everyone forget. Sometimes it's better just to keep private lives private.

Safe haven. These subjects include travel, cooking, and current events that aren't hot-button topics. Everyone loves these subjects as long as you avoid bragging or being a know-it-all. Truly, as the hostess, you should have read that day's paper, have recently read a good book or two, and be prepared with thoughtful opinions about a couple of items you think your guests might be interested in hearing about.

Death by dreadfully boring conversation. Real estate and taxes. Just . . . ugh.

Plain old tacky. Here we have whining and gossiping. These are the conversational equivalents of overhead lighting—everyone comes out looking ugly.

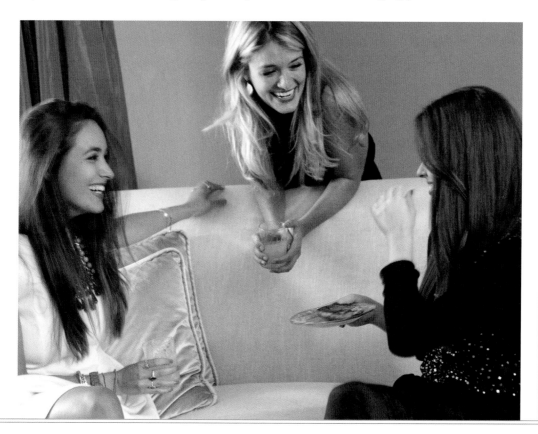

No-shows. You cooked for twelve and only ten showed. If it's their first case of absenteeism, you may choose to give them a pass. But if they're repeat offenders who never have a good excuse, cross them off your guest list next time. If you feel the need to confront them, you can let them know that you worked hard to include them in your plans and were disappointed by their lack of respect. But my experience has been that anyone rude enough to either bail without notice or show up in time for dessert only won't pay much heed to your words. I would save my breath and remember that more may be merrier, but fewer guests make for intimate gatherings, which is also a treat. So be merry with the guests who made it—and this week, you can enjoy extra leftovers.

The uninvited. You cooked for six and seven people showed up, because your friend Ursula assumed it would "be cool" if she brought Adam, who she "met at the bar down the block" this afternoon. You may not know Adam from Adam, but once an uninvited guest is dropped at your table, it's easier to make room than invite them to leave. Once they're there, be gracious; if you ever invite Ursula again, let her know clearly that her invitation does not include a plus-one unless she asks in advance.

Control-freak freak-out. Remember to try to be a guest at your own party. Allow yourself to plan for perfection up to the hour, but once the party starts, plan to have fun.

Leave a Great Impression

I'm a big fan of always letting guests leave with a little something. Generally, I entertain at night, so it's fun to have guests go home with a small item for breakfast the next morning or a snack for the ride home. A signature granola mix, like my Vanilla, Date, and Pistachio Granola on page 26, can be tucked into a cute cellophane bag and tied with a ribbon for a Martha-worthy score that will have your guests remembering you fondly the following morning. Same goes for mini-muffins, and an assortment of homemade cookies is always well-received. If you're feeling extra crafty, and have the time handwrite or print up some labels for your treats, all the more professional and special.

Another favorite of mine is this Spiced Nuts mix, which I love to put out as a snack at the party and bag up to give to guests as they go, in case they're peckish on the ride home.

SPICED NUTS

makes about 2 cups

6 garlic cloves

¾ teaspoon coarse sea salt

2 cups mixed raw nuts (cashews, almonds, walnuts, hazelnuts, pistachios)

2 tablespoons chopped fresh thyme

1 tablespoon chopped fresh rosemary

1 tablespoon Nigella seeds (optional)

1 tablespoon soy sauce or shoyu

1½ tablespoons brown sugar

1 tablespoon olive oil

½ teaspoon cayenne or more to taste

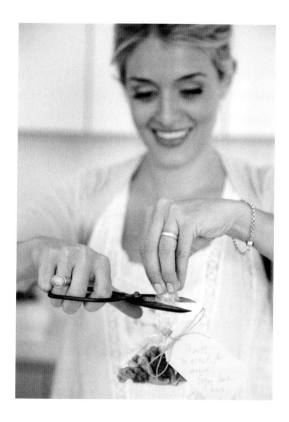

1. Preheat the oven to 325°F.

2. Mince the garlic cloves and sprinkle the salt on top. Use the flat edge of your knife to drag over the mixture a few times, smoothing the garlic to a creamed paste.

3. In a large bowl, toss all the ingredients together thoroughly. Spread the mixture in a thin layer on a baking sheet. Bake for 12 minutes, toss the nuts with a spatula, and bake for another 10 minutes, until the nuts are light golden brown and a cooled nut is firm and toasted. Cool the nuts on the baking sheet before packaging them in gift bags or boxes.

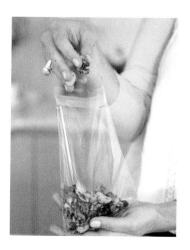
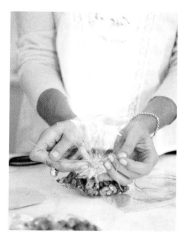
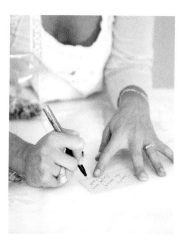

HOW TO BE A GRADE-A GUEST

Throwing a party is lots of fun, but going to one lets you enjoy the fruits of someone else's labor! Want to be invited back? Be the belle of the ball with these simple tips for charming your way through any situation:

Talk to strangers. Talking to strangers is one of the great joys of being at a party. Ask lots of questions and pay attention to the answers. Make eye contact! Have some funny, insightful, or kind things to contribute. If you meet someone wonderful, you might make a friend or learn something new. Don't be afraid to make the approach: At a party, people are already in the mixing mood and are usually pretty excited if they don't have to be the one to make the first move but still get to enjoy good conversation.

But . . . don't be rude. If you've met someone at a party whose every sentence makes you have to hold back a yawn, take action delicately. He may be boring, but that doesn't make him stupid. Even if Mr. Painfully Dull shows no signs of wrapping up his story on the day's trades, you must rise to the occasion. When you have the chance, excuse yourself politely to refresh a dwindling drink or take a bathroom break, but don't do that awful thing where you nod blankly as they ramble on and peer over their shoulders to see who else is there that you'd rather

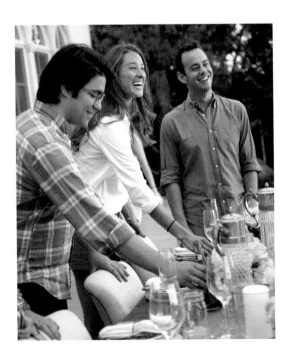
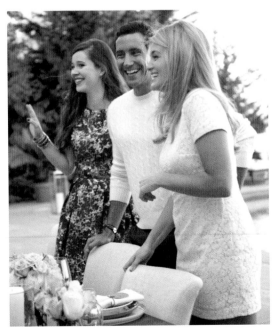

be talking to—or who could come to rescue you. If your White Knight does miraculously show up to whisk you away, well, then, I consider that divine intervention, and you're free to run! But in all other cases, being bored may not be delightful, but it's preferable to being rude.

Put your phone away. You're at a party, for crying out loud. Do you really need to tweet your impressions of the chocolate cake, check your stocks, or send that drunk text to your ex-boyfriend? No, you don't. Photos with friends are a worthy excuse to bring it out. Otherwise, leave your digital world in your purse and focus on the action around you.

Don't drink too much. Yes, have a drink. Have two, in fact. But when the tequila shots start going around, politely decline. There's a time and a place for everything, but it's not usually when you're hoping to make a great impression. This is actually true whether you're hosting or guesting: The last thing you need is to be the host who doesn't remember the party, or the guest who gets sent home by taxi . . .

Don't eat all the snacks. Tempting though it may be to scarf all the lovely canapés your host prepared—and though I'm sure he or she will be glad to hear you enjoyed!—resist the urge to spend more than 25 percent of your time at a party hovering over the snack table. Not only is party snacking one of the easiest ways to mindlessly pack in the calories, it will also prevent you from enjoying all the human interaction you could be having.

Laugh easily. If you're having a good time, let it show! Flash that beautiful smile, let your hair down, and throw your head back if a joke really was all that funny. People will love to see you happy, engaged, and full of life. Don't fake it, but don't try to hide it either. The more you enjoy someone's company, the more likely they are to be enjoying yours—so make sure they know how you're feeling!

Give Thanks

Taking a gift with you to a party can be cumbersome and potentially presumptuous: Who knows whether your host will appreciate your thoughtful pecan pie on her spread when she's planned a Chinese banquet and already has fortune cookies for everyone? Even wine can be seen as pushy if you expect your host to serve it that evening. In both these cases, the gift is more about you the giver being appreciated, whether for your baking prowess or your wine purchase, than about expressing gratitude.

Best to make it clear your gift is for the hostess to enjoy at her leisure by wrapping it or delivering it in a bag and placing it discreetly wherever gifts are being left. In addition to wine,

HOW TO TAKE A GREAT PICTURE

What with today's technology, everybody has a photo booth in their back pocket. Encourage guests to pose for "candids," and email them the next day as a reminder of just how much fun your soiree was. Simply hold the camera up high and shoot at a slightly downward angle and those awkward double-chin photos will be a thing of the past.

When you're the subject, remember that taking a great picture is as easy as tilting your chin slightly down and smiling genuinely but softly (overeager doesn't look good on anyone) without letting your teeth touch. Most people look better from three-quarters view as opposed to straight on, so figure out your best side and snap a few shots in the mirror with your smartphone to see where the angles of your face play best. Fifteen minutes and a few erased digital shots later make for a life of great pictures. And don't be afraid to have your picture taken as often as someone else is willing to take it. You can always destroy evidence, but the more pictures you take, the more likely you'll be to see a beautiful one you love!

chocolates and flowers are typically the safest hostess gifts you can give. All very generous . . . but how boring! Why not a more thoughtful gift, such as . . . a personalized gift basket!

Gather your desired personalized items tailored to your hostess (I like to do a small selection of vitamins, favorite all-natural cosmetics, chocolates, essential oil perfumes, booze, books, or candles—I like the mix of healthy and not; how cheeky!), fill a galvanized bucket (you can pick these up online in bulk or at floral wholesale supply stores) with stuffing like crepe paper, Irish moss, or even shredded newspaper, arrange your items on top, and then wrap loosely in cellophane tied with a ribbon—or ask a local florist to do it for you. The buckets come in all different sizes, or you could use wicker baskets, a pretty box, or any container you like. Any way you choose, you'll be giving a gift that will be ultra-personalized, chic, and unique—all things we want to be!

Party On/Party Off

The best guests know when to leave, and hosts need only know this: When the party's over, music off, lights on, and poof! They're gone.

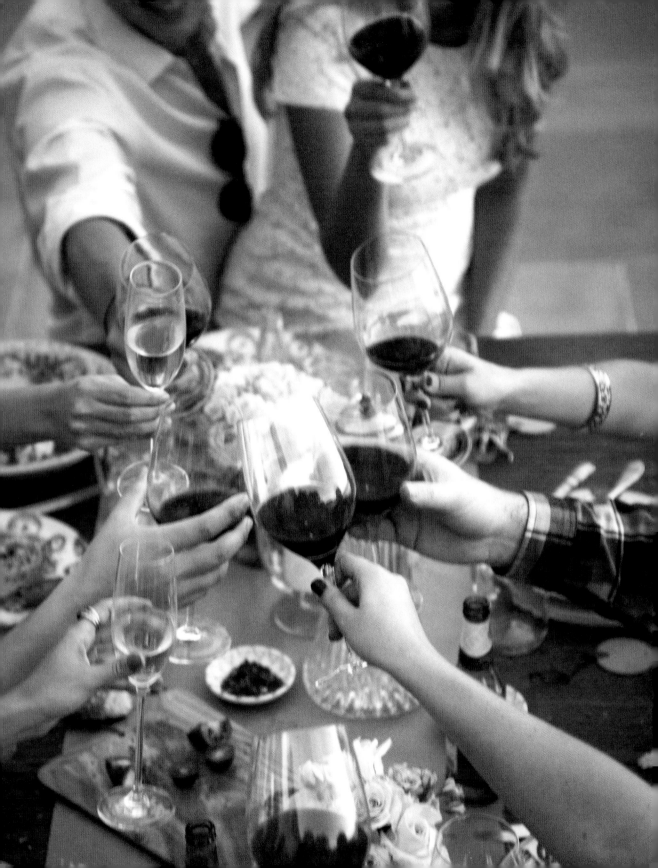

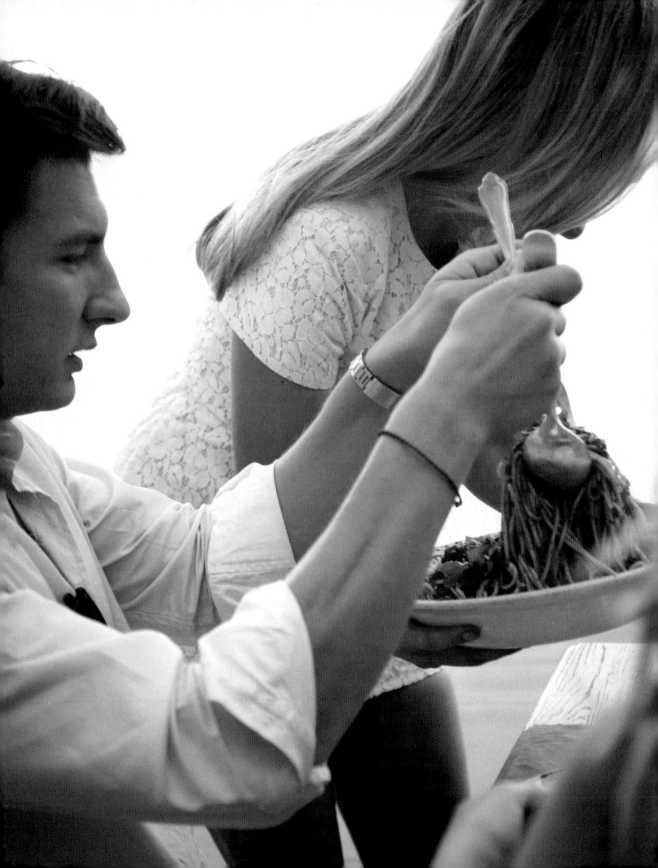

TEN

PARTY OF 1, 2, OR 12

dinner

There is a difference between dining and *eating*. Dining is an art. When you eat to get the most out of your meal, to please the palate, just as well as to satiate the appetite, that, my friend, is dining.
—YUAN MEI

PACK AWAY THE CARTONS, THE TINS, THE BOXES WITH INSTRUCtions for oven or microwave warm-ups. Tonight we don't just eat, stuffing our faces full of the nearest frozen burrito. Tonight we dine, on Roasted Veggie Whole-Wheat Mac 'n' Cheese—as irresistible as the classic but with a healthy, colorful twist—Chile Jam Chicken with Caramelized Sweet Potatoes and Peaches, Homemade Mint-Ricotta Ravioli, or Veggie, Bean, and Cheese Enchiladas to feed a few or lots more. Even the pickiest princesses will embrace the tastes of your menu when market-fresh fish and meat, seasonal produce, delicious cheeses, and fine herbs meet simple, easy technique. And then maybe you can persuade one of them to do the dishes.

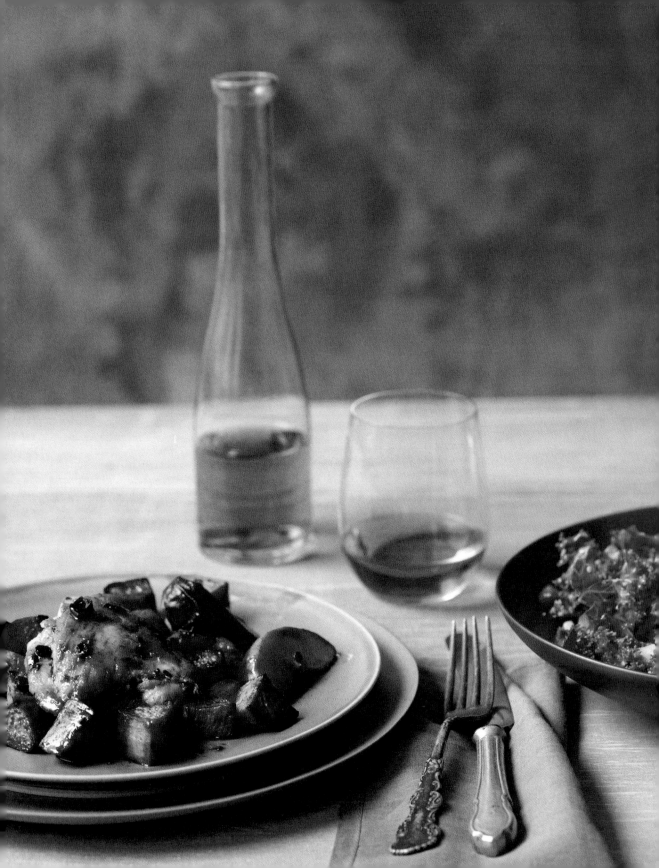

CHILE JAM CHICKEN WITH CARAMELIZED SWEET POTATOES AND PEACHES

serves 2

THIS IS NOT YOUR AVERAGE chicken dinner. Chile jam adds spice and sweetness, and the accompaniments of caramelized sweet potatoes and peaches take it out of this world. Let the chicken thighs continue to crisp in a cast-iron pan as the jam glaze reduces around them, and it will naturally create a crisp sticky-crunchy coating that is to die for!

1. Pat the chicken dry and season both sides liberally with salt and pepper. Heat the oil in a large skillet over medium-high heat and arrange the chicken thighs inside (cast iron works really well to get a nice crispy crust). Brown the chicken on one side, giving the chicken time to unstick itself from the pan surface and form a good, crispy coating, about 10 minutes (you can give it some help with your tongs or spatula if needed). Flip the chicken thighs and brown for 6 to 10 minutes, or until you can insert a knife to the bone and no red liquid emerges.

2. Lower heat to medium-low and spoon a quarter of the chile jam over each thigh. Melt the jam over the chicken and on all sides, using tongs to flip and swirl the thighs in the pan. Cook for 1 to 2 minutes to allow the jam to form a glaze. Remove the thighs to a serving plate and spoon the glaze on top. Scrape up any bits sticking to the bottom of the pan—these will be the crispiest and the first to go!

3. Just before serving, squeeze fresh lemon juice over the chicken to brighten its flavors and heighten the sweetness and spice. Serve with Caramelized Sweet Potatoes and Peaches.

4 skinless, bone-in chicken thighs

Sea salt

Fresh-cracked black pepper

2 tablespoons olive oil

4 tablespoons chile jam (some of my favorites: Hell Fire Pepper Jelly from Jenkins Jellies or INNA Jam's Plenty Spicy Jalapeño for heat seekers)

Juice of ½ lemon

Caramelized Sweet Potatoes and Peaches (recipe follows)

CARAMELIZED SWEET POTATOES AND PEACHES

serves 2

1 tablespoon organic coconut oil, melted

2 tablespoons pure maple syrup, room temperature (if it is cold, the coconut oil will solidify on contact)

½ teaspoon ground cinnamon

Iodized salt

1 medium sweet potato, scrubbed and cut into 1-inch chunks

2 medium peaches, pitted and sliced into 4 wedges each

1 medium sweet onion, peeled and quartered

THIS IS ONE OF THOSE RECIPES that sort of just popped into my head as a possibility and then became a luscious reality once I got into the kitchen and started experimenting. The peaches caramelize and burst with juice in every bite, while the sweet potato gives this side dish some hearty, vitamin-packed substance. And if you've never tried a roasted onion before, well, my friend, you are in for a treat—as they roast, they turn subtly sweet and tender, adding tons of flavor without overpowering the dish.

1. Preheat the oven to 450°F.

2. In a small bowl, whisk the coconut oil, syrup, cinnamon, and salt. Put the potato and peaches in 2 separate bowls. Pour three-quarters of the syrup mixture over the sweet potato and one-quarter over the peaches and toss. Spread the potato in an even layer in a large baking dish and roast for 10 minutes. Toss the potato and roast for 5 minutes more. Add the onion and roast for 15 minutes. Toss the potato and onion, add the peaches in an even layer, and roast 10 minutes, or until the potato and onion are fork tender and the peaches have caramelized.

LADY GREMOLATA Don't worry: It sounds fancier than it is! Our mouths crave excitement, which is why we get bored with one-note dishes and probably why I enjoy going back and forth among chocolate, sour candies, and popcorn at the movies. If you can find a way to put multiple different pockets of flavor in a single dish, your mouth will enjoy it that much more!

This is one of my cohost Michael Symon's specialties: In his cooking, he always knows how to pair complementary opposites—like acid and fat, savory and sweet—to make the overall effect that much more satisfying. He'll add a raw, crunchy salad bursting with citrus or vinegar to an otherwise, rich, fatty cooked dish (often meat), and they balance each other out with a result that's always divine.

Think about ways to add different pops of flavor for your mouth to discover. One of my favorite tricks to help balance the rich sweetness of this particular dish is to add a quick salad of mixed greens or kale with a lemony dressing as a side dish. To go a little fancier, toss together a quick gremolata, or herb condiment. Take the zest of 1 lemon and half its juice, 1 to 2 tablespoons grated fresh horseradish (if you have it; you can substitute 1 grated garlic clove if you don't), 2 to 3 tablespoons orange juice, and a big handful of torn parsley and toss together with a pinch of salt and 1 to 2 tablespoons chopped toasted nuts (walnuts, almonds, hazelnuts, or whole pine nuts work best) to add some crunch and texture. Use this mix to add a bright hit of acidity that will make all the flavors of a rich, bold meal more fun to eat!

ROASTED VEGGIE WHOLE-WHEAT MAC 'N' CHEESE

serves about 12

2 medium carrots, peeled

1 medium turnip, peeled

1 sweet potato, peeled

8 tablespoons olive oil

Pinch of sea salt

Grindings of fresh-cracked black pepper

8 garlic cloves, unpeeled

1 onion, diced

¼ cup all-purpose flour

1 cup whole or 2% milk

1 cup shredded cheddar cheese, or a mix of cheddar and Monterey Jack

1 pound whole-wheat penne or elbow pasta, cooked

BREAD CRUMBS

½ cup whole-wheat bread crumbs

2 tablespoons grated pecorino or Parmesan cheese

2 tablespoons olive oil

2 garlic cloves, minced or pressed

1 small handful fresh parsley, finely chopped

EVERYBODY LOVES MAC 'N' CHEESE. Seriously, it's a rule. No one will be any the wiser that this version is packed full of roasted veggies and uses whole-wheat pasta. And the best part: Mac 'n' cheese this good and good for you means you can eat twice as much!

1. Preheat the oven to 425°F.

2. Chop the carrots, turnip, and sweet potato into equal-size pieces so that they cook evenly. Place the veggies in a bowl and toss with 4 tablespoons of the oil, the salt, and pepper. Toss to coat evenly. Pour onto a rimmed baking sheet, add the garlic cloves, and bake for 20 to 25 minutes, or until tender, tossing periodically so that all sides brown and caramelize.

3. Squeeze the roasted garlic out of the peels. Add the garlic and roasted veggies to a food processor or blender and blend until smooth, working in batches as needed.

4. In a large sauté pan over medium heat, combine the remaining 4 tablespoons of oil and the onion and sweat, stirring constantly, for about 3 minutes, or until the onion is tender. Sprinkle the flour over the onion and stir to combine. Cook 2 minutes, stirring frequently. Add the milk and cheese and stir until you have a smooth mixture, add the pureed vegetables, and stir to combine.

5. Take the mixture off the heat and stir in the cooked pasta to combine. Pour this mix into an oiled 9 x 13-inch baking dish.

6. Toss all the bread crumb ingredients together and sprinkle on top of the casserole. Bake at 400°F for 20 minutes, or until the casserole is bubbly and the bread crumbs are browned.

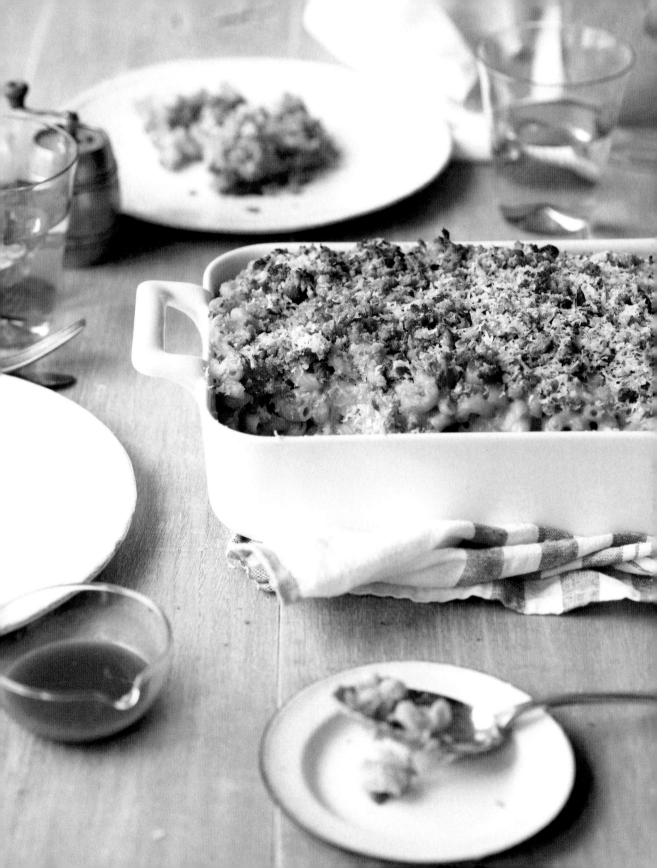

10-MINUTE GLAZED ARCTIC CHAR

serves 4

1 pound wild line-caught
Arctic char fillets (¾ inch to
1½ inches thick)

¼ cup olive oil

¼ cup low-sodium soy sauce
or tamari

2 tablespoons pure
maple syrup

2 tablespoons fresh lime juice

4 garlic cloves, peeled and
minced

1½ teaspoons Tabasco sauce
(optional)

2 tablespoons thinly sliced
scallions (white and light
green parts)

THIS RECIPE WORKS REALLY WELL with any tender, flaky fish—salmon and halibut are also good choices—and is equally great as an easy weeknight meal or dinner-party dish. I generally opt for line-caught wild fish, though an organic, nongenetically modified farm-raised fish is also a good choice. Check out the Monterey Bay Aquarium's website (www.montereybayaquarium.org) for their Seafood Watch list. It's a great resource to help keep consumers up-to-date on best practices when it comes to choosing the most healthful and sustainably raised fish.

You can ask your fishmonger to clean the fish, but keep the skin on. You'll want to purchase about ¼ pound of fish per person.

1. Place the fish skin side down in a dish or bowl to marinate.

2. In a medium bowl, use a whisk to blend the oil, soy sauce, syrup, lime juice, and garlic. Pour the marinade over the fish, cover the dish with plastic wrap, and marinate in the refrigerator for at least 15 minutes and up to 45 minutes, periodically spooning the glaze from the dish onto the fillets.

3. Preheat oven to 400°F. Place a baking sheet in the oven to get it hot.

4. Remove the fish from the marinade (reserve the marinade) and place it on the hot baking sheet, skin side down. Dash the Tabasco sauce over the fish (if desired), sprinkle it with half the scallions, and bake for 5 minutes. Spoon the reserved marinade over the fish, then bake 5 minutes more. Remove the baking sheet from the oven and let the fish sit for 10 minutes. You'll know it's done when the fish is easy to flake apart with a fork. If you cut into the fillet, you will see that the flesh has started to turn from translucent to opaque, but remove it from the oven before the thinnest parts become tough and dry. I like to keep it so I can still see a bit of translucence at the center of the fillet. Top with the remaining scallions and serve warm.

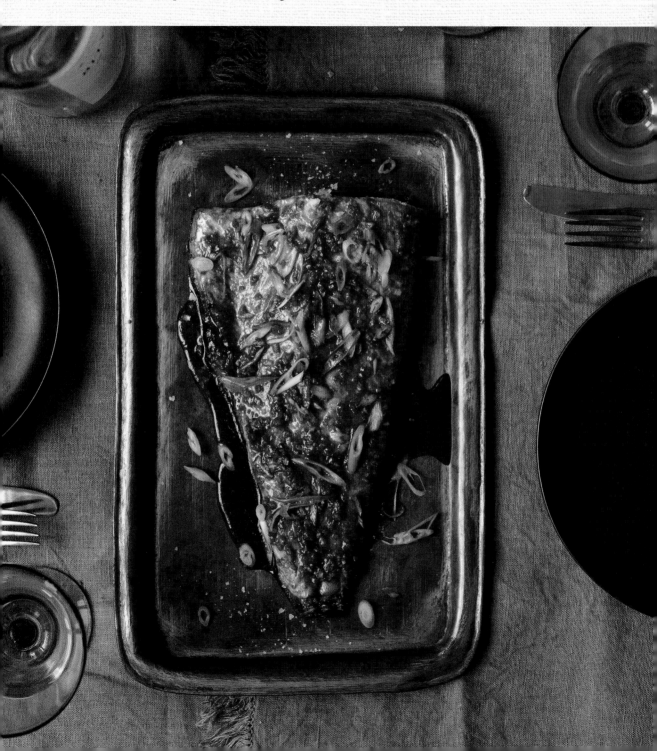

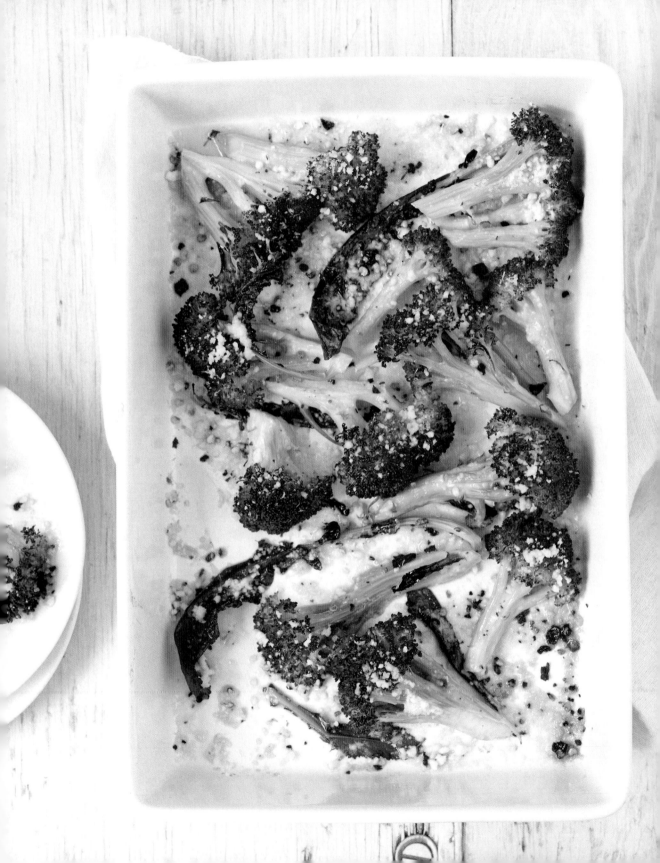

CHEESY "PIZZA" BROCCOLI

serves 4

THIS IS ONE BROCCOLI DISH *that has kids and grown-ups alike demanding seconds. Tastes like pizza, acts like health food! It makes a perfect side or vegetarian main with a nice grain to go alongside.*

1 head of broccoli

2 tablespoons olive oil

6 tablespoons grated pecorino or Parmesan cheese

½ to 1 teaspoon dried chile flakes

1 teaspoon dried oregano

Juice of ½ lemon

Sea salt and fresh-cracked black pepper

1. Steam the broccoli whole for a lovely presentation, or speed the process along by breaking or cutting into bite-size florets. Steam the broccoli until you can easily insert a knife into the center of the broccoli head (about 20 minutes) or a fork into the larger florets (5 to 6 minutes).

2. Preheat the broiler. Drain the broccoli and place it in a baking dish. Drizzle it with the oil, and sprinkle it with cheese, chile flakes, and oregano. Broil the broccoli until the cheese is golden brown, 2 to 3 minutes. Squeeze some lemon juice onto the broccoli, season with salt and pepper to taste, and serve.

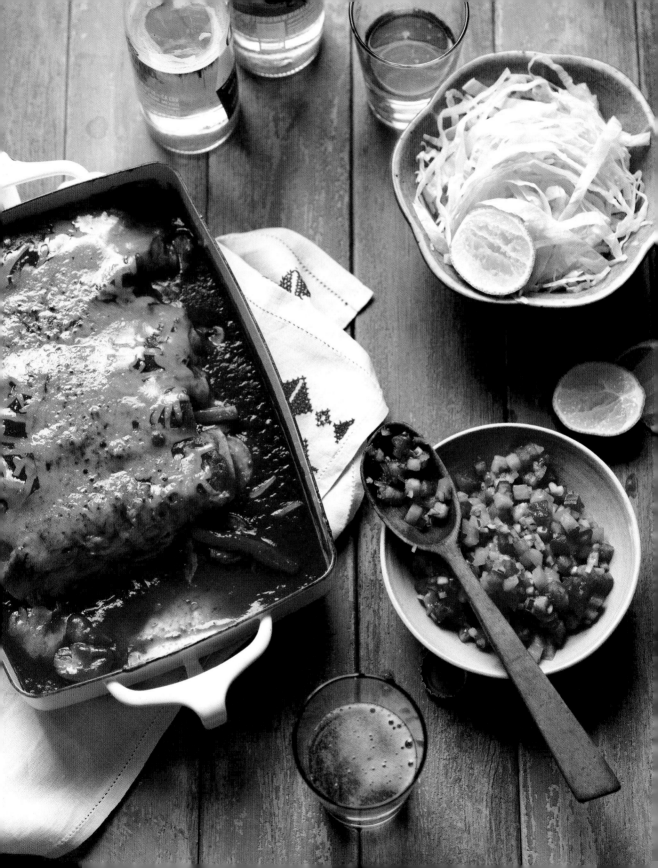

VEGGIE, BEAN, AND CHEESE ENCHILADAS

serves 4

SINCE WE ATE MOSTLY VEGETARIAN *meals growing up, my mother had to develop some clever ways to satisfy my father's carnivore taste buds without the main ingredient: meat. Hearty and packed with layers of flavor, this is one dish that never failed to have everyone at the table excited—it's equally great as tomorrow's leftover lunch. Give it a try for your next Meatless Monday meal or at-home fiesta.*

1. Preheat the oven to 350°F.

2. In a large skillet, melt 2 tablespoons of the coconut oil and 2 tablespoons of the olive oil over medium heat. Add the onions, reserving ½ cup, and sauté until translucent, about 3 minutes. Reduce the heat to medium-low. Stir in the garlic and sauté 1 minute. Add the chipotle powder, beans, ¼ cup water, and the habañero (if using). Cook about 3 minutes, then remove from the heat.

3. Using a potato masher or two forks, mash the bean mixture into a chunky paste. If necessary, add more water to keep beans from drying out. Add 1 tablespoon of the coconut oil and stir to combine. Set aside.

4. In a medium skillet, heat 1 tablespoon of the olive oil over medium-high heat. Add the mushrooms and cook until most of the liquid has evaporated and the mushrooms are beginning to brown, 6 to 7 minutes. Using a slotted spoon, remove the mushrooms from the pan and set them aside in a medium bowl.

5. In the same skillet, heat the remaining 1 tablespoon of olive oil over medium heat. Add the zucchini, squash, bell pepper, and salt until the veggies are tender but not mushy, 4 to 5 minutes.

½ cup plus 3 tablespoons organic coconut oil, softened

4 tablespoons olive oil

2 medium sweet yellow onions, peeled and minced

2 garlic cloves, peeled and minced

1 teaspoon chipotle powder

One 15-ounce can pinto beans, drained and rinsed

½ habañero pepper, minced (optional; discard the seeds and ribs if you want less heat)

½ pound button, cremini, and/or shiitake mushrooms, rubbed clean with a damp cloth and thinly sliced

1 medium zucchini, cut into ¼-inch-thick rounds

1 small yellow squash, cut into ¼-inch-thick rounds

1 red bell pepper, cored, seeded, and cut into ¼-inch-thick strips

Pinch of sea salt

2 cups Enchilada Sauce (recipe follows), or one 14-ounce can

Six 6-inch corn tortillas

1½ cups grated Monterey Jack or cheddar cheese

1 avocado, pitted, peeled, and cut into ¼-inch-thick slices

(list continues)

½ head of iceberg lettuce, shredded

½ cup pimento-stuffed Spanish olives, sliced thin

½ cup sour cream

1 cup Salsa Fresca (see page 25)

2 limes, cut into wedges

Transfer the vegetables to the bowl with the mushrooms and stir to combine. Discard any remaining oil in the skillet and wipe it out with a paper towel.

6. Pour half of the Enchilada Sauce into a 7 x 11-inch baking dish. Return the skillet to medium-high heat and melt the remaining ½ cup of coconut oil. Fry each tortilla 20 seconds on each side (this will help keep them from cracking when you roll them around the beans and cheese). Pass the fried tortillas through the enchilada sauce to coat. Place the tortillas on a clean work surface.

7. Spread 3 tablespoons of bean mixture onto each tortilla, leaving a 1-inch border. Top with cheese and ⅓ cup of the vegetable mixture. Roll the tortillas like a cigar and place them seam side down in the casserole dish, nestling them into the Enchilada Sauce. Pour the remaining sauce on top, sprinkle any remaining grated cheese on top as desired, and bake until the enchiladas are heated through, the cheese is melted, and the sauce is bubbling, 20 to 30 minutes.

8. Serve with the avocado, the remaining ½ cup onion, lettuce, olives, sour cream, salsa, and lime wedges.

DASH

FREEZING FOR THE FUTURE If you're planning on having company over and want to make this dish a few days ahead of time, assemble everything and put it into the baking dish. Wrap tightly with aluminum foil and freeze for up to 2 weeks. When you're ready to bake, defrost in the refrigerator and bake as usual.

ENCHILADA SAUCE

makes 4½ cups

1. In a heat-resistant bowl, cover the chiles with boiling water and let stand until soft, about 30 minutes. Drain and press out the excess water. Cool the chiles, then remove the stems and seeds. In a blender or food processor, puree the chiles, onion, and garlic until smooth.

2. In a large saucepan, combine the tomatoes, stock, chile puree, oregano, cumin, and salt and bring to a boil over medium-high heat. Reduce the heat to medium-low, cover, and simmer the sauce for 30 minutes, or until it reaches a tomato-sauce consistency (add water or more stock if it gets too thick). Cool and refrigerate until needed.

3. You can make this sauce ahead of time and store it frozen in an airtight container for up to 3 months.

4 dried ancho chiles, seeded and stemmed

½ large yellow onion, peeled and quartered

3 garlic cloves, peeled

One 28-ounce can pureed tomatoes

1 cup chicken or vegetable stock

½ tablespoon dried oregano

½ teaspoon ground cumin

½ teaspoon sea salt

—— DASH ——

HOT MAMA **When handling superhot peppers such as habañeros, be very careful not to touch your eyes, lips, or any open skin. As soon as you're done handling them, wash your hands with soap and warm water to remove the oils, paying particular attention to under the nails.**

MINT-RICOTTA RAVIOLI WITH SNAP PEAS AND ASPARAGUS

makes 30 ravioli, to serve 4

4 tablespoons olive oil

3 tablespoons butter

2 scallions (white and light green parts), sliced thin

1 garlic clove, peeled and minced, plus 3 garlic cloves, peeled and sliced thin

1 cup ricotta

Leaves from ½ bunch of fresh mint, sliced thin

Sea salt

1 package wonton wrappers (see Note)

1 cup snap peas, trimmed and halved

9 medium asparagus spears, woody ends removed, sliced thin and tops left whole

1 to 1½ teaspoons dried chile flakes

Fresh-cracked black pepper

½ cup grated pecorino

Note: You could also use strips of fresh lasagna if your supermarket offers them. Just layer one on top of the other to seal the ravioli packets or cut the sheets into squares or circles and fold in half taco-style to form rectangular or half-moon packets.

IF YOU'RE CRAVING HOMEMADE RAVIOLI, you could make your own pasta or use fresh lasagna sheets cut down to size, but using pre-made wonton wrappers as we do here works like a charm and saves you tons of time. You can find them near the tofu at your grocery store. Filling these ravioli seasonally with whatever fresh ingredients are at the market is the way to go, but this light and fresh spring combination of mint, peas, and asparagus is spectacular.

1. In a medium sauté pan, heat 1 tablespoon of the oil and 1 table-spoon of the butter over medium heat. Add the scallions and minced garlic and sauté over medium heat, stirring constantly, until the scallions are translucent and garlic is just golden brown, about 2 minutes. Remove from the heat and place in a medium mixing bowl to cool. Add the ricotta, mint, and a pinch of salt and mix to combine.

2. Keep the unfilled wrappers covered with a damp paper towel while you work. Place ½ tablespoon of the filling onto the center of a wonton wrapper, wet the edge lightly with a fingertip dipped in water, and fold the wrapper in half over the filling, pressing to seal it shut with a finger or fork. Be careful to remove all air bubbles. Set the filled ravioli on a baking sheet lined with parchment paper and keep loosely covered with plastic wrap. Repeat with the rest of the filling.

3. Meanwhile, bring a large soup pot three-quarters full of water to a rolling boil over medium-high heat. Add 1 tablespoon salt. Gently drop the ravioli in a few at a time, keeping the water at a rolling boil. Do not crowd the pot or the ravioli will stick together. When the ravioli rise to the surface, after about 2 minutes, cook them 1 minute more. Use a slotted spoon to remove the ravioli and place them on a clean dish towel to drain. Reserve a scoop of the pasta water for the sauce.

4. Heat 1 tablespoon of the olive oil and 1 tablespoon of the butter in a large skillet over medium heat and gently toss all the ravioli to coat. Set aside.

5. In a skillet large enough to fit all the ravioli (or you can work in batches), heat the remaining 2 tablespoons of olive oil and 1 tablespoon of butter over medium-low heat. Add the sliced garlic and sauté 1 minute, being careful not to burn it. Add the snap peas, asparagus, chile flakes, and a pinch of salt and cracked pepper and sauté until the vegetables are just softened, 2 to 3 minutes. Add the ravioli and 1 or 2 tablespoons pasta water and toss gently to heat through. Top the ravioli with grated pecorino just before serving.

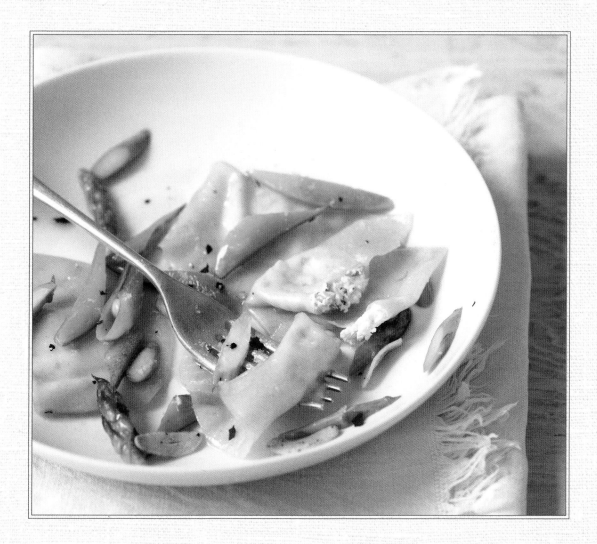

LINGUINE WITH CLAMS AND CURRANTS

serves 4

15 littleneck clams

4 tablespoons extra-virgin olive oil

6 garlic cloves, peeled and chopped

½ to 1 teaspoon dried chile flakes

1 cup dry white wine

15 medium shrimp, cleaned and deveined

⅓ cup dried currants

2 tablespoons (¼ stick) unsalted butter (optional)

Sea salt

½ pound linguine

½ bunch of fresh flat-leaf parsley, minced

THIS IS PROBABLY MY ALL-TIME FAVORITE PASTA—I love the garlic-butter goodness of the white wine sauce, the salinity of the clams, and the bright sweetness of the plumped currants that make this dish a standout. Try to get your hands on some delicious New Zealand cockles, the tiniest, most tender, and mild clam to use. I will say this: If you don't have clams on hand, the sauce is mighty wonderful with just the shrimp, or omit both for a vegetarian option!

1. Most clams have already been cleaned by the time they get to the market, but you can give them an extra scrub to make sure you don't end up with any grit in your dish. First, debeard the clams: Scrub them with a vegetable or nail brush and pull or cut off any hairs sticking out of the shell. Then submerge them in cold water, covering them with a damp cloth if you like, and soak for 20 minutes to give them time to spit out any dirt or sand they're holding on to. Lift the clams out of the soaking basin and rinse them well under running water. Any open clams that don't close when you tap them gently on the counter should be discarded.

2. In a large skillet that can be fitted with a lid, heat the oil over medium-low heat. Add the garlic and heat it through without browning (burned garlic will make the whole dish bitter). Add chile flakes to taste and turn the heat up to medium, then add the wine, shrimp, and currants. Cover and simmer 2 minutes. Uncover, transfer just the shrimp to a bowl, and set aside. Add the clams to the uncovered pan. The liquid should be simmering. Steam the clams open slowly so they don't get rubbery; they should all be open within 12 to 15 minutes. As they steam, swirl the pan and move the sauce around so that no garlic sticks to the bottom or

SHELLFISH WISDOM Don't forget that shellfish like clams and mussels are alive when you bring them home, so they must be kept cold at all times. The best way to store them is in a strainer with ice over a bowl to catch melting liquid until you're ready to use. Make sure you check the shells for any cracks, chips, or holes that could signal a dead animal—and food poisoning, yuck! You want solid shells, and any open ones should close right up if you tap them lightly on a countertop. If one doesn't, toss it in the trash.

---

sides and browns. As each clam opens, remove it from pan and set it aside with the shrimp. When all the clams have opened, return them with the shrimp to the skillet. If you want an extra rich and creamy sauce, stir in the butter.

3. Generously salt a pot of boiling water; pasta water should always taste like the sea. Add the pasta and cook for 1 minute less than the package instructs. Take the pasta out of the water and throw it directly into the pan with the seafood and sauce. Add a little extra pasta water if needed to stretch and loosen the sauce. Toss with fresh parsley and serve.

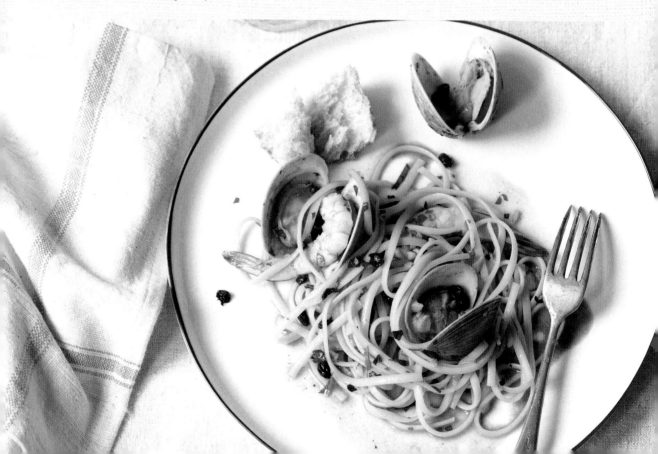

SPAGHETTI WITH STATEN ISLAND SPECIAL (MARINARA) SAUCE

makes about 5 1/2 cups sauce

1½ tablespoons extra-virgin olive oil

1 white or yellow onion, diced

5 garlic cloves, peeled and chopped

1 teaspoon dried oregano

½ to 1 teaspoon dried chile flakes

One 28-ounce can crushed tomatoes

One 28-ounce can whole tomatoes (or use a second can of crushed tomatoes if you prefer a smoother sauce)

¼ cup dry white or red wine

2 tablespoons (¼ stick) butter

2 teaspoons sugar

Leaves from ½ bunch of fresh basil

Sea salt and fresh-cracked black pepper

1½ pounds of your favorite pasta

½ cup grated Locatelli (pecorino) cheese for garnish

MY CHILDHOOD smells like this sauce cooking. We ate it at least once a week growing up, my mom or grandpa making double batches so everyone in the kitchen could happily drink it by the spoonful or scoop up steaming tastes on torn hunks of bread as it simmered away. The recipe has been in our family for years, and it's a staple at every family gathering. These days, I'll make a huge pot one Sunday a month and freeze smaller portions for easy weeknight eating.

If you're planning to use pasta, figure about ¼ pound per person for an entrée portion, or ⅛ pound for appetizer servings.

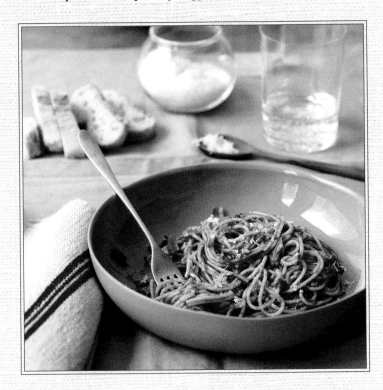

PASTA WITH INTEREST We all know what white pasta tastes like. It's delicious, but there are a whole slew of pastas made from other sorts of flours. Even just whole-wheat pasta is worth a try, but other alternative-flour pastas would be great under this sauce. I love artichoke flour or quinoa spaghetti. Often, these types will be more nutrient dense and contain more fiber than traditional semolina pasta, and many have the added benefit of being gluten-free. Though I'm not normally an advocate for hyperprocessed gluten-free products if you don't need to avoid gluten, I am a fan of naturally reducing the amount I eat by choosing foods that naturally don't contain gluten. It turns out many of us have an adverse reaction, ranging from sensitivity to allergy to immune response (as with celiacs) to gluten, a protein found in wheat and some other grains. The response at the low end of the spectrum can be anything from digestive trouble to foggy thinking and headaches. If you have celiac disease or an allergy to gluten, the effects are much more dangerous and it's important to avoid gluten altogether. But there are plenty of certified gluten-free pastas for you to enjoy even if this is the case, and the Staten Island sauce is safe, too!

1. In a large pot or Dutch oven, heat the oil over medium-low heat. Add the onion and sweat it for 2 minutes, stirring so it doesn't brown. Add the garlic, oregano, and chile flakes and cook for 1 to 2 minutes, stirring occasionally, until the garlic is slightly golden and the onion is softened. Add both cans of tomatoes and use a potato masher to crush the whole tomatoes and stir to combine (you could also use your hands to crush the tomatoes in a separate bowl ahead of time). Cook over medium-high heat for 5 minutes. Add the wine, cover, and bring the mixture to a boil. Reduce the heat to low and simmer the sauce for 90 minutes, partially covered, stirring occasionally.

2. Add butter and sugar and stir to combine. Add the basil. Continue simmering, uncovered, for 30 minutes. Add salt and pepper to taste.

3. Bring a large pot of water to a boil and salt it well. Add the pasta and cook it 1 minute less than the package instructs. You can either place the pasta in a serving dish and spoon the sauce on top, or heat portions of sauce in a skillet and remove the pasta from the cooking water directly into the pan with the sauce and toss to combine, adding pasta water to loosen the sauce if necessary. Serve with grated cheese.

4. You can make this sauce ahead of time and store it in an airtight container in the freezer or in a glass jar in the fridge for up to 3 months.

OZ FAMILY STIR-FRIED RICE

serves 8 to 12

3 tablespoons organic coconut oil, softened

1 pound medium shrimp, cleaned and deveined, or one 8-ounce package tempeh

1 medium yellow onion, chopped

6 garlic cloves, peeled and minced

1 tablespoon minced fresh peeled ginger

1 cup sliced shiitake mushrooms (3 ounces)

⅓ cup low-sodium soy sauce or tamari

2 tablespoons sriracha chile sauce

2 tablespoons toasted sesame oil (optional)

1 cup snow peas

2 cups chiffonade-cut kale (long strips)

1 large carrot, peeled and shredded

4 cups cooked short-grain brown rice (day old is best)

3 eggs

2 tablespoons rice wine vinegar

2 tablespoons mirin

2 tablespoons pure maple syrup

Sea salt and fresh-cracked black pepper

2 scallions (white and light green parts), sliced thin

4 tablespoons toasted sesame seeds

THIS IS A GREAT MEAL to help you clean out your fridge. Use whatever veggies you have on hand! A cast-iron skillet will help the rice brown and fry to a crispy coating at the bottom of the dish.

1. Add 1 tablespoon oil to a large cast-iron skillet over medium-low heat. Add the shrimp and cook them on both sides until they are pink and completely opaque and cooked through, about 5 minutes. Remove the shrimp from the pan and set them aside in a bowl. (If you're substituting tempeh, thaw if frozen, then place in a large cast-iron skillet with half the coconut oil over medium heat. Use a wooden spoon to break the tempeh brick apart into small pieces and fry them until cooked through and some pieces are crispy, 5 to 8 minutes. Set aside.)

2. Increase the heat to medium, add 1 more tablespoon oil, and sauté the chopped onion for 2 minutes, until softened but not browned. Add the garlic and ginger. Stir continuously to make sure the garlic does not burn. After 2 minutes, add the mushrooms and sauté until the mushrooms are softened. Add the soy sauce, sriracha, and sesame oil (if using) and stir to combine. Add the snow peas, kale, and carrot and cook until the kale is slightly wilted, about 3 minutes. Add remaining tablespoon of oil and the rice and toss in the pan until the rice is heated through. Chop the shrimp into bite-size pieces and add them to the rice mixture.

3. In a small bowl, whisk the eggs. Push the rice to one side of the pan and pour the eggs onto the pan surface, moving them with a spatula to scramble and cook. Stir the cooked egg throughout the rice. Drizzle the rice with the vinegar, mirin, and syrup and give it a final toss before serving with a sprinkle of salt and pepper, sesame seeds, and thinly sliced scallions.

VEGAN CAULIFLOWER PESTO MASH

serves 4

PRESTO PESTO! This is a great alternative to mashed potatoes. Easy to whip up, even easier to devour. If you're planning on kissing anyone tonight, make sure they have at least a bite, as it's very garlicky!

1 head of cauliflower, trimmed and cut into medium florets

8 fresh basil leaves

1 or 2 garlic cloves, peeled

2 tablespoons olive oil

¼ cup pine nuts

Sea salt and fresh-cracked black pepper

1. Bring 2 inches of water to a boil under a steam basket and steam the cauliflower until it is tender, 5 to 8 minutes, depending on the size of the florets. If you want to steam the cauliflower whole, it will take a bit longer, usually 25 to 35 minutes.

2. Coarsely chop the basil leaves and garlic. Add the cauliflower to a blender or food processor and pulse once or twice. Add the basil, garlic, oil, and pine nuts and puree or process until smooth. Add salt and pepper to taste and serve.

GRANDDADDY'S STUFFED ARTICHOKES

serves 6

6 artichokes, leaf tips removed and outer part of stems trimmed

1½ cups Italian bread crumbs

1 cup grated Locatelli (pecorino) cheese

2 or 3 garlic cloves, peeled and minced

1 teaspoon dried oregano

1 teaspoon sea salt

½ cup olive oil

1½ cups chicken or vegetable stock

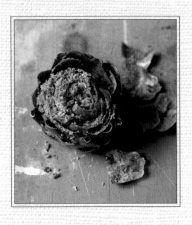

ARTICHOKES ARE *like little pieces of art you get to eat! They're quite the statement appetizer, and people have to eat them with their hands, so they're an immediate icebreaker with everyone getting messy and enjoying themselves.*

This particular version comes from my mother's family on Staten Island, and they have become my grandfather's specialty—he makes them for every big party, and there are never enough. The original family recipe probably called for half the bread crumb, cheese, and stock mixture we now use, but we think ours is twice as nice. The little teeth marks you see on the artichoke leaves in the picture are mine! ☺

1. Fill a large pot fitted with a steamer basket with 2 or 3 inches of water and bring to a boil over high heat. Drop the heat to medium-high and add the artichokes to the basket and steam until you can easily insert a knife into the center of each, about 30 minutes. Slice the stems off the artichoke and mince them. Set the artichokes aside.

2. Preheat the oven to 350°F.

3. In a large bowl, combine the bread crumbs, cheese, garlic, oregano, and salt. Add the minced artichoke stems and stir to combine.

4. Loosen the leaves of the artichokes by gently pulling them away from the center and drizzle with ¼ cup of the olive oil and ¾ cup of the stock. Pack each artichoke with one-sixth (about 3 tablespoons) of the bread crumb mixture. Place the stuffed artichokes in a large baking pan and drizzle with the remaining ¼ cup oil and ¾ cup stock to moisten the bread crumbs and wet the bottom of the pan. Cover with aluminum foil and bake for 30 minutes.

5. Preheat the broiler. Remove the foil and carefully broil the tops of the bread crumbs for 1 to 2 minutes, taking care not to burn them. Enjoy hot out of the oven or cold, no dipping sauce needed.

6. To store, place any remaining artichokes in a baking dish and cover it tightly with aluminum foil. Refrigerate for up to 3 days.

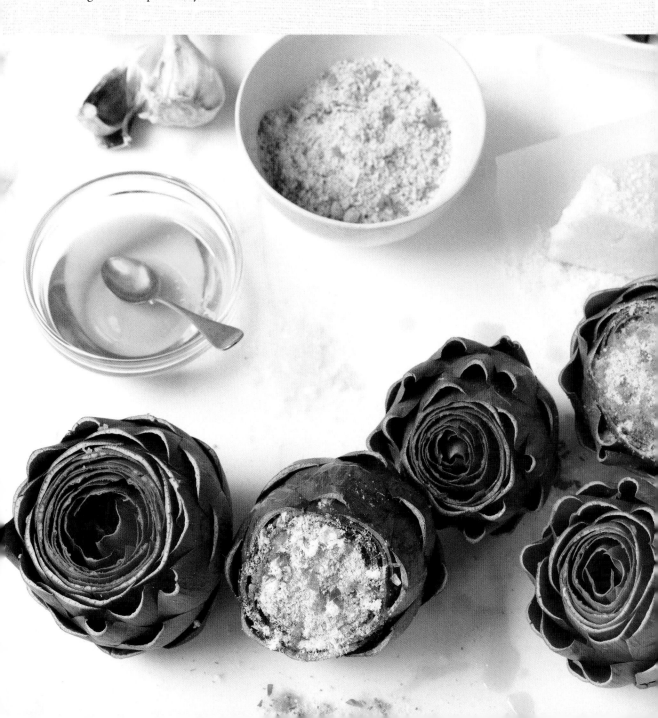

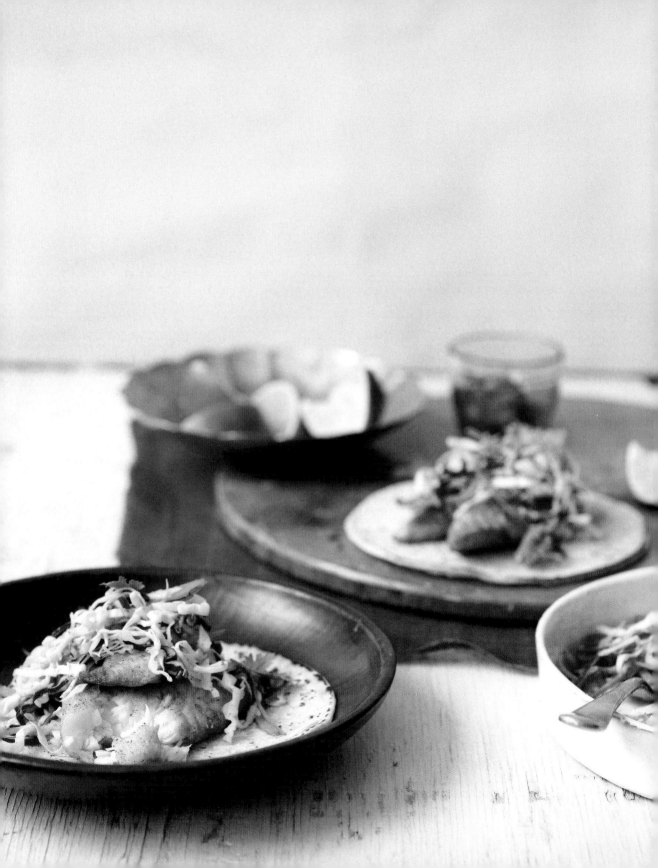

FISH TACOS WITH CREAMY CHIPOTLE CABBAGE SLAW

serves 4

A FEW YEARS AGO, John took me to Hawaii for my birthday. We ate lunch on the beach every day, and every day I had the same perfect dish: just-caught fish tacos served up with pineapple and pickled veggies, fresh guacamole, salsa, and crisp onion rings. This is my homemade version of the comfort food I love. I took out the onion rings so I don't have to feel guilty about eating this once or twice a week, but with the sweet-tart crunch of the Creamy Chipotle Cabbage Slaw on top, I don't even miss 'em. Feel free to add guac and salsa to yours at home for extra cram-packed deliciousness!

4 tablespoons olive oil

1 medium yellow onion, sliced thin

1 red bell pepper, cored, seeded, and sliced thin

Sea salt and fresh-cracked black pepper

⅓ cup all-purpose flour

1 teaspoon chipotle powder

1 pound mild fish (tilapia, halibut, or cod) cut into 4 fillets

8 small corn tortillas

4 cups Creamy Chipotle Cabbage Slaw (recipe follows)

Cilantro for garnish (optional)

1. In a medium skillet over medium heat, heat 1 tablespoon of the oil. Add the onion and bell pepper and cook until the onion is translucent and the bell pepper is softened, about 5 minutes. Season with salt and pepper to taste. Reserve the mixture in a bowl.

2. In a shallow bowl, combine the flour, chipotle powder, and 1 teaspoon salt. Pat each fish fillet dry and lightly dredge in the flour mixture, shaking off any excess flour. Heat 1 tablespoon of the oil in the skillet over medium heat and place 2 fillets at a time in the pan. Gently panfry for 3 to 6 minutes, until the underside of the fish turns opaque. Use a rubber spatula to flip the fillets and finish cooking to your desired doneness. Remove to a paper towel–lined plate, remove the remaining oil from the pan, and repeat with 1 tablespoon oil and the remaining 2 fillets.

3. To serve, for each fish fillet, heat 2 tortillas in a clean pan with the 1 remaining tablespoon of oil, then set them on a plate. Cut each fillet in half and divide the fish evenly among the 8 tortillas. Top with a helping of the sautéed veggies and a good amount of cabbage slaw and serve with cilantro, if desired.

THE TRICK WITH NONSTICK Using a nonstick pan will help make sure the fish doesn't stick to the bottom, but you also want to make sure the oil doesn't smoke when you're using a nonstick pan. The heat at this temperature risks releasing hazardous gases from the nonstick coating. Stainless-steel and cast-iron pans do not carry this risk of off-gassing, but they are a little bit trickier to maneuver as things tend to stick a bit more, so you may need to add a little extra olive oil to the pan to make sure the food you're cooking comes off easily.

CREAMY CHIPOTLE CABBAGE SLAW

makes 6 cups

4 cups shredded green cabbage

1 cup shredded purple cabbage

2 medium carrots, peeled and shredded

1 small red onion, sliced very thin

3 large scallions (white and light green parts), sliced thin

1 jalapeño, minced (discard the seeds and ribs if you want less heat)

½ cup mayonnaise or Vegenaise

½ cup plain Greek yogurt or sour cream

¼ cup fresh lime juice, or ⅛ cup fresh lime juice plus ⅛ cup champagne, white wine, or apple cider vinegar

2 tablespoons sugar or honey

1 teaspoon ground cumin

1 teaspoon chipotle powder

Sea salt and fresh-cracked black pepper

1. Combine the cabbages, carrots, onion, scallions, and jalapeño in a large bowl. In a medium bowl, whisk the mayonnaise, yogurt, lime juice, sugar, cumin, and chipotle powder together until smooth and creamy. Pour the dressing over the cabbage mixture and toss to combine. Season with salt and pepper to taste. Allow to marinate at least 20 minutes before using.

2. To store leftovers, cover with plastic wrap and refrigerate for up to 3 days.

ELEVEN

BUY THE TICKET, TAKE THE RIDE

work smart, play hard, skip town

When he worked, he really worked. But when he played, he really *played*.
—DR. SEUSS, *THE KING'S STILTS*

WHEN YOU WERE A KID, YOUR PLAYDATES, DOCTORS' VISITS, homework assignments, and vacations were overseen by older, wiser people who had your best interests at heart. In college, your roommate, friends, and boyfriends helped think of fun stuff to do on the weekends and for spring break. But now you're a sharp-minded adult, not a child who needs to be told what to do or a teenager who needs to be invited along. The proof: You can read. You know how to make soup. You have an app that balances your checkbook.

I take this as a clear sign that you're ready to create a schedule based on your values, your purpose, and your priorities, not just what your mother thinks you should do or what's playing at the Film Forum at four. It's too easy to postpone enjoyment in favor of our daily to-do lists. But travel and extracurricular accomplishments are just as important as your other responsibilities, so stop waiting! Buy the ticket. Make the plans. Take the ride. Create your happiness. Life waits for no (wo)man.

Bottom line: In order for life to bloom and grow, the work-play-go equation must remain in balance. Everybody's personal equation is a little bit different. Some of us need more social time; others thrive on time alone. Some need to see the world, others just want to explore their own backyard. Some of us need dance music, some of us need Beethoven, and some of us need total and absolute silence when we're trying to figure things out. So crank up the stereo or slip on those noise-canceling headphones, and let's get down to business.

WORKING SMART

Having a job is an unavoidable fact of life, but having a pencil-pushing, mindless job that just pays the bills is not the only option. When I talk to my parents and their friends, I see people who chose one career path and stuck with it. When I talk with my peers, I don't hear the expectation that any of us will stay with one job forever. A career switch is something that used to be almost frowned upon, but these days, we're practically encouraged to have multiple professional reincarnations, so we can explore different joys and different skill sets at different stages of our lives. That's the good part.

The challenge is that having too many options with no one to force our hand can lead to inertia. Experts call it the paradox of choice. On the one hand, we're lucky to have so many options, but on the other, too many choices can be paralyzing! How do we know which move is the right one? We don't. If the first job you have after graduation is what you want to do for the rest of your life, you're lucky. It took trying a whole bunch of different jobs in order to find the one that was right for me. And what I've learned so far is that being successful at work requires curiosity, excitement, and drive, an awareness of the rules, and the willingness to sometimes ignore them.

I am convinced that our parents' generation is much more likely to go through a midlife crisis than ours is, because by virtue of all the choices we have available to us now, we're forced to do the soul-searching and find our happiest path right from the outset. Everyone likes to talk about the recent surge of so-called quarter-life crises as if it's a bad thing, but it's not! It just means we're putting in the overtime now and investing in a solid foundation to build our lives on rather than rushing off in one direction and possibly regretting it later.

This may mean more growing pains right now, more months and even years spent feeling anxious to get on track and frustrated as we try to find a path that fits us perfectly, but once we've found it (and yes, there will be sidetracks and backtracks along the way), we're cruising, and we're that much better established to deal with curves in the road ahead—career changes, changes of heart—because we've already experienced that period of self-examination and discovery right out of the nest.

Our parents may have to do this tough introspective work much later in life if they were forced into one career right out of school and take the time to examine whether it's making them happy only when they hit fifty. So consider yourself lucky! Do the work now, and maybe you'll get that fire-red Porsche a little earlier in life and without all the emotional baggage in the trunk.

Stay on the field. The biggest mistake I made when I lost my way along my career path was quitting my first job because I didn't 100 percent absolutely love it. I was working as a story coordinator at a television show, putting in long hours sourcing news stories from every outlet and then trying to book the relevant in-studio guests before any other program. I was tethered to my phone at all times, constantly checking breaking news and being on high alert for incoming leads. Every day, we had the mad dash to the finish line to pull the show together. And then, after it aired, the madness started again for tomorrow's program. It was a very exciting job, and no two days were ever the same, but I looked at my boss and realized I did not want her job down the line. I thought quitting would give me the time to think about what I did want to be doing with my life. You know where that move took me? Nowhere.

I was spinning my wheels for months before I got back on track. Who's to say where I would be today if I had stayed at that job? That could very easily have been the wrong move, too. The only real mistake I made was that I spent a lot of time *thinking* about what I could possibly enjoy doing, what I would possibly be great at, but very little time actually *doing* anything. Feeling stuck led to being stuck; feeling overwhelmed led to being overwhelmed.

I'm a huge believer that things happen for a reason—we all have lessons to learn, and new doors do open when old ones shut. I only wish that I'd been able to see that six-month period as an incredible once-in-a-lifetime opportunity to do anything and everything that might enrich me! Instead, I spent that time wallowing and worrying about what I would do next. The problem wasn't that I didn't know where I wanted to be; it was that I didn't have an attitude in place that could have helped me see the opportunities around me.

I had to make a drastic change to break the cycle of feeling impotent, so I threw myself into a busy schedule. I volunteered and took French classes and made a bunch of new friends with their own varied life experiences to share with me. I gained certification as a holistic health counselor from the Institute for Integrative Nutrition and put out a new expanded edition of *The Dorm Room Diet*. I began doing speaking tours again, which led to more television and media exposure. I started blogging, which eventually led to my own syndicated newspaper column and features in *Glamour* magazine.

I found ways to feel stimulated and stimulating. I put myself out there, met people, connected, and started to remember what I wanted to be able to contribute. Part of the reason ABC took notice of me when they were looking to cast *The Chew* was that I'd stayed active in the national discussion about learning to balance a healthy lifestyle with limited time and budget. When I think about the fact that I now get paid to eat delicious food and hang out with great friends, I have to laugh about all the days I spent holed up in my bedroom, hoping answers were going to surprise me during the commercial breaks between *Forensic Files* reruns.

What I learned is that taking advantage of opportunities is about being ready when they appear. As my parents love to say, you can't catch the ball if you're not standing on the field.

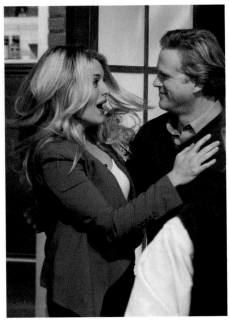

Fun days on the job! In addition to eating and hanging out with my great friends and cohosts every day on *The Chew*, I've gotten to meet some incredible guests. I'm a diehard fan of *The Princess Bride*, so when my cohosts surprised me by bringing on Cary Elwes (Wesley himself!), I totally played it cool . . . not.

Keep moving forward. If you feel stuck, keep going. Actions lead to reactions, but inertia only leads to more inertia. Do research, ask questions, and ask for help. Once you make an informed decision, take a step. At least you'll be learning from experience, which is always preferable to sitting idly in a single spot, no better off and possibly worse off for the wasted time.

The trick is to make a choice, any choice. Any motion is forward motion. You can always change direction—change the rules, change the goals—but don't get out of the game entirely. It doesn't have to be painful. Not every job is about paying your dues, but you have to spend time getting your footing so that you can make real moves.

Everybody has to start somewhere. So pick your go spot, and get going!

Commit to things you love. If you've found a path you love, commit to it. I grew up in a house where commitment to work was the bottom line. My father is a surgeon, and I still remember the nights when he was a resident at the hospital and couldn't come home at all because he had patients to tend to. On many evenings, we would wait to eat dinner at nine or ten when my dad finally got home.

My mom and grandma chose to stay home to raise their brood of children, but they simultaneously achieved higher education degrees, wrote books, even served in government. My family definitely agreed with the saying "idle bodies make idle minds," and I still respect what strong minds can accomplish when they commit to a goal and focus their energy.

Pay attention to quality of life. Once you've achieved some success, you'll have to make an effort to pull back and save some energy for your personal life. Seeing how hard my parents work taught me the pride and accomplishment that hard work brings but also the value of knowing when to commit to enjoying life in the moment. The prize should be as much about the journey as the destination.

Work smart. We all need to make a conscious commitment to be at work when we're at work and at home when we're at home. The more hectic my career gets, the more I take care of my precious free time. When

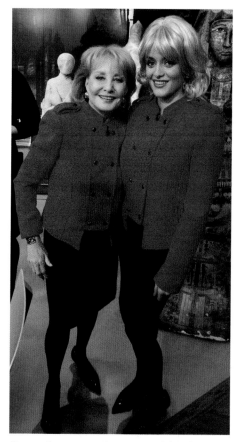

One of my most memorable days on set was our 2012 Halloween spooktacular, when *The Chew* crew dressed up as . . . *The View*! Clinton was Elisabeth Hasselbeck; Michael was Joy Behar; Carla was Sherri Shepherd; Mario was Whoopi Goldberg; and I was Barbara Walters. The ladies made a surprise visit to our set wearing our exact costumes—here Barbara and I are in our matching outfits, having a ball!

I'm on, I'm 100 percent on. But when I'm off, I don't have my cell phone on me at all times. I don't check my emails frantically. I give myself time to just be me and be away. To pay attention to my thoughts, to get dinner ready, to hang with my honey when he gets home.

Instead of working hard, I'm working smart. Working too fast, for too long, ultimately becomes counterproductive. If you're always ticking things off that to-do list without taking a moment to let the dust settle, you know how exhausted and burned out it can make you feel. That kind of

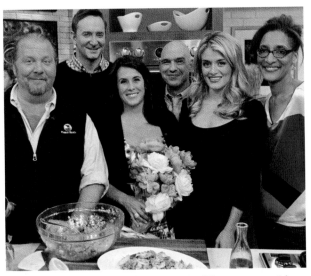

My cohosts and I hanging on set with my mom, Lisa, when she joined us for Mother's Day to whip up some delicious Oz Family Stir-Fried Rice (page 260)!

exhaustion will just make it more challenging to keep creating top-notch results in the long run and it makes it easier to miss the forest for the trees.

Working smart is about appreciating *value*: Value your time, value your effort, and value your creativity. Instead of giving 75 percent for twelve hours, give 100 percent for nine and get the heck out of the office so you have time for the gym and to enjoy a leisurely dinner, soaking up wine and good conversation, before hitting the sack for a restful night's sleep and getting up for another full-throttle day! Doesn't that sound better?

Know where to draw the line. We all want to make more money, be more successful, get more, have more, do more, give more. How much is enough? What lines won't you cross for the beaucoup bucks? I have friends who will move across the country for a job, and friends who will move around the world for love, and they aren't necessarily the same people. What's your bottom line?

PLAYING HARD

Playdates aren't just for kids. Time together is just as important as time alone when you're looking to unwind and replenish. I definitely need that alone time to just sit in bed and read or have a couple hours where there's nothing I "need" to do. I love exploring a new part of the city, strolling around streets, discovering it like a tourist. But after I've had time to decompress, it makes me so happy to have dinner with John or have one of those nights surrounded by my friends where conversation flows freely, you learn something new, you're reminded why you love these people, affection is reaffirmed, and you leave feeling totally filled up.

Throwing a great party has this same effect on me. I love entertaining, making people feel taken care of—well fed, well hydrated, jubilant and gregarious and free. And I *loooooove* being able to curate what's on the menu. Brainstorming the theme, menu, music—these are all totally relaxing and fun for me, probably because I don't take any of it too seriously. If you're not coming to my party to have a good time, I don't want you there, and if you need irritatingly formal canapés to have a great time, then you're probably not that much fun anyway.

Figure out what makes you feel filled up and replenished, and then make plenty of time for it.

Cultivate hobbies, not just have-tos. What do you do for fun? Do you garden? Paint? Do you have a growing pillbox collection? What charities are you involved with?

Asking other people about their interests is a great way to get to know them and learn about fun things that may be happening in your city or in the world at large. And learning what you do for fun is how people get to you know the real you.

Consider the kinds of questions you might be asked on a great first date. Those are the questions you want to have really good answers for. "What do you do?" doesn't have to be answered with "I'm an accountant" or "I'm a nautical engineer." You might say, "I visit flea markets in every city I go to" or "I make quilts." A hobby is something that you do for fun because you're curious about it. Because you love it. Because you just can't help it. Because you want to be great at it. Because it's fun to be an amateur. Hobbies don't have to be expensive or what all of your friends are into. It just has to be something that you really love purely because you find it interesting and it gives you joy.

Improve your cocktail conversation skills and give yourself something to talk about with your nosy cousins, on dates with the new guy, or at dinners with your husband's family by trying new things. Having fun makes you more fun. That may not be a truism, but it should be.

Say yes. From button collecting to beer tasting, if you have a friend who loves it, chances are they'd love to inspire you with their passion. If they invite you, go. Say yes. Have that experience, even if you never want to hear another word about an antique closure ever again.

People rarely look back and say, "Gee, I wish I'd said no to that." Saying yes opens up a whole new slew of possibilities. Saying yes means that you can join a club, whether it's a city club sports team or a botanical society or an art-appreciation group.

If nothing else, your death-defying spelunking trip will make for great stories!

Get excited to be a beginner again. After childhood, we can easily forget how to learn, and being bad at something can be read as failure. It's too easy to fall into the "expert" trap, where we only want to do things we've practiced enough to be virtuoso at. But bad is the first step toward mastery. How else are you going to learn to do something new?

Being a beginner gives us a chance to feel young and playful again, which we always need more of. It's wonderful to be a prodigy at the piano, but if you've never done a water sport and you want to learn how, you're going to have to be okay with falling over about a million times before you're an accomplished surfer or a sailor. And so what if you never reach professional status? Having fun with something is about being open to imperfection, not an obsessive need to get an A in everything you do.

Hobby for one, hobby for all. Some hobbies are group activities; some are more solitary pleasures. When considering your new hobbies, try to have one of each: one interest that introduces you to new people and allows you to develop relationships as you go, and one that requires calm, quiet, and concentration. That way, you'll always have something fun to do with others and on your own.

GROUP ACTIVITIES

Join the Roller Derby.

Learn how to play field hockey.

Join a band.

Make a short film.

Start a book club.

PLAYTIME FOR ONE

Sew a change purse.

Stand on your head.

Paint a sunset.

Plant some herbs.

Read Proust—or Harry Potter.

Indulge your voyeuristic side. It's great to create, but sometimes we've got to push back the laptop, sketch pad, or easel and go admire the fruits of somebody else's rich and creative mind. So go spy on a play, a concert, or a comedy show. Watch a magic show. Go to the zoo and admire the lions, the tigers, and the bears. Or just go to the movies! I *loooove* movies—darkness, no distraction, surround sound and cushy seats, naughty snacks, the experience of seeing a movie at that scale. I don't get to go as often as I like, but that makes it a treat.

Looking is a great way to learn, and learning can rejuvenate us creatively and energetically. And events make great answers to the common Monday morning question: "How was your weekend?"

Party like a rock star. Early to bed may make us healthy, wealthy, and wise, but some kinds of fun necessitate staying up late, sleeping in, and nursing a Sunday morning head thumper. Sometimes you just have to let your hair down. So tear up the dance floor. And every now and then enjoy the sunrise by staying up late instead of waking up early.

SKIPPING TOWN

Your career feeds your wallet and hobbies feed your heart. And travel? Travel feeds your soul—and your imagination. Travel doesn't have to mean hopping a plane to Phuket. It's just about getting outside your comfort zone, seeing a part of the world that's unfamiliar, and learning a little something. Oh, and eating delicious food, of course! But a day trip to a different part of town can be just as fun and fulfilling as a voyage abroad, as long as it gives you a break from your normal routine. I make travel a priority because I know that if I want to live in the world fully, I need to experience it firsthand. I think of it as my opportunity to see what other people find interesting, what they love, what they consider beautiful, and what they care about. Their new perspective informs my own.

Regardless of where you're headed, don't waste a minute of your valuable time away: Do your research ahead of time and figure out the choice restaurants, bars, dance halls, museums, art galleries, boutiques, concerts, sporting events, arcades, and bespoke hatmakers (or whatever else floats your boat!) you want to make sure you see while you're away. Explore the cities around where you live that you take maybe for granted—if you see them with a tourist's excitement, they take on a totally new light. Make the most of your time and a forty-eight-hour trip can be as full to bursting as a week away.

THESE ARE A FEW OF MY FAVORITE THINGS

I love to cook, I love to go out to dinner—but I also love things that have nothing to do with food. And it's important that I do, or else I'd only have one thing to talk about. The following are just some of the things that I enjoy doing when I'm not on the clock.

Floral arranging. I learned how to arrange flowers by asking tons of questions of experts like my wedding planner, Kate Parker, and surfing the web for tutorials—you'd be

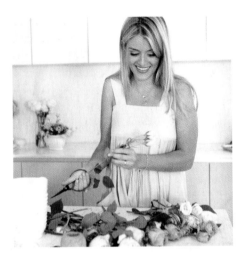

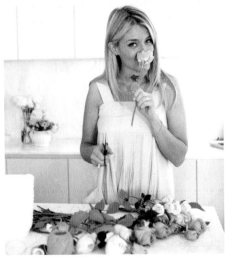

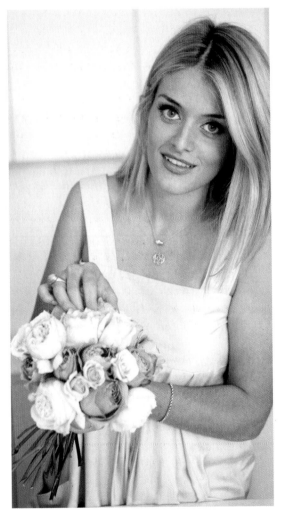

shocked (or maybe you wouldn't) by how much you can learn from YouTube! By doing it myself, the arrangements look exactly the way I want, and I can tailor them for any occasion. Even better, I can usually get a much better price by buying in bulk from local floral wholesalers, meaning more fresh flowers for me!

Collecting lists of restaurants and bars I want to try in different cities. I pull reviews and recommendations from blogs, newspapers, magazines, local press, Twitter, and friends, and I keep a running list on my iPhone of different things to see, eat, and do.

Keeping inspiration on file. I pack my file cabinet with tearsheets of beautiful interiors, vacation destinations, gorgeous dresses/makeup/hair color, inspirational lifestyle and people, quotes I want to remember, great gift ideas, and so on. Inspiration boards are wonderful—but inspiration cabinets are a private getaway!

Buying books. One of my favorite childhood memories is going to the backyard woods of my grandmother's farm and reading fantasy books like the *Chronicles of Narnia*, *Harry Potter*, or *Dune* in the hammock hidden among the trees. I still love to be surrounded by paper and words and ideas.

Discovering new beauty products. I'm obsessed and therefore a marketer's dream. In the past few years, I've gotten really diligent about checking for harmful chemicals and toxic colors/perfumes on my label packaging. I don't use products with any of the silicones (like dimethicone), and I avoid artificial dyes and perfumes as much as possible except for a few generic staples that I simply cannot live without, such as CoverGirl LashBlast mascara and Giorgio Armani high-precision retouch concealer and foundation. I'm all about finding the most effective, all-natural cosmetics, but I still make allowances for the essentials that give me that I-got-eight-hours-of-sleep-last-night—even if I didn't!—look.

Cycling indoors. I've never been very coordinated, so I love the fact that with every class I go to, I feel a little bit better able to keep pace, do the dance moves on the bike, find the rhythm, break a sweat, and really get into it.

Taste-testing croissants. My obsession: finding the best croissant ever. Perfectly tender and flaky on the inside, with crisp, golden exterior. Extra butter. Plain is perfect, but real almond filling (no amaretto flavoring!) is great, too. There are two places tied for first right now: Blue Provence in Palm Beach, Florida, and Le Moulin Rose in Paris.

Discovering your travel style is like reading a guidebook about yourself. Everything has a place on your personal totem pole, and figuring out how you travel best and happiest is mandatory if you want to come home nourished, exhilarated, and relaxed. So invest in making a game plan, prioritize the travel experiences you care about, and spend time looking forward to a trip you will remember for years.

Start fresh. Seeing how we operate in an unfamiliar place can teach us wonderful things about ourselves that we may not even notice when we're on more familiar ground. For instance, as a junior in college I went with friends to Madrid. We planned our days around walking excursions where we could get lost, wander, explore, and enjoy memorable meals in great restaurants. We explored and then we ate. Went to a museum and then ate. Got lost and ate again. It was perfect.

That week, I realized some things about my nature that might have been obvious to my friends but felt like news to me: (1) I like to plan and (2) I like to plan around food. My family has always been big on food, the kind of people who talk about lunch at breakfast and dinner at lunch, so that shouldn't have surprised me—but this trip was the first time I realized how much of that attitude had transferred to me.

When we're navigating our daily routines, we tend to do things by rote, not even realizing why we've made the choices that we play out every day. But when you're on vacation, when your schedule is free and clear and wholly yours, when you've got nothing but time to fill, seeing how you spend yours can give you great insight into what you're truly passionate about.

Cherish traditions. Every summer when I was a kid we made the six-hour road trip from New York City up to my grandparents' place in Maine, stopping at all our favorite little haunts along the way—an old bookstore with delicious hot chocolate in Connecticut; Faneuil Hall in Boston and Sturbridge Village; our favorite restaurants in Portland. But by far the best part was pulling up to the house and feeling the rush of having arrived for a week of total Maine revelry.

The anticipation of reliving all the things we'd loved best from last year—wild games of capture the flag and kings in the corner and charades with my mom's six siblings and all their children—was half the fun of traveling up there. But even better was bringing someone new into the fold. When I took John there for the first time, I was even more excited to experience everything like new through him—his first Sunday morning pancakes! His first loss at the Ping-Pong rally! His first overturned canoe! And then he and I added a few of our own traditions—lobsters on the dock at J's or Harraseeket! Coffees, pastries, and newspapers by the bay—no phones allowed! We started going back up for New Year's every year, and pretty soon we had a whole tradition instituted for that, too. Eventually, we ended up getting married at the house in Maine because we both saw it as the place where our relationship had blossomed while we created so many happy memories together.

The beauty of traditions is it doesn't matter what they are so long as you get to enjoy them over and over, even better with people you love.

Go back. When John and I planned our honeymoon, we imagined ourselves in Bermuda, thinking that an island visit, complete with blue waters, starry skies, and romantic walks on the beach would be ideal. Just our luck: Hurricane Earl had the same idea. We got rained out of our dream stay, with only one afternoon to plan an alternative. So we chose Paris (or rather, ticket availability twenty-four hours in advance chose Paris for us—we didn't mind)!

Since we'd both already been a few times before, there was no need for a complex itinerary. We had already seen the typical tourist spots—Eiffel Tower, check; Notre Dame, check. And after spending three months nonstop planning for the wedding, the idea of having no plan at all was absolutely marvelous. Suddenly, whimsy and adventure were the order of the day!

Instead of the ocean, we had the Seine. Instead of starry skies, we had the City of Light. And instead of long walks on the beach, we traipsed around every corner and arrondissement, ate three crepes a day (no wedding dress to fit into, woo-hoo!), had falafel in the Marais, took picnics by the river with little baskets we packed ourselves full of fresh baguettes, local butter and cheese and produce (oooh, the berries!), and had Nutella, Champagne, and macarons for dessert. It could not have been a more relaxing or enchanting way to begin our lives together. In fact, it was bliss.

New vistas beckon, surely, but a return trip is a marvelous way to explore pressure-free. No must-sees, no must-dos, and the only items on the agenda are exactly what you feel like, when you feel like it. So you can visit your favorite spots, find some brand-new ones, and have the best time ever.

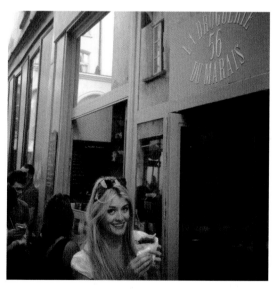

Leave it to me to attempt to eat every crepe in Paris so I could find my favorite one. This is it! The *beurre et sucre* at La Droguerie in the Marais.

YOUR HAPPINESS LIST

What makes you happy? When I think about the moments that spark my inner joy, these are some of the many things that pop into my head:

1. The good times I've spent with my husband, family, and friends, laughing till we cry, crying till we laugh
2. Doing something really well (even better, doing something terribly and then working hard to get great at it)
3. Eating an amazing meal—times two if in an amazing place with my favorite people, or discovering a little hideaway to get a local dish and drink prepared perfectly
4. Visiting a market in a foreign place, making a great find, getting a good deal, and then discovering the perfect place for it at home
5. Being able to help someone else
6. Seeing adults get giddy
7. Seeing kids understand for the first time
8. Feeling powerful and valuable

People often make lists of things they want to do—bucket lists, if you will. Instead of thinking only about what you want to put in your bucket, think about what's already in there, what makes you feel great when you remember it, and that will clue you in to the kinds of experiences you should continue seeking and embracing.

When we were kids, every vacation we took as a family began with us all getting off the plane so jet-lagged that all we wanted to do was crash at the hotel. My parents, however, would announce that *they* were going out for a walk around our destination, and who knows *what* they might find! Well, that was enough to have all of us traipsing along behind them, dragging our feet and exhausted but determined not to miss the discovery or experience of a lifetime. It was always well worth it when we stumbled upon an incredible site, delicious restaurant, or beautiful new path, or just had some wild adventure. The answer to "Aren't you glad you came?" was always a resounding "Yes!"

There was the time my dad convinced us all that Oz family capture the flag was just what we needed, never mind that our playing field was to be a deserted island littered with boulders, shrubs, and no medics on standby; we survived . . . barely. And the time we went out on New York City's East River on the Fourth of July in a friend's boat and my then-two-year-old brother accidentally put the boat on autopilot, leaving us stranded in the middle of a thunderstorm with no splash lights, nearly being run over by giant cruise boats out to see the fireworks. And the time we discovered a little gem of a restaurant on a family bike ride that we've never been able to find again—like some magical experience meant only for that one moment in time.

It's not that these experiences were always the most enjoyable while we were living them, but they are crucial memories in our family fabric, so much more than napping at the hotel could ever have been.

For me, connecting to inner joy is still about feeling as if I'm maximizing my potential and taking advantage of every opportunity. My wonderful parents instilled a psychosis in all their children that no amount of therapy could erase (nor would I want it to): We all worry that to pass up an opportunity is to risk missing the most important experience of our lives. And who knows? The one time we decide to stay home may be the one time that proves the rule.

It's because of this fear that I'll miss out on something valuable that I've found myself jumping out of planes; taking last-minute trips cross-country; eating fish eyeballs; rapping about vitamin D on television; taking the leap of faith to get married at twenty-four; skinny-dipping in the ocean (even though I'm deathly afraid of sharks); and so many other embarrassing, crazy, and totally enlivening things that make me who I am.

For me, accessing my joy has shown me that every time someone offers me a chance to learn, explore, and see something new, I leap. And I'm going to keep on leaping, because I want a life rich with memories—happy, scary, sad, dangerous, exciting, fulfilling, unbelievable—and the things that make me happiest are those that give me the most opportunity to build these pictures for my mental scrapbook.

So throw an impromptu dinner party. Order in, or better yet, cook it yourself. Invite someone you love to share it with you, or invite the neighbor you've only just met but want to befriend. Be a little reckless. Invest in you and realize that all the little things that go into building your life are only as important as you make them. Choose well, choose grandly, and choose "yes!" as often as possible. That's the *Relish* way.

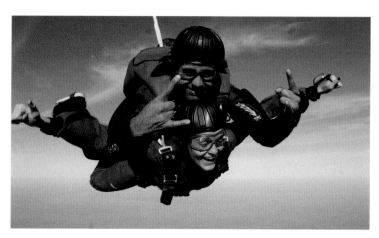

Me, 13,500 feet over Miami Beach, leaping out of a plane! I was utterly terrified the entire time. Then I jumped, and the rest was easy!

Follow your pleasures. Our travel itineraries should be a mixture of our favorite fascinations and some brand-new pleasures. Because food is a hobby of mine, when I travel, the first thing I do in any new place is to go and see their supermarkets and farmers' markets. That's why I know that every grocery store in France has a huge cheese refrigerator and walls of fresh bread, even though they have *boulangerie* on every corner. And that in Turkey, there are giant ice cases on the sidewalks filled with fresh-caught seafood and crates of watermelon straight from the farm.

For me, as a visitor, these glimpses of the local diet tell me what life is like for the people who live here every day. It's a new experience, something special and real and inspiring. If you can score an invitation to someone's house for a home-cooked meal, even better. It's incredible to eat a meal that's cooked by someone who has been making the same dishes over and over for fifty years. You can see it in their hands—the recipe is in their fingers. Watching a grandmother who has been kneading the same dumpling dough for a thousand batches or stirring the same pot of tomato sauce a thousand times—that's the kind of skill you can't learn from books.

By using travel as an excuse to learn more about what you're already interested in, you can pad out your itinerary and broaden your horizons.

Hunt for treasures. When my dad and mom would go traveling without us, they would always bring home treasures. A set of Russian nesting dolls, glass bead necklaces, a Chinese fan.

Once after a trip to Venice, they brought home a Venetian marionette. But my dad wasn't content to just hand it over. He gathered us up and told us a wonderful story about how the marionette had found him (not the other way around, of course), embedding his fairy tales with magic and intrigue, princes and princesses, and a dose of art and culture and history.

What a memorable childhood experience! It was a great way for him to share his travels with us and for us to learn and connect as a family. As kids, it gave us a glimpse of the world around us and instilled a lifelong wanderlust I haven't been able to shake.

Now when I go away with my husband or on my own, whether it's just to the next state over or to faraway lands, I love wandering into spaces that are full of the unexpected. I always hit up a flea market, because I love coming home with inexpensive little tchotchkes that remind me of my adventures. I look for mementos that I'll want to share with my kids, ones that inspire me: a piece of artwork, an article of clothing, a teacup and saucer, a set of old Champagne coupes, a twenty-five-pound carved wooden elephant that I lugged home from a market in South Africa but that will be in my living room forever even though I dropped him (well, technically I tripped up the stairs and fell *on* him) within moments of purchasing him and broke his delicate tail.

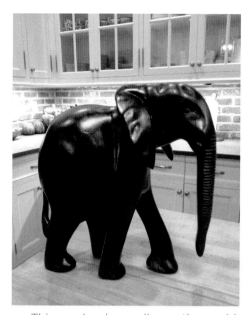

This guy has been all over the world: I found him at a market in South Africa, fell on him and broke his tail on the trek home (I've always been a klutz), glued him back together, and now he's one of my favorite decor items and travel mementos—all the better for his achy-breaky tail!

While I am constantly trying to weed clutter out of my life, I almost never shed something I picked up on one of my travels. Seeing and touching these objects, like the treasures my parents brought home from their adventures, ties me to my experiences, to other people's cultures, and to the world—and that kind of inspiration is something I want to keep with me always.

Speak in tongues. Every year, we visit family in Turkey. When it came time to choose courses in college, I decided to study Turkish, and after a year of language classes, I spent eight weeks in Istanbul as part of an immersion course. I was blown away by how powerful the experience was. Knowing the language made it feel completely different from all the other times I'd been there. Instead of feeling as if I was on vacation in a foreign place, I felt as if I was returning somewhere familiar, a new place that felt like home.

I'm actually terrible at languages, and I've lost most of what I learned because I don't speak regularly, but the catchphrases and bits of conversation I can still pick up give me a thrill—it's the kind of mental exercise I plan to keep pushing myself to do for as long as there is traveling to be done. You never want to find yourself in a new country without the ability to say a few very basic and important things. Learn how to say:

Hello, good-bye, and thank you

I don't speak French/Japanese/Swahili. Do you speak English?

May I please have a cup of coffee/a glass of white wine/red wine/beer?

Can I have a taxi, please?

Where is the bathroom?

Remember that terrible trips make great stories. Not every vacation is going to go smoothly. Luckily, terrible trips make for great stories later on (sometimes much later on). Even a trip that includes sunburns, insect bites, food poisoning, awful hotels, stolen tickets, and the loss

NEAR AND FAR

Adventure sometimes means traveling for hours on planes and trains to far-flung destinations that require a passport and a pocketful of malaria pills—but it doesn't always necessitate doing battle with tsetse flies. Just driving to another town or city, no time change required, is sometimes all we need to expand our world and learn how to do something new.

So roam far or stay close. Either way, you can do what you love, love what you do, and try something new.

Here are some local and far-flung ways to have a new experience:

Have some wine and cheese.................San Francisco/Napa Valley or Tuscany, Italy

Go skiing...Tahoe or Austria

Take a surfing lesson ....Maui or Sydney

Drive on the wrong side of the road.....U.S. Virgin Islands or London

Dance salsa..Miami or Bogotá

Cook like the French................................New Orleans or Paris

Go hiking ....Adirondack Trail or New Zealand

of a driver's license or passport can be an incredible experience. In all likelihood, these are the trips you'll be talking about—and laughing about—years later. So whether you find yourself puking in Peru, covered in calamine lotion in Costa Rica, or stranded at a market in Marrakech, remember that one day you'll be safe at home with a lot of Technicolor memories.

Bring the party home. Travel is great for experiences—and for the experiences we can bring home with us. So don't hesitate to get into the import/export business—legally, of course. Head out into the world to learn and explore, and on weekends when you'd like to get out of town but your schedule (or bank account) won't accommodate, you can bring the party *a su casa* with the following tricks:

VISIT PARIS, OR . . .

Buy: Brie, crusty loaf, grapes
Drink: Côtes du Rhône
Listen: Edith Piaf
Eat: near a river

VISIT MADRID, OR . . .

Buy: olives, Iberico ham or salami, crusty bread or Tomato Toast (page 105)
Drink: Rioja
Listen: *Vicky Cristina Barcelona* sound track
Eat: at midnight, after a nice long nap

VISIT ISTANBUL, OR . . .

Buy: feta cheese, honey, watermelon, pita and hummus
Drink: Efes Pilsen
Listen: Tarkan
Eat: in the backyard

VISIT LONDON, OR . . .

Buy: scones, clotted cream, strawberry jam
Drink: Earl Grey tea
Listen: put the Beatles on replay
Eat: at 4 p.m. in the library

VISIT ROME, OR . . .

Buy: thin-crust pizza and gelato
Drink: Chianti
Listen: Pavarotti
Eat: at lunchtime and then have an espresso

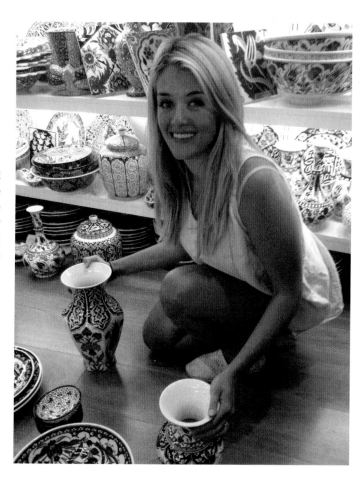

Me bargaining for Iznik plates and vases in the Turkish bazaar. They're great to hang on walls or use as serving platters and decorative items around the house.

TRAVELING WITH OTHERS

Whether they're old buddies or new acquaintances you've only just met, traveling with other people bonds you together through common memories. It's the sort of thing that forces everybody outside their comfort zone and brings true colors to light very quickly. Usually, this only serves to strengthen existing affection for people; it's fun to see what they would do outside the usual world you see them in!

My friend Bianca and I have a history of enduring massive logistical drama every time we travel together. We've been bumped off planes, delayed for hours, trapped on a rickety tin-can boat in Jamaica that almost capsized during crossing. It is always exceedingly unpleasant in the moment, but it's also provided some of our most memorable moments together. Even though we were both exhausted, frazzled, and seasick by the time we got off the boat in Jamaica, we perked right up at the sign of a local vendor selling freshly picked papaya with lime; we devoured one whole using plastic knives and our hands, letting the juices run down our arms. It's moments like that that feel both exotic and familiar—the best thing you can take away from traveling with friends.

One thing to keep in mind is that traveling in packs can necessitate a bit of finessing if you don't want to just be swept along in the tide of what everyone else wants to do. People have a tendency to revert back to acting the way they would within their family unit—probably the period in their lives when they spent the most amount of time having to cater to, or at least consider, the needs of others. People who are planners, people who are adventurers, people who are only concerned with the happiness of the group, and people who are only interested in martyring themselves—you'll be sure to get an earful about all the things they didn't get to do because they were prioritizing your itinerary at some point before the trip is over—will all quickly identify themselves.

Then again, this isn't much different from office politics, except this time you're supposed to be trying to get away from it all—which is precisely what you should do if need be. I'm normally a big fan of compromise, and though there is certainly a time and a place for it with group travel, this is actually one of those scenarios where I think it's most important to put yourself first.

Even the best of friends can have conflicting goals for a trip, and if you don't want to wind up feeling like you only got to do an eighth of the things you'd planned for Mexico, you should make a list and prioritize the things that are most important to you and make another list of the things you'd be okay to skip if the group isn't into the idea. Invite everyone else to come along for your important stuff, but don't be afraid to go it alone if you need to (within reason—you always want to have a buddy along if you think it's anything potentially unsafe). The beauty of traveling with a group is that you can share tips and knowledge and find out about a ton of adventures you might not have even known to take. But groups are equally good as friendly faces to meet up with for epic catch-up dinners after you've spent the day taking full advantage of your vacation the way you want to.

Traveling with significant others is a whole different ball game. Here the goal is not to distance yourself, and certainly compromise comes back in a big way. But it's also a much more important opportunity to grow a budding romance, so you'll want to pay close attention! When John and I had been dating for six months, he came on my family trip to Turkey. He was thrown right in the mix—everything from the savage bargaining we engage in at the covered bazaar to the dinner conversation, including my aunt's commentary on everyone present. Letting him experience my family, unfiltered, at length, on vacation in a foreign place really gave him an inside look at the people who raised me—and thereby a better understanding of me.

Travel experiences, especially those with family exposure, help you develop an understanding of someone you thought you already knew everything about. After we were married, John took me to Serbia and Croatia for a week to see where his family was from. He took me to the farm where his father grew up. We ate at the restaurants by the sea where his mother took vacations. We had pastries at the shop down the street from where his grandparents lived. These were the things he loved about a region dear to him, and by sharing these little experiences with me, he made his happy memories and associations visceral for me, too.

Seeing a new country for the first time but through the lens of someone who has been many times and loves it teaches us about the place and the person. So try to see every experience as an opportunity to keep your eyes open, and remember that even breakfast can be a teaching moment. (He loves pastries? Note to self.)

It also isn't necessary to go transatlantic in order to see someone you love in a different light. Bed-and-breakfasts make wonderful habitats for a weekend, and you can easily indulge your need for adventure and exploration without looking for your passport. A vacation does not need to be large scale or extravagant to be perfect. A night away or a weekend adventure—even an afternoon jaunt when you're playing hooky or dinner in a new district—can make for the most exquisite memories.

One more thing: Don't wait for someone else to do all the work. If you're hoping to break away from your routine, or you want a little adventure, get your fingers tapping and do a little search. Plan it out and surprise a buddy or your partner with the details! Especially with significant others, they will learn what you want from how you act. Seeing you plan a trip that you would like might inspire them to take the initiative next time—as long as you don't squash every idea they come up with. And for friends: Invite them along on something you plan this trip, and maybe they'll take the reins next!

Act on the things you want and let the people in your life learn from you. Then let them take the lead and see where it takes you! (Yes, every now and then you might have to grin and bear a fishing weekend if you don't want to crush that impulse to plan nice things for you. And who knows: There might be a fly-fishing master locked inside you yet.)

PACKING FOR THE GOLD

There are some women who manage to look good even when they've just stepped off a twelve-hour flight. How? They know what to put in their carry-on to freshen up after being strapped in a seat for a day, and they know what to pack to keep looking effortlessly chic all trip long. Whether you're traveling to a luxe city, the most glamorous of islands, or the rustic, rugged environs of the Adirondack Trail, when you pack well, you'll feel comfortable no matter where you end up.

Start your packing by creating your own list of must-brings, taking into consideration where you'll be going, the situations you'll find yourself in, and what you won't be able to pick up on the road. While items like sunscreen are always readily available (unless you'll be in the middle of nowhere), prescriptions may not be, so be sure to bring the essentials along.

Destination known. Creating a list of needs is a great way to make sure you get everything in your bag, but your needs must come from where you are going, not what you usually use at home.

The first thing to consider is what your destination demands. Fancy parties require fancy dresses; work meetings require work appropriate shoes; the beach calls for flip-flops and sunscreen.

Comfort station. Think about what makes you comfortable. If you're someone who doesn't care about what products you use and you're staying at a reputable hotel, then you can rely on the shampoo the staff will leave in your room. If you're the kind of girl who breaks out at the hint of an unfamiliar scent, you'll want to make sure to bring your own moisturizer, no matter what you have to leave behind in order to fit it in. Consider what you won't be able to get once you're there. If you're traveling to a major city, a quick stop at the pharmacy will net you shampoo, conditioner, sunscreen, and the like,

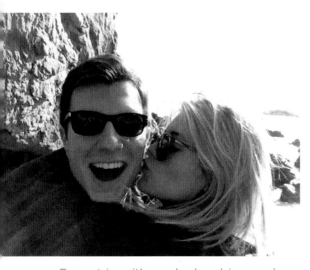

Every trip with my husband is an adventure. As much as I wish there were someone else to have taken this picture, we were the only ones visiting El Matador beach in Malibu, California, in the dead of winter! So we took a shameless selfie instead.

so there's no need to crowd them into your backpack. But things like medication and contact lenses probably won't be available so pack those first.

The perfect ensembles. When it comes to clothes, be choosy. It's worth spending the extra hour to style the actual outfits you'll wear so you don't bring unnecessary items. Where possible, have overlaps—such as a cardigan that pairs well with multiple clothing combinations. Shoes are probably the hardest to choose, because they have to be comfortable enough for walking but stylish enough that people won't know you're a tourist. Flats are good for this but lack support if you're an all-day walker like me. I usually cave and bring along one pair of lightweight walking sneakers, especially because I somehow always find myself scaling ruins or walking ten miles to find a hidden gem.

Must-haves. A plastic bag or pillowcase for dirty laundry. Room spray or a travel candle for potentially musty quarters. Travel packets of laundry detergent and stain remover for that favorite shirt that can't wait for the cleaners after its run-in with the pasta carbonara. Light reading to help you fall asleep or whittle away the jet-lag hours (I also upload books on tape on my iPod). A guidebook. A pocket diary to keep track of places you want to remember, little sketches, postcards, receipts, pressed flowers, and so on. A camera with film or a memory card or your smartphone. Chargers and adapters. The hairbrush and swipe of lipstick you know make you look three times better in 30 seconds. A good scarf to block burned shoulders from the sun, dress up outfits, hold your hair in place on a windy road in Monaco, and generally give you the aura of intrigue that every well-heeled, well-traveled lady should strive for.

Room for souvenirs. Vacation is my favorite time to shop, so I bring an extra collapsible bag with me on every trip for the inevitable moment that I realize I've purchased more than will fit into my bag (and John's).

BON VOYAGE, BUON VIAGGIO, HAVE A GREAT TRIP!

Whatever language they speak when you get there, the important thing is to get up and *go*. To wake up and *do*. To open your eyes and your heart to all of the places and the people in the world that you might fall in love with . . .

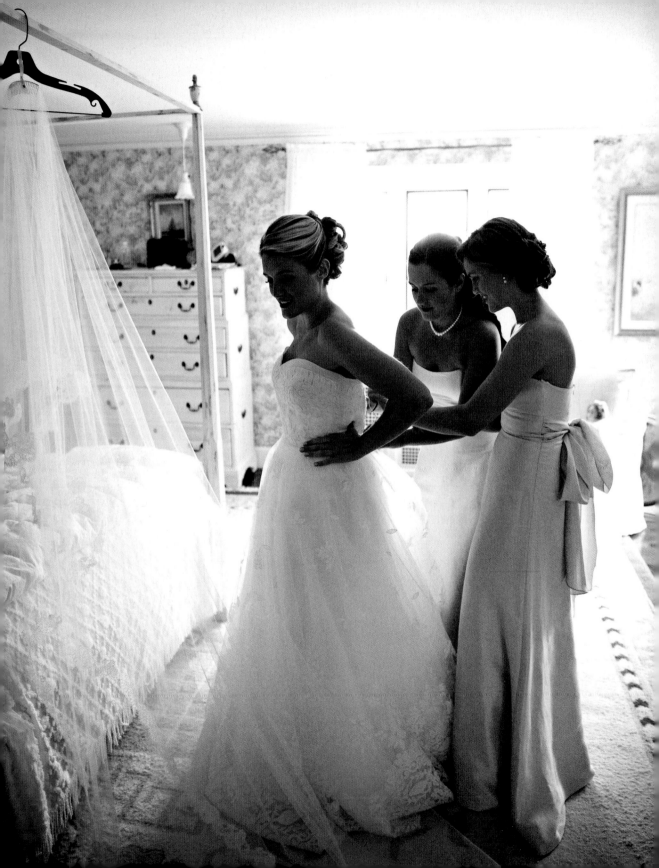

TWELVE

I HEART YOU

DNA, BFFs, and the one

Nobody has ever measured, not even poets, how much the heart can hold.
—ZELDA FITZGERALD

I AM IMAGINING YOU IN YOUR CLEAN, LOVELY HOME WHERE, having just made and eaten a most delightful meal, you are satisfied and mindful and ready to read the final phase of this book: the one that focuses on the people around you. Who are the costars in the comedy-drama-romance of your life? Whose birthday is highlighted on your calendar? Whose names appear in your best stories? Who is your bridge over troubled water? Who is the wind beneath your wings? (Cue music . . .)

Your nearest and dearest are the ones who keep you grounded, who have your best interests at heart, who know you better than any-one. You need them, no matter what. And they're the ones who will truly make your life worth relishing—so keep them close!

We're living in the age of connection, but I hear a lot of people wishing they were more part of a community—locally, not globally. We have the ability to communicate with thousands of people with a few swipes of a finger, but we're suffering from a curious kind of *dis*connection—because we're going too big instead of focusing our attention on the people who really matter. Even if you have more Twitter followers than anyone else you know, it's your real-life friends and family—the in-person, come-over-for-dinner, let's-hang-out-on-weeknights-and-weekends kind of people—who create your emotional landscape. Even though our phones can give us definitions, translations, and directions, it's the people we love who give us true (emotional) support and (personal) feedback.

WATERING THE FAMILY TREE

Family are (or can be) the friends you're born with—just like friends are the family you choose. Maybe you and your family are close as can be; maybe some of your relatives don't fall squarely in the center of your relationship Venn diagram of perfect family and perfect friend, and that's okay. As long as you know the difference between DNA and BFF, you'll be able to better enjoy family gatherings and reframe the way you see your family dynamic. A sister may be sweet and generous, but she can also be your nemesis! A brother may be solid and supportive, or he might totally ignore you. If your siblings are jerks, don't be fooled by their resemblance to you, and protect yourself. If they're the coolest, sweetest, funniest people around, count yourself lucky and don't take them for granted!

If you're close with your parents, don't abuse the privilege by treating them kindly only when it suits you. If you call your mom to update her on your life, make sure you ask about hers, too. And don't stop calling just because you've suddenly had an uptick in the activity on your social calendar. Good family—family you take care of and who take care of you—will be the rock under your foundation if you invest in those relationships. Remember: They knew you when you were pooping in diapers, popping pimples as an ugly teenager, struggling to make friends in college, dating your first boyfriend—they know everything! And they probably have the pictures to prove it.

If you want your family relationships to work, you've got to put the work in. Time represents values. So make room in your life for what matters.

Participate in family holidays, birthdays, and reunions. If you have brothers and sisters, as kids you knew that they were *always* around. Even when you begged them to get lost. Then, one day, everything changes, and your sister is in school in California while your brother is in New York becoming an actor (by which he means bartender). Instead of bickering and playing all the livelong day, there are friendly phone calls and emails and not nearly enough hang time. And what about your uncle Bob, who taught you magic tricks when you were a kid and still sends you cards on your birthday? When is the last time you saw him?

Yes, I know you have deadlines to manage and limited time and money to spend, but in the meanwhile, tell your friends you'll go dancing another time and book that ticket to Philly, or Tulsa, or Brooklyn so you can go to the family reunion. And wear the darn T-shirt.

Remember the good times. When I was a kid, we spent every Friday night driving an hour and a half from our home in New Jersey down to Philadelphia to visit my mother's parents. My friends teased me for missing all the fun with them every weekend, but looking back, I wouldn't trade those family weekends with my clan for all the slumber parties in the world. There were raucous game nights and plenty of family dinners. My grandmother's house was where I learned to cook and ride ponies bareback. It was where we ran around outside and played in the stream and ate hoagie picnics, and then my siblings and I all piled on to the foot of my grandparents' bed to watch *Abbott and Costello* movies until way past bedtime. Those visits grounded me and showed me that I was part of a community. Those weekends made it possible to develop a deep relationship with my grandparents and see them as role models.

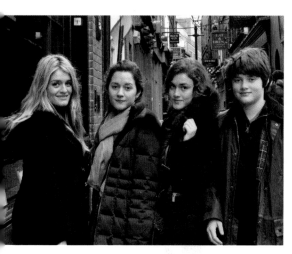

Travel is better with family to share it! Here are the Oz siblings (aka Ozlings) wandering a new part of town. If I had to guess, we're likely searching out our next meal. . . .

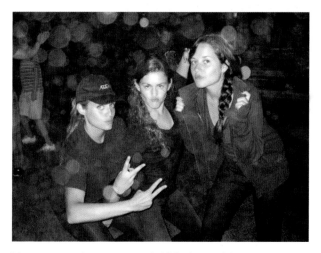

You can run but you can't hide from this gang! A team picture with my two sisters from an epic game of Oz family capture the flag: nighttime edition!

Who I am today was grown in those Philadelphia weekends. I count myself very lucky to have such a supportive family; not everyone feels the same way. There's a reason the word *family* is so often offered along with an eye roll—because family can get too close and step on feelings and over boundaries. It's so easy to get annoyed at the people you're stuck with, or be extra harsh on them because you know you're tied by blood, and it can be just as easy to overlook the good stuff. So think back. What are some great experiences you've had with your family? Channel those positive feelings the next time your little sister calls to say the dry cleaner couldn't get the stain out of the designer dress you loaned her.

Forgive the not-so-great stuff. Dads who are too strict or are always at work or are threatening to marry their girlfriends. Moms who dress too young for their age, are obsessed with their yoga studio, ask too many questions. Brothers who flirt with your friends, sisters who make more money than you. And let's not forget Cousin Ike, who swam in one Olympic tryout and still hasn't stopped talking about it. Did Cousin Melinda tell everyone in your elementary school that you had a crush on Stevie Fisher? Get over it. They might be more suited to being characters in a science-fiction movie, but they've got your DNA (or they married it) and they aren't going anywhere, so try to forgive them their trespasses, at least this once.

Dodge awkward questions. It can be scary to evaluate family relationships with a critical eye, because you can't just break up with your parents or cousin or uncle without ramifications. Luckily, being stuck with people in your family doesn't mean you have to get stuck in awkward conversations. The good news is that it is possible to love your family, be a supportive member of the clan, and still find a way to avoid the clutches of nosy Aunt Matilda.

We've all got an Aunt Matilda. When I was trying to find my career path, some of my relatives could not stop themselves from asking me indelicate questions about my "situation." "What do you want to do?" "Have you figured it out yet?" They may have been trying to be helpful, but instead of inspiring me, it made me feel as if I wasn't good enough because I was still working out the answers—and that wasn't the kind of help I needed. I had plenty of self-doubt and anxiety all on my own, thanks.

If you're feeling ambushed by relatives during a period of change, or fielding awkward questions about your desire to go back to school, quit drinking, lose weight, start a band, learn computer programming, end a relationship, date someone new, get married, have a baby, or the opposite—you're happy where you are and others are clamoring for a change you'd rather avoid—stay strong. If you're being pressed about sensitive subjects, take action. Be vocal. Unless someone's truly evil, they're just looking to connect with you, not give you high blood pressure. So give them a different way to connect: Ask them about their lives. Ask them about the weather. Or just steer them toward the hummus plate and go talk to somebody else.

Don't be afraid to change roles. We all have a part to play in the family drama, and when we go home we often regress to the role we were assigned when we were kids, whether it's the bossy eldest, the annoying baby brother, or the über-responsible second mother. But you're a grown-up lady now, and your family de-

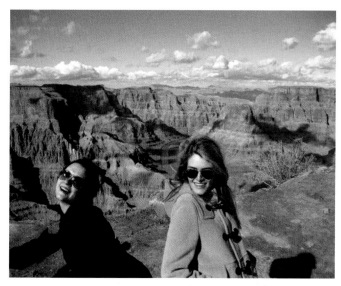

Me and my sister Arabella goofing around at the Grand Canyon on a family trip.

serves to get to know the mature, confident, settled woman you've become, so don't be afraid to shift your role—and give others room to grow into their starring roles, too—meaning your baby sister doesn't always have to take your word as gospel now that she's got a baby of her own.

FRIENDS, WONDERFUL FRIENDS

Friends are a different story all together. We collect them, choose them, keep them close, and sometimes have to let them go. They are the people we laugh with, the people we go dancing with, the people we can be goofballs with and never worry they'll judge us. They're the family we choose, and hopefully we choose them for life.

I don't know what I would do without my best ladies and gents, and I never plan on finding out. Some I met forever ago, some I've met more recently, and all of them are an integral part of my life.

We learn from our friends, we talk issues out with them and we make personal decisions based on their feedback. In the best of worlds, they are people with characteristics you would be happy to emulate, people who draw out the qualities about yourself that you like best. Don't underestimate how important loyalty, compassion, and sound advice can be. You'll be happier in the long term if you choose wisely when you invite people into your inner circle. And being a good friend is a sure way to have good friends.

My mom always tells me to have standards, not expectations. The difference is that one sets what is acceptable for you and how you want to be treated; the other is demanding that someone act the way you want them to. We have no control over other people, so we might as well get used to not having expectations for them. Instead, surround yourself with people who consistently meet the standard of friend you want to be to them, who make you feel appreciated and happy. And make sure to appreciate them right back.

Show up—even if you're running late. Being a good friend takes energy and effort. For a true friendship to evolve, for real closeness to develop, you have to be willing and ready to invest in your friend's life and to let her invest in yours. To do that, you have to show up. Showing up ranges from dinner parties (we all remember those people who never emailed to let us know they couldn't make it) to baby showers (that are more than an hour away in the middle of nowhere) to helping her pack up after divorce or move into a new home after marriage. We make

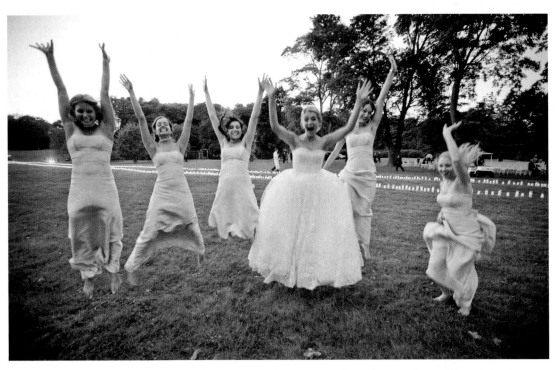

This is one of my favorite pictures from our wedding. I loved getting to share this celebratory moment with some of my bridesmaids, barefoot and jumping in the grass like kids!

RANDOM ACTS OF REACHING OUT **Every now and then, send your friends funny, random, or generous emails, voice messages, or even just texts. Congratulate them on a recent promotion or compliment a beautiful pic they posted. Remind them of that hilarious outing you had to Coney Island. Send a picture you stumbled upon in your photo library of the first night you went out all together and the ridiculous costumes you wore—you look so young! Include a link to an article that made you think of them—or just something that made you laugh.**

My friends and I do this all the time, and it's an easy and effective way to keep in touch even when we don't have as much time as we would like to see each other. Everyone likes to know you think of them sometimes and that you know them well, and to be able to share common memories is always a great way to build on a solid friendship. Gandhi said we should be the change we wish to see in the world, so flood your inner circle with happiness, kindness, and fun—and change the world that feeds your soul!

---

friends with people when our paths cross. Later, as our paths diverge, it can become more confusing to navigate back to a feeling of closeness. Showing up means staying interested and in touch. Remember to think about them where they're at, not where they used to be. If Susie just started nursing, no, she doesn't want to do tequila shots with you at the club on Saturday night. And if Marguerite just got dumped, no, she doesn't want to hear about your magical night of romance on Valentine's Day. Being a friend means seeing what your friend is going through, not just projecting your situation—or who they used to be—onto them. And nobody wants a fair-weather friend. You have to be there to help her pick up the pieces just as eagerly as you were there to celebrate the good times.

Learn how to listen. Is it just me, or has everyone around us gotten extra snarky? It's great to be clever and witty, but too many attempts at crafting the perfect punch line can make you miss the message. Your friends know that you're really cool and fun and funny, but sometimes they don't want a stand-up act: They just want you to be there. If you want close friendships, you have to be willing to have candid discussions. So pay attention. Listen. Share. Don't sit there clicking on your phone. Stop checking your newsfeed. Be there fully. Being a friend is as much about listening as talking—maybe more.

That said, part of being a good listener is being a trustworthy audience. If someone shares something personal with you, put it in the vault. If you overhear a juicy piece of gossip, keep it to yourself. Keeping someone's confidence is of the utmost importance. We all want to be seen as people with integrity who deserve our friends' trust. If you damage that, it's really hard to earn it back. And remember: A dog that brings a bone, carries a bone, so don't expect any trust or discretion from your gossip buddies. Better to steer clear.

Know when to forgive. One of my best friends in the world lives abroad and is truly awful about keeping in touch, but because I know that about her, I don't take it personally or feel insulted by it. If I really needed something from her, I know she'd be here in a heartbeat. Another of my best friends is superb about keeping in touch but often expects the same level of attention in return—and I don't always meet her ideal, especially when it comes to remembering birthdays. Luckily for me, she's come to understand that my forgetting her birthday is not because I don't love and cherish her. It's just one of my shortcomings, and one that she forgives.

Be honest—and kind. If a friend asks for your direct advice, you may tell the truth, but be gentle. Think productive, not mean. If you observe her doing something hugely stupid, out of character, or physically dangerous, you may tell her even if she has not asked for your opinion, but you must tell her nicely. Warning! Beware the moping trap. If you've got a friend who is constantly wondering if she should dump her (jerk of a) boyfriend or a brother who's always complaining about his girlfriend, tread carefully. Should you unthinkingly offer back a casual "You're so right, they suck," odds are that a week later, they'll be back together and you'll be stuck with your stiletto in your mouth. The best advice I can give you is to ask questions and sympathize, because everybody needs to be heard. Chances are if you let them talk out the issue they're facing, they'll work through to the answer or solution they really want. People often just need a forum and a trusted pair of ears. Then again, if they're always inviting you to a pity party, never an actual party, you might want to turn that kindness on yourself and cut loose. If Eeyore just wants to continue a twenty-four-hour whining loop despite your best advice—boring for you, not helpful for her—keep reading: There's more below on distancing yourself from friendships that just aren't working.

Offer to help. Childhood is full of droplets of wisdom that work just as well for adults, if we could just remember them. One great little droplet is this: Look for ways to help without being asked. People who need help are often too overwhelmed to know that they need help, or they're too embarrassed—or overloaded—to ask. So pay attention to conversations with friends, and try to figure out what you can *offer* to do.

HOW TO TELL THE DIFFERENCE BETWEEN A CONFIDANT AND AN ACQUAINTANCE

Don't hesitate to draw distinctions between your social groups. A social acquaintance and, for that matter, an online "friend," is not the same thing as a best friend. An acquaintance can certainly become a friend, but simply going out for a drink with someone does not make them a confidant.

So don't go running around telling everyone you meet about your messy breakup, no matter how many rounds of margaritas you've shared or how many of your Instagrams they've liked. Trust me, you do not want to spill all to the boss's new assistant over French fries in the cafeteria, even if she's buying, unless you want the CEO to know exactly what you do when you're off the clock.

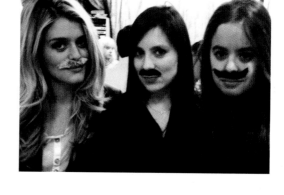

CONFIDANTS

A confidant always calls you back.

A confidant comes to your birthday parties.

Your confidants know about your last breakup because they watched you bawl your face off.

A confidant tells you when they're feeling sad, depressed, angry, or disappointed.

A confidant knows that you're from Connecticut, that your parents are divorced, that you highlight your hair, and that you're going to break up with your boyfriend at the end of the summer.

ACQUAINTANCES

An acquaintance is someone you've only ever emailed or texted.

An acquaintance leaves a "happy birthday" note on your wall.

An acquaintance only knows that your "relationship status" online has changed.

Online acquaintances tell you when they've been to a new restaurant and what they ate.

Acquaintances know that you're from the Northeast.

FOUR-LEGGED FRIENDS

This is me with my baby cat, Babycat, who is now more like four, but he's the punk of all punks, and so he remains "baby." When in doubt, turn to the four-legged for solid, unconditional, unwavering love and companionship—they can teach us a lot about how to love openly, ask for the affection we need, and return it!

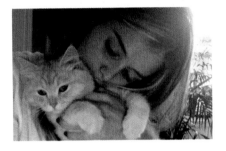

If a friend who lives down the block has the flu, take her dog when you go running in the park. If a friend is bogged down at work, drop off a tray of lasagna or have dinner delivered. Yes, life is busy. And yes, the busier we are, the more work it takes to make room in our schedules for others. But if we want to be part of a loving community, we need to take action and create it by caring and doing, not by purchasing a membership card.

The Skinny on Friend Breakups

How do you know the people you think of as friends? Are they old friends whom you've known for years, who really knew you as the ugly duckling before the swan, the girls you went to soccer camp with? Are they newer friends who can better relate to you as you are right now, friends who have similar jobs or hobbies or live nearby? Or are they leftover friends, the ones you probably shouldn't have in your life anymore but who manage to stick around by proximity, habit, or sheer persistence? The relationships you're cultivating should offer depth as well as convenience, because we're all affected by the people we keep company with.

Are your friends the kind of people who want to grow and evolve and who want to see you grow and evolve? Or are they the kind of people who like you best when you regress, falling back into bad habits you've worked hard to escape? Some people want you to stay the same so that they can stay the same. Others don't understand why you'd want to change at all and resent the time you no longer have for them. Others may feel stuck in their own lives, and seeing your evolution may feel like a judgment on their own intransigent habits. The truest friends, the ones you should want to keep forever, are the friends who can support you wherever you want to go, whoever you want to become.

As you consider who your true friends are, the ones who really merit your attention and energy, consider how little time you have for yourself and the people who really matter the most. And then ask yourself why you would bother wasting another precious minute with someone who's not doing it for you.

Crushes, Beaus, Live-ins, The One

Family is forever and friendship should be easy, but romantic relationships are where many people find bliss. They take work—and that's not a bad thing! Cultivating a loving, trusting, supportive bond; uniting with someone, valuing them as your equal, and having them feel the same way about you; this is what we're all looking for.

Maybe you want a marriage just like Mom and Dad's; maybe the idea of marriage makes you cringe. Maybe you've had a ton of relationships; maybe you're a serial lone wolf. Most people have to kiss a lot of toads before they find a prince, and making mistakes is okay (so long as you don't know it's a mistake when you're making it—knowingly making bad choices leads to bad results).

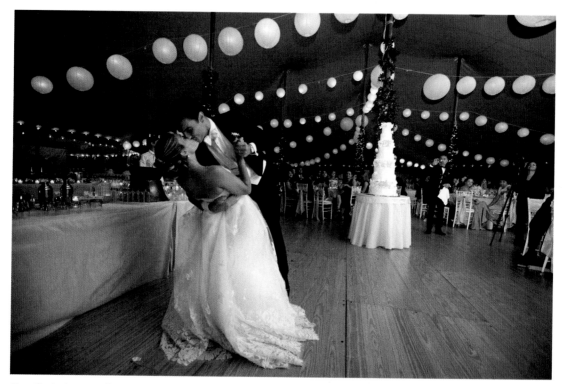

Our first dance after "I do!"

When you're young, you might think you have time to spend with people you know you don't have a future with. It can be fun for a while, something to pass the time. Or maybe you are convinced you've struck gold—and then things go south. Your twenties and thirties are about having the meaningful experiences that shape you, and you should have fun! But as you get to know yourself better, you'll naturally want to preserve yourself more, treat yourself better, and let go of people and things that aren't working. The more we focus on being true to ourselves and letting our best selves shine, the easier we will find it to shed bad habits (yes, people can be habits, too) and feel that their absence is a gift rather than a loss.

When it comes to growing up, the goal is to learn from our lapses of judgment so we can relish all the right moments that are to come. The main thing is not to waste time worrying that we're not playing it right because, for now, the whole game is to learn by trial and error. The goal is to not wake up in twenty years and think: *I don't like who I'm with* or *I don't know who I am*, or *I don't like who I am, and I haven't spent the time to really cultivate the person I want to be.*

Invest now, play now, be honest, try new things now, and greet that future morning comfortable in your own skin and with a whole lot of life experience. The more full our own lives are, the more obvious it is that we're not relying on someone else to give us our identity or purpose or happiness, the more people will want to be a part of our lives and create joy together. So let them! Put yourself out there unafraid and let them flock.

Whether you're on your own, just starting something new, trying to take it to the next step, happily married, or working through a rough patch, start with you. What's your goal? Where are you happiest? What can you do to make sure you're heading toward this place? A more centered, complete you is the best place to start any loving relationship. And a more centered, complete you is what this book is all about!

Being Open to Loving Relationships

If you've found yourself somehow "undateable," ask yourself whether you've been keeping your mind open to being in a loving relationship. So many of my friends who have either jumped from one bad relationship to the next, or can't seem to find someone to spend their time with, are in one way or another sabotaging this chance at happiness. Whether it's self-doubt that undermines your confidence, or the tendency to see fault first to protect yourself from feeling hurt later, the only person you're denying is you.

Wake up to the fact that there is lots and lots and *lots* to love about you! Think about the things that you are attracted to: humor, kindness, and intelligence, interesting things to say and cool life experiences. Now think about how you do or do not emanate the things someone

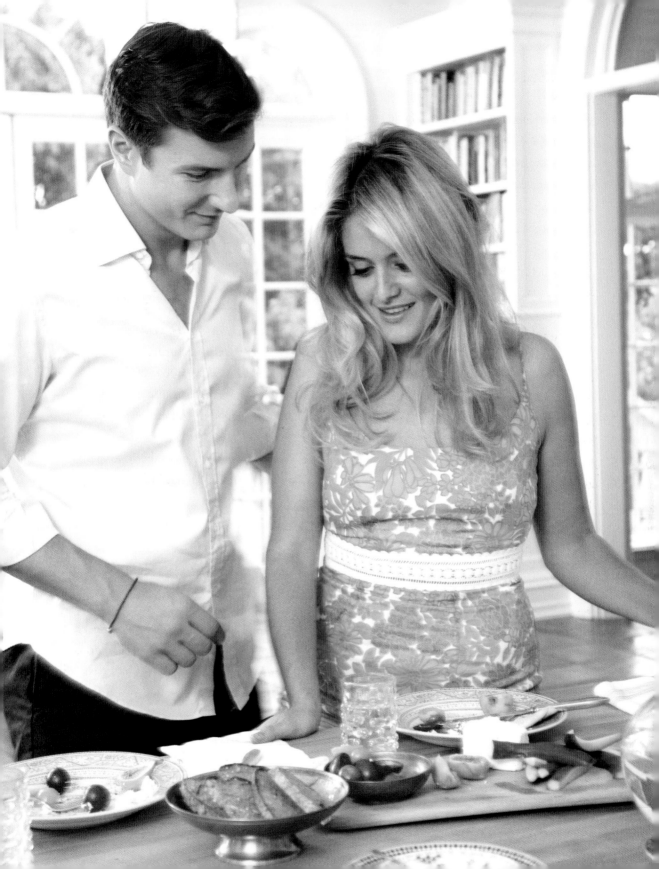

would find attractive about you. For starters, whether you're skilled or still learning, you can cook, create a gorgeous home, and throw sensational parties all while investing in your long-term happiness—you're a straight-up catch! Don't let any little voice—even the one in your head—tell you otherwise.

Take the desperation away, take the anger and fear away, and instead start focusing on feeling complete just as you are. Radiate with self-love and confidence; glow with independence. Know that you are a whole person, with a whole lot to offer. An emotionally evolved, beautiful-inside-and-out kinda gal. I promise you, if you believe these things for yourself, it's the most attractive thing you can do.

Making Good Relationships Great

Relationships need a whole lot of care and attention and effort—and it's all worth it. I've been married for only three years, and I've already learned that while love feels like magic, being sprinkled with long-term pixie dust requires long-term investment and a healthy dose of fun.

Paying the mortgage and deciding who takes the trash out is part of a relationship, of course, but you can't let responsibilities suck all the air out of the room. You and your partner fell for each other because you enjoyed spending time together, so make sure to keep a sense of play in the equation by planning date nights where you don't talk about taxes, cozy mornings during which nobody does the dishes, and the occasional bout of teasing, tickling, and otherwise goofing around. If you can see each other as friends always, the rest is bound to be fun.

Here are some fail-proof ways to keep the romance alive and kicking happily ever after!

Remember that little things count big time. Getting flowers on my birthday is really nice. But when John brings me a bodega bouquet in the middle of July just because he thought of me and they were my color (blush pink!), that means the world. So show appreciation. Send sweet notes. Say thank you! Teach him how you want to be treated by treating him that way. What you do often is what you will do always, so practice like you play.

When you're together, give each other your full, undivided attention. "We" time isn't "Wii" time. Put the phone down. Hide your iPad. You can't gaze lovingly into someone's eyes if you're reading emails and he's checking the scores.

Fight well, with honesty and kindness. There's no place for mean in a healthful relationship. Arguments are normal. Fighting dirty is unacceptable. If an issue needs to be worked out, put down the boxing gloves, pick up the box of tissues, and show him where it hurts—nicely. And then listen to him, hear out his injuries (do not belittle them), and do your best to fix them without feeling attacked. Take off the armor and approach the situation with compassion and an ear for understanding. It takes practice, but you will both be much happier if you can learn to fight nicely.

Learn to compromise. Being in a strong, loving relationship sometimes means doing things you don't want to do (or at least that wouldn't be your first choice), whether it's eating at a restaurant you don't love or choosing where to live based on someone else's career or needs. There's no formula to use, and sometimes it will feel like all the sacrifices are being made on your end (this is actually a psychological phenomenon—people always think they're doing the most work in a group project). The trick is to remember that your partner's happiness is as important as your own and that you should both be pursuing them equally. If your kindness and generosity are being taken advantage of, that's something to talk about. But try not to keep tabs—love is not tit for tat.

Have your own lives. We want to be happy together, and so we learn to be happy apart. Happy couples work to find a balance between their independent lives and their lives together. Sometimes all I want is time alone with my husband. Other times, doing things solo is wonderful, because when we each have our own sense of happiness and fulfillment, we can share that with one another. Just because you're partners doesn't mean you have identical needs, wants, and likes. Having time apart gives you both a chance to fulfill those individual desires without feeling imposed on or resentful for being dragged along to the eightieth hockey game this year. Plus you'll have great stuff to share when you meet up for dinner. As long as you keep teaching each other, feeding your passions and cultivating your own interests keeps the love alive!

Kicking Bad Relationships to the Curb

Plenty of us waste precious time in relationships that, if we are truthful with ourselves, we know aren't right. We're paralyzed by the fear that we won't find anyone we'll like as much, that we won't know how to fill the gap, that we won't know what to do on our own. We can tolerate all kinds of nonsense—from forgotten birthdays to forgotten phone numbers—under the misguided belief that "this is as good as it gets." But you don't know what you don't know, and the longer you spend bound to someone who isn't right, the longer you'll be closed off to the possibility of meeting someone who is.

Here's the truth: You have to demand the respect you deserve and remember that people will treat and see you how you treat and see yourself. So prioritize your needs, the things that make you feel stable and secure and fulfilled. But also remember that people only have as much control over your life as you give them. Unless they're really worthy of the honor and the privilege, don't give them access. More important, tell them to take a hike if they can't treat you kindly, with respect, and with honesty at all times.

Relationships Teach You About You

Whether it's family, friends, or the salt to your pepper, the funny thing about relationships is that they actually teach us much more about ourselves than about other people. Why do we need certain things from certain people? Why do certain things they do make us feel upset, undervalued, unloved? Why do we want to test them rather than give them the answer key and get straight to the good part?

The deeper you go emotionally with someone, the more you uncover not only about the way you like to exist in a relationship but also about the ways you need to grow as an individual.

The most intimate relationships we have bring up the issues outstanding in our lives that we need to work on, and we are (sometimes inexplicably) drawn to people who shine a light on those potential growth areas over and over again. Say you're someone who's always said you want to be taken care of and never have to worry, which is another way of saying never have to have responsibility. That may be your identity, but it may not. If you are meant to grow into the capable, self-reliant, independent person your subconscious knows you need to be, you'll probably find yourself ending up in relationships with people who force you to stand on your own.

We can resist this growth, and often we do, choosing to look outward and see the things that cause us irritation and upset rather than looking inward and recognizing the opportunities for growth that these interactions are giving us. Plenty of relationships have ended because we refuse to be honest with ourselves and try to justify where and how we are (this is the "I'm right!" mode that traps us in the status quo) rather than seeing what might be missing. It is often easier to say "He is so needy!" rather than looking inward and seeing that potentially, his neediness was an opportunity for you to become more intimate, more emotionally developed because this was a gap in your life. The thing is that we will keep getting pushed to grow until we do. Our lessons might take different forms, but they'll always be propelling us toward the higher self our subconscious wants us to become.

So learn the lesson already and get on being happy with all the wonderful people in your life by being happy, first and foremost, with you!

The most important relationships we have feed our lives in a way even the most perfect meal never could, so we should treasure them like gold. Below, I've pulled together my five favorite tips for maintaining happy, healthy relationships in all the areas of your life.

1. The best relationships are based on good health and bad memory.

2. Choose your attitude.

3. Remember the value of standards and the danger of expectations.

4. Set them up for success.

5. Never go to sleep angry.

Read on if you want all the juicy tidbits of how these tips will work for you!

5 SECRETS FOR RELATIONSHIP BLISS

Secret 1—The best relationships are based on good health and bad memory. First things first: Would you rather be right or happy? Now, think back on all the petty arguments that have ruined time together over practically nothing—were they worth it?

If the fight is only a short-lived outburst where you say things you don't mean, it probably doesn't need to happen. If it's the kind that is long, festering, and sticks in your craw days and weeks later, then it needs a long-term solution, not the short-term relief that venting affords. I am all about airing grievances and speaking my mind, but it has to be solution-oriented. Holding grudges, as tempting as it is, hurts you more than anyone else by bottling up the negative energy and souring you from the inside out—like a pickle!

On the flip side, recalibration and reconnection can happen in an instant. Being kind, and supplying emotional and physical nourishment (help keep each other healthy from the inside out!) brings you together and drives away bitterness, resentment, and hurt. We all need to be heard, and we all want to be with someone who makes us feel safe enough to share exactly what makes us tick and what makes us boil. So take a walk together or set the table for two and hash it out, keeping the affection you feel for each other front and center. Take what you can learn and forget the rest. You'll both feel better afterward.

Secret 2—Choose your attitude. This one comes from my grandmother and sums up her personality in a nutshell. She's a firm believer in the idea that you can only control your own attitude—and that attitude is key to how you feel: If you think you feel good, you start to feel good! Likewise, if you tell yourself you're tired or old or mediocre at life, you will start to be all those things. We were never allowed to say "I'm bored" under her roof. Her response: "Only boring people get bored."

Think about it this way: Part of creating a life worth relishing is making a commitment to focus only on things that make your life better and more full somehow. When choosing your attitude, you're deciding what your outlook on life will be. Habitually happy people are not that way because only good things happen to them. Instead, they simply decide that no matter what happens outside their control, their attitude will be a positive one. Their circumstances don't change—but how they see those same circumstances does. Choosing to do the best you can with what you can control, and make the best of what you cannot, seems like good life advice all around.

Secret 3—Remember the value of standards and the danger of expectations. This is one of the most valuable things my mother ever taught me, and it follows perfectly from my grand-mother's tip above. When you focus on standards of your own rather than expectations for somebody else, you're choosing an attitude of power—power to change your surroundings, power to change yourself, and power to pursue happiness rather than waiting for someone else to make you happy.

Standards define how you value yourself, and they are the bare minimum you require in order to be in a relationship—for instance, no cheating, no stealing, no lying. You control where these standards are set, and if someone is not able to meet them, then it's simple: They don't get to be part of your life. Compromising on your standards doesn't do you or anyone else any favors—and it certainly won't make you happy if even this lowered bar can't be met.

Expectations are another thing entirely. These are little tests you give people to see if they will react how you want them to, whether it's expecting your boyfriend to call five times a day or expecting your friend to cancel her plans because your calendar just opened up. Sometimes what you want and what the other person wants are aligned and you'll be happy. Sometimes he will bend to your will, but he'll probably resent you for it. And sometimes she will do what she wants instead and you'll be disappointed.

Whenever you base your happiness on someone else's behavior, the power is no longer in your hands because the choice isn't yours to make. The only choice you do have is whether to adjust your expectations or not. Unlike standards, adjusting expectations does not in any way diminish you. In fact, it's a worthwhile exercise to see how you can create positive change by focusing on your own behavior. In all likelihood, getting to the root of the issue will show you how little of what you expect of other people actually has to do with them and how much of it is really about things you need—and can probably give yourself.

If you would like to read more on this point, go straight to the source. My mom's book on precisely this topic, and all matters of the happy heart, is called *Us: Transforming Ourselves and the Relationships That Matter Most.*

Secret 4—Set them up for success. No matter how close you are to someone, she can't get it right all the time unless you tell her what you want—and even then, she'll sometimes want to do things her way instead (shocking!) and you'll just have to live with it, or not. Rather than testing her ability to guess, set her up for success by being clear and open about what you need: It's much easier, and you'll both be happier. And treat others the way you want to be treated—they'll learn from you!

Secret 5—Never go to sleep angry. This little droplet of wisdom seems to be the most commonly held tenet of happy couples everywhere. I don't know if there's a biological reason why going to sleep angry is bad—other than it's actually difficult to fall asleep if one is in a rage about something—but it always seems as if I wake up with renewed resentment. Like my subconscious solidified all the petty ways I knew I just had to be right and so-and-so was obviously in the wrong (this goes for partners, friends, coworkers, and the random dude who body-slammed you on the subway).

Let it go. If it really needs to be hashed out, reach someplace to pause and approach it again in the morning with a clear head. Going to sleep in the heat of an argument only fuels the fire of the fight. If it lingers over long periods, chances are you're focusing more on getting a confession or proving someone wrong than you are on finding a solution.

And while you're at it, everyone knows to pick battles, but I've found it even more important to pick your timing. It may seem like an opportune moment to bring up a contentious subject as your partner is sinking into his or her pillow after a long day at the office, but in all likelihood, the response will not be a desired one. Cranky people are seldom rational, and tired people are seldom forgiving. It won't always be sunshine and rainbows, but learning to forgo the blowout fights as often as can be means less time cleaning up the mess and more time enjoying the party.

Now, who wants dessert?

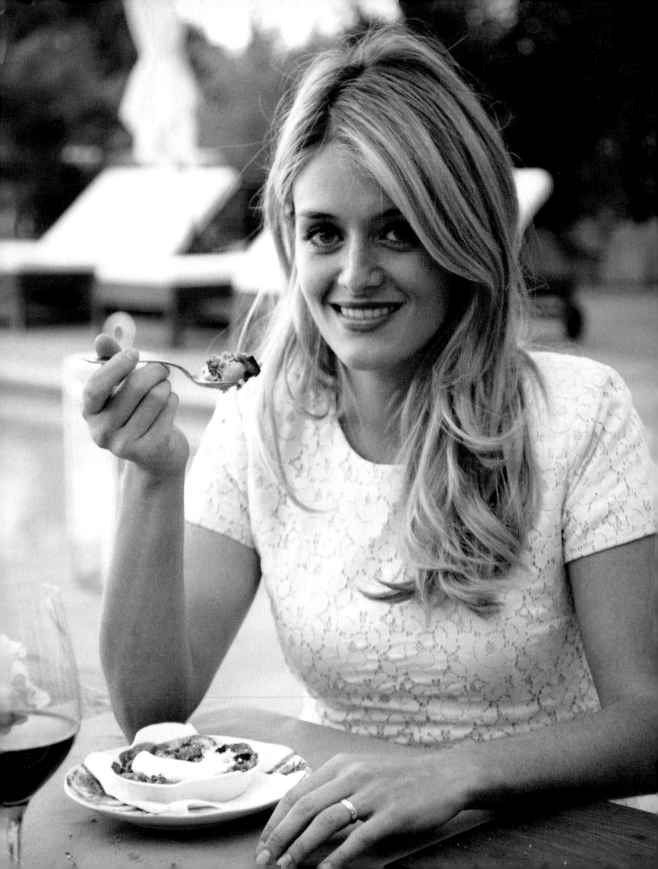

THIRTEEN

YOU'VE EARNED IT

dessert

Cookies are made of butter and love.
—NORWEGIAN PROVERB

A DELICIOUS DINNER IS DIVINE, BUT DESSERT MAKES IT A MEAL. PART of my style of eating is making sure to leave room for confections that are made from scratch, refuse to be ignored, and are blissful to enjoy. This chapter is dedicated to the desserts I look forward to—the sweet somethings that signal the end of a grand dining experience and the beginning of postprandial fun!

From the exotic comfort of Persian Brown Rice Pudding to the coziness of Chocolate Chip Oatmeal Cookies, these desserts will knock your socks off. If all you need is chocolate, the creamy Chocolate Fudge Pops await. Or maybe you're craving cake, be it decadent Coconut Pecan or the equally tempting Strawberry with Caramel Fleur de Sel Whipped Cream Frosting. There's no shortage of inspiration here for the simply extravagant or extravagantly simple dessert.

You started smart—now you get to finish happy!

RED FRUIT MINI CRUMBLES

makes six 4-inch ramekins

OATMEAL TOPPING

1 cup rolled oats
(not quick-cooking)

½ cup light brown sugar

½ cup whole-wheat flour

½ cup chopped walnuts

½ teaspoon salt

8 tablespoons (1 stick)
unsalted butter, cut into small
cubes and chilled

FRUIT FILLING

2 tablespoons organic coconut
oil plus extra for oiling the
ramekins

½ cup sugar

¼ cup honey

1 tablespoon fresh lemon juice

5 apples (Gala or Pink Lady),
peeled, cored, and thinly sliced

1 tablespoon cornstarch

1 pint strawberries, hulled and
cut in half lengthwise

1 pint raspberries

1 teaspoon pure vanilla extract

Whipped cream (optional)

FRESH FRUIT IS GREAT. Fresh fruit cooked down to a sweet-tart, saucy goodness and topped with an oatmeal cookie crumble is divine. This is one of my favorite desserts to serve at dinner parties because it looks so beautiful presented in individual ramekins for portioning and can be customized to whatever fruit is in season.

You'll think I'm crazy, but try this recipe with a sprinkle of sea salt and fresh-cracked black pepper over each crumble before serving. The salt actually wakes up your taste buds to all the sweet-tart flavors, and pepper pairs beautifully with strawberries.

1. Preheat the oven to 350°F.

2. To make the oatmeal topping, in a medium bowl, combine the oats, sugar, flour, walnuts, and salt and mix well. Add the chilled butter cubes and work the mixture with two knives or your hands until clumps form.

3. To make the fruit filling, in a large skillet over medium heat, melt the oil. Add the sugar, honey, and lemon juice and cook until the sugar is melted. Stir in the apples, raise the heat to medium-high and cook, stirring frequently, about 4 minutes, or until they begin to soften and release their liquid. Stir in the cornstarch and cook, stirring frequently, until the apples are tender but not mushy and the liquid is clear, about 4 minutes. Remove from the heat and stir in the strawberries and raspberries and the vanilla.

4. Divide the mixture among six 4-inch ramekins, filling them about three-quarters full. Top each with a generous 2 tablespoons of the oatmeal mixture. Transfer the ramekins to a baking sheet. Bake until the fruit is bubbling and the topping is golden brown, about 35 minutes. (Keep an eye on 'em! Cooking time may vary.) Let stand to cool slightly, and serve with whipped cream, if desired.

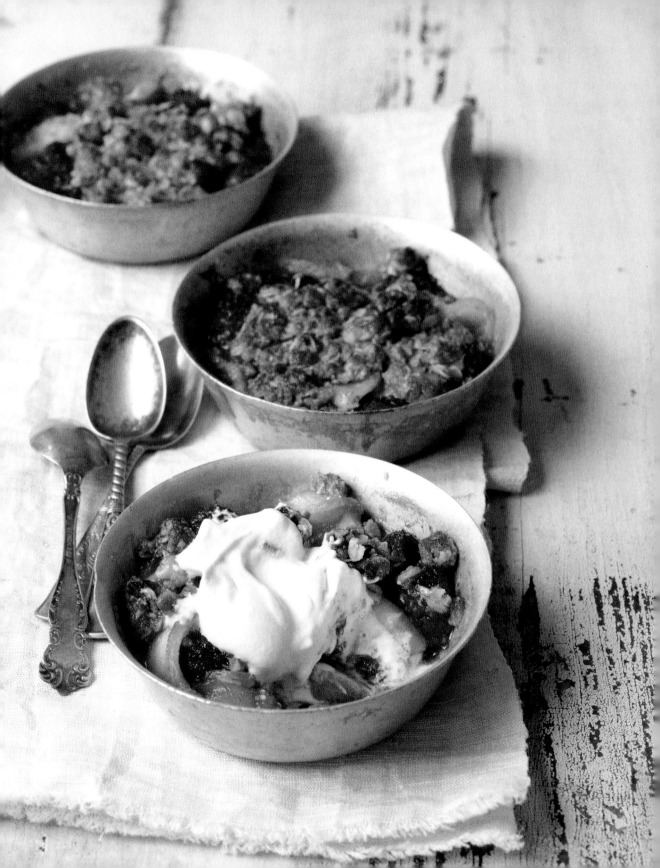

CHOCOLATE CHIP OATMEAL COOKIES

makes about 3 dozen 3-inch cookies

2 cups rolled oats
(not quick-cooking)

²⁄₃ cups whole-wheat flour

½ cup all-purpose flour

1 teaspoon baking soda

1 teaspoon salt

8 tablespoons (1 stick) cold
unsalted butter, cut into pieces

½ cup organic virgin coconut
oil, softened

²⁄₃ cup granulated sugar

½ cup packed light brown
sugar

1 tablespoon vanilla extract

2 large eggs

½ cup chopped walnuts or
pecans

½ cup unsweetened shredded
coconut

1 cup semisweet or bittersweet
chocolate chips

THESE ARE NOT YOUR TYPICAL chocolate chip oatmeal cookies. For one thing, they're made with coconut oil and butter, yielding an especially tender cookie with a uniquely delicious coconut flavor, complemented by plenty of shredded coconut. For another, I'm using rolled oats and some whole-wheat flour for a great chewy texture that also makes these a treat you can feel good about loving. The nuts and chocolate chips don't hurt either.

1. In a food processor, pulse 1 cup of the rolled oats to a grainy powder. Add the processed oats to a large bowl along with both flours, the baking soda, and salt and whisk to combine well.

2. In a standing mixer or with a hand mixer in a large bowl, cream together the butter, oil, and both sugars until the mixture is light yellow and fluffy. Beat in the vanilla, then add the eggs one at a time, beating for 10 seconds between each addition.

3. Add a third of the dry mixture to the wet mixture at a time, beating to incorporate after each addition. Fold in the remaining oats, nuts, coconut, and chocolate chips. Roll the dough into 2-inch balls and place them on a parchment-lined baking sheet. Cover with plastic wrap and freeze for 2 hours or overnight. Chilling the dough will help your cookies cook evenly and limit spread so you get chewy results rather than thin, lacy ones.

4. When you're ready to bake, preheat the oven to 375°F. Transfer the frozen dough balls onto a parchment-lined baking sheet, keeping them 1½ inches apart. (Do not put a frozen sheet pan in the oven!) Bake for 14 to 17 minutes, banging the sheet onto the open oven door at the 9-minute mark to help deflate the cookies; this will help you get a chewy cookie with a crispy rim. Rotate the pan front to back when placing it back in the oven so all sides cook evenly. The cookies are done baking when the rims are golden brown and crispy and the center is still slightly moist. Cookies will continue baking as they cool.

5. You can store the frozen dough balls in double-layered plastic zip-top bags for up to 1 month. Alternatively, roll the dough into a log, wrap it in parchment paper and then aluminum foil, and freeze—you can cut cookies off the log and bake them as needed.

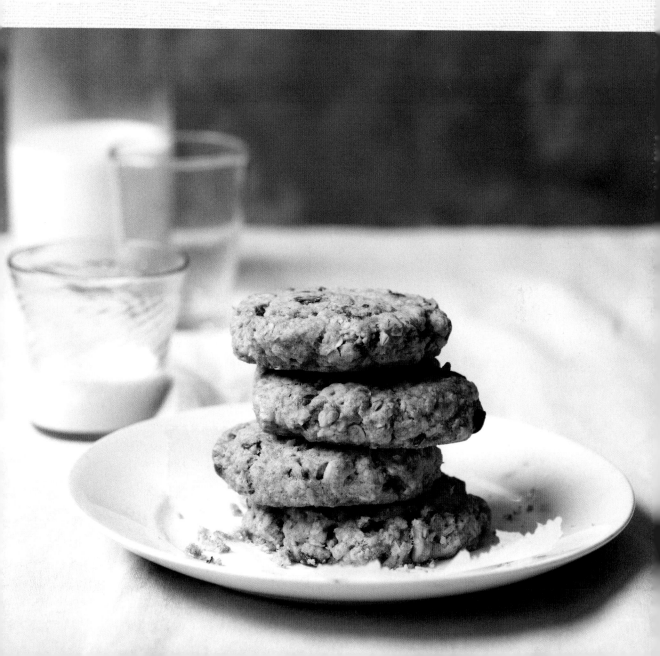

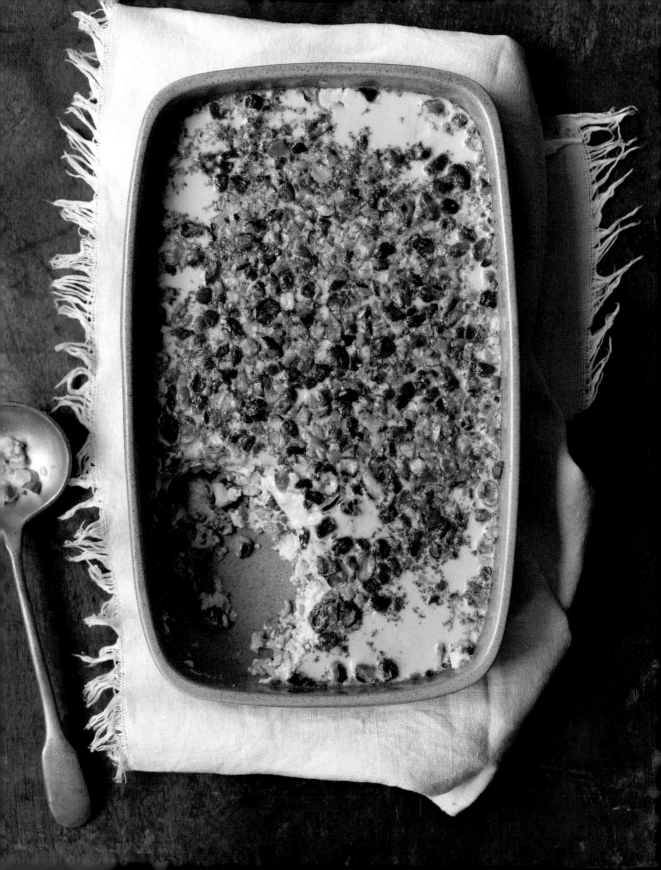

PERSIAN BROWN RICE PUDDING

serves 6 to 8

RICE PUDDING is pure comfort food. I love it in every form, but the Persian spices in this version make it a standout.

1. Preheat the oven to 300°F. Grease a 9 x 9-inch casserole dish with butter.

2. In a small saucepan over medium-low heat, scald the milk, taking care not to boil it. Remove it from the heat and add the cardamom, cinnamon, salt, orange zest, and sultanas. Cover and steep for 10 minutes.

3. In a medium bowl, whisk together the eggs, syrup, and vanilla. Add in pistachios and stir. Slowly temper the eggs by adding a small amount of the hot milk mixture to the eggs at a time, whisking to combine to prevent eggs from cooking. Once both liquids are combined, add the rice and stir to coat.

4. Pour the rice mixture into the casserole dish and cover it with aluminum foil. Place the dish inside a larger roasting pan and place the roasting pan in the oven. Carefully pour water into the roasting pan until it reaches halfway up the side of the casserole dish to form a water bath.

5. Bake the pudding for 1½ to 2 hours, or until a knife inserted into the center of the pudding comes out clean.

Butter or organic coconut oil, for greasing the dish

3 cups whole or 2% milk or coconut milk

1 teaspoon ground cardamom

1 teaspoon ground cinnamon

¼ teaspoon salt

Zest from ½ orange

½ cup sultanas (yellow raisins)

4 eggs, beaten

2 tablespoons pure maple syrup

2 teaspoons pure vanilla extract

½ cup pistachios, chopped

1¼ cups cooked brown basmati rice

CASHEW COOKIES WITH PEACH MAPLE SORBET

makes about 36 single cookies or 18 sandwich cookies

SORBET

3 cups fresh or frozen peaches (if using fresh, 6 to 8 medium peaches)

1⅓ cups almond milk

3 tablespoons pure maple syrup

1 teaspoon pure vanilla extract

¼ teaspoon salt

CASHEW COOKIES

6 tablespoons organic coconut oil

⅓ cup sugar

1 teaspoon pure vanilla extract

1 cup rolled oats, ground fine in the food processor

½ cup raw cashews, ground fine (just to the texture of the oats—pulse 10 to 12 times, taking care not to turn them to butter)

3 tablespoons all-purpose flour

2 tablespoons ground flaxseed

1 teaspoon salt

MY AUNT AND UNCLE who live out in L.A. came up with the recipe for this vegan sorbet out of desperation one day when their then toddler son, Dylan, was going through an obsessive ice-cream phase—a combination of teething and the fact that ice cream is generally worthy of obsession.

To feel good about letting him have a treat with every meal, they developed this insanely delicious frozen blend of fruit, almond milk, and the natural sweetness of pure maple syrup. I slapped it between two (decently healthful) cookies and thereby created a guilt-free confection totally worthy of obsession by eaters of all ages. Then again, if you don't feel like making the cookies, the sorbet comes together with about 5 minutes of work and is one of my favorite refreshing desserts all on its own.

1. To make the sorbet, if using fresh peaches, peel them, pit them, and cut them into 6 wedges. Combine the peaches, almond milk, syrup, vanilla, and salt in a blender and puree until smooth but not warm. Pour the mixture into a plastic or glass container and freeze for 2 to 4 hours, until set.

2. When ready to serve, remove the sorbet from the freezer and let it rest at room temperature to soften for 5 to 10 minutes before scooping.

3. To make the cashew cookies, preheat the oven to 350°F.

4. Use an electric mixer or forks to cream together the oil, sugar, and vanilla until smooth and creamy. In a separate bowl, whisk together the oats, cashews, flour, flaxseed, and salt. Add the wet ingredients into the dry ingredients and stir well to combine.

5. Line a baking sheet with a Silpat mat or grease with coconut oil. Roll the dough into balls 1 inch in diameter and place them 1½ inches apart on the baking sheet. Flatten with three fingers to about ¼ inch thick. Bake for 14 to 18 minutes, until the cookies are crispy on the edges and soft toward the middle. Allow to rest for 1 minute, then use a spatula to remove the cookies from the baking sheet to a rack to cool.

6. To make the sandwich cookies, place a scoop of the sorbet between 2 of the cashew cookies. Enjoy immediately!

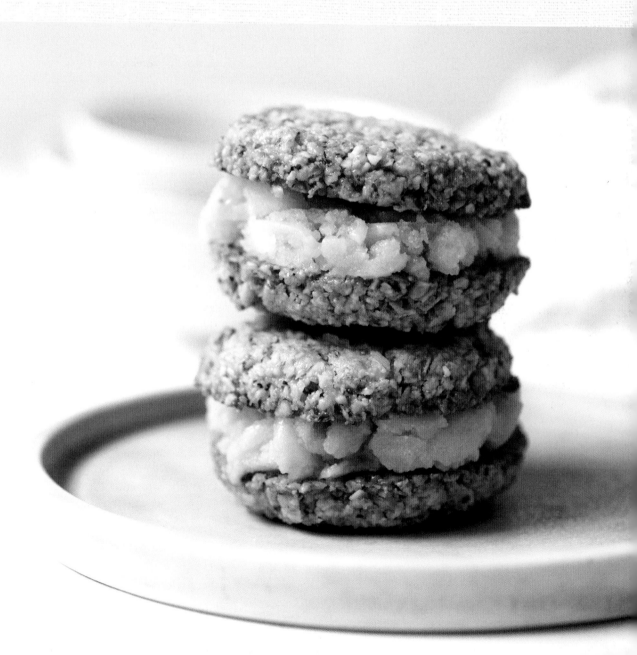

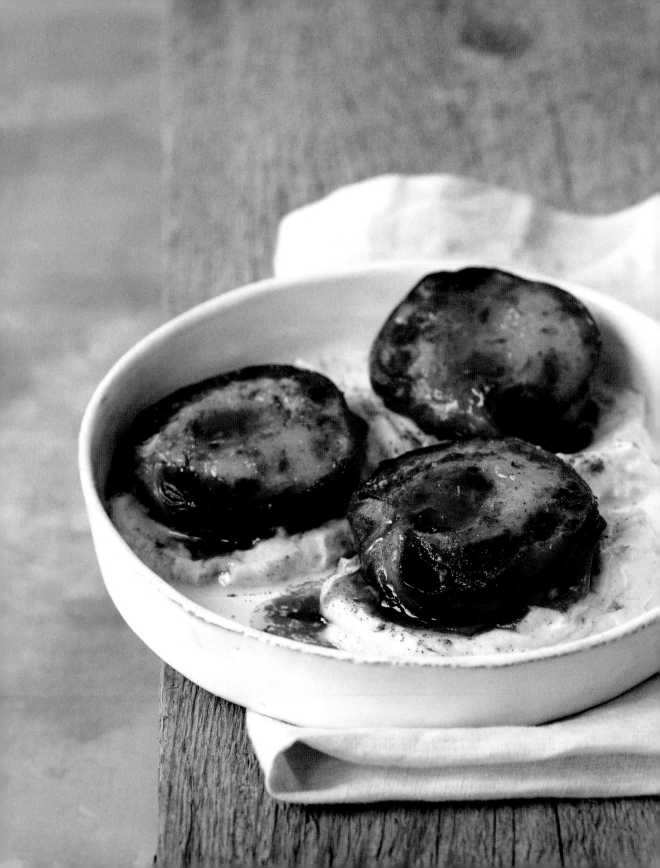

ROASTED PEACHES WITH MAPLE MASCARPONE

serves 4

FRESH PEACHES, plump and fragrant right off the tree, are what I most look forward to about summer farm stands. We always stop off on our drives down to the Jersey Shore to pick up a huge bagful; half of them are gone by the time we get home. But on the occasion when one isn't quite as juicy as it should be, roasting is the perfect way to give it the boost it needs. It caramelizes all the sweet sugars, draws out the natural juices, and paired with maple mascarpone, it is pure summer in every bite.

1. Preheat the oven to 425°F and oil or butter a baking sheet.

2. To make the peaches, brush them lightly on all sides with the oil. Place them, cut side down, on the baking sheet. Roast 20 minutes, or until they are soft.

3. To make the mascarpone, in a medium bowl, combine the mascarpone, syrup, lemon zest, cinnamon, cardamom, and salt.

4. To serve, dollop a heaping tablespoon of the mascarpone mixture onto a plate and nest 2 peach halves on top. Drizzle with maple syrup and dust with cinnamon and cardamom. Garnish with mint leaves (if using) and a squeeze of fresh lemon juice. Serve warm.

PEACHES

¼ cup melted organic extra-virgin coconut oil or unsalted butter

4 large ripe peaches, halved and pitted

MAPLE MASCARPONE

1 cup mascarpone cheese

¼ cup pure maple syrup plus ¼ cup for drizzling

½ teaspoon fresh lemon zest

½ teaspoon ground cinnamon plus more for dusting

½ teaspoon ground cardamom plus more for dusting

¼ teaspoon salt

8 mint leaves for garnish (optional)

Juice of ½ lemon

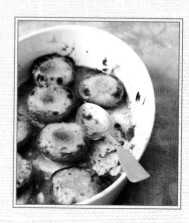

COCONUT PECAN POUND CAKE

serves about 10

CAKE

16 tablespoons (2 sticks) unsalted butter, at room temperature, plus more for the pan

4 large eggs

2 cups sugar

1 tablespoon pure vanilla extract

3 cups all-purpose flour plus more for the pan

½ teaspoon baking powder

½ teaspoon iodized salt

1 cup buttermilk

1¼ cups unsweetened shredded coconut

1 cup chopped pecans

GLAZE

½ cup water

1 teaspoon pure vanilla extract

2 tablespoons (¼ stick) salted butter (if using unsalted, add ¼ teaspoon iodized salt to the mix)

1 cup sugar

Salt (optional)

Powdered sugar for dusting

THIS GLAZED BUNDT CAKE is far and away my most requested dessert, and the one I most look forward to eating—especially on Christmas Day, still in my nightclothes with a hot mug of Earl Grey tea. It's pure indulgence, and that's just how this cake is supposed to be enjoyed.

My grandmother's friend Mrs. Henderson (who actually taught my very first cooking class at camp one summer!) makes us this cake every year at Christmas. We eagerly await its arrival—whenever that may be—and a swarming horde of family devours it within the hour.

In her original version, Mrs. Henderson sometimes included variations with a rum or lemon glaze, and a lighter-textured cake made with oil. Since she was kind (or evil) enough to share the recipe, I've adapted it to my tastes, substituting real butter for a denser pound cake and simplifying the glaze to a basic sticky sugar syrup that moistens the cake even more.

I dare you to resist this. Warm out of the oven and wafting its intoxicating blend of toasted coconut and pecans. If by some miracle any is left on the plate long enough to cool, you'll have to let me know how it tastes.

1. Preheat the oven to 350°F. In a large bowl, beat the butter, eggs, and sugar with an electric mixer until light and fluffy, about 3 minutes. Beat in the vanilla.

2. In a separate large bowl, whisk together the flour, baking powder, and salt.

3. Beating by hand or with the mixer running on low, incorporate the dry ingredients and buttermilk into the butter mixture in three parts. Mix until just combined, then fold in the coconut and pecans.

4. Butter and flour a Bundt pan. Pour the batter into the pan, using a spatula to evenly smooth the surface. Bake for 60 to 65 minutes, or until a knife inserted at the center comes out clean or with only a few crumbs.

5. About 5 minutes before the cake is finished baking, make the glaze. In a small saucepan, combine the water, vanilla, butter, sugar, and salt if using and bring to a boil over high heat. Reduce the heat to medium-low (gentle simmer) and cook for 5 minutes, or until it coats the back of a spoon. Remove from the heat, but do not allow the glaze to cool too much.

6. As soon as the cake comes out of the oven, pour half the glaze on top—it will bubble and sizzle. Let the cake cool for 2 minutes, then carefully invert it onto a serving plate and pour the remaining glaze on top (you could also reserve some to spoon over individual slices if you like). Dust with powdered sugar. Some would say you should let the cake cool for 10 more minutes—though we never manage to.

7. If there are any leftovers, wrap in plastic wrap and keep on the counter for up to 3 days.

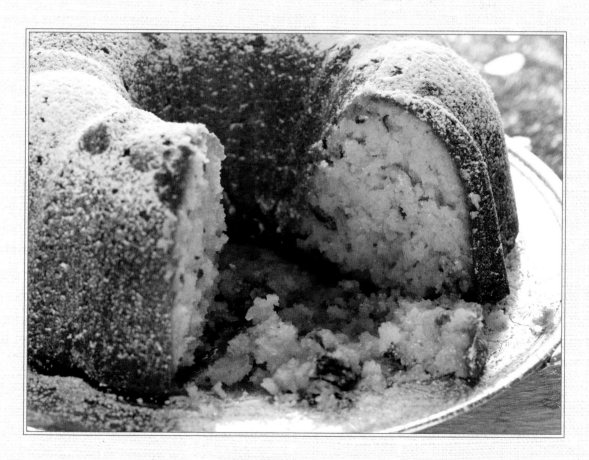

STRAWBERRY CAKE WITH CARAMEL FLEUR DE SEL WHIPPED CREAM FROSTING

makes one 8-inch 2-layer cake

3 pints fresh strawberries, hulled

2¼ cups all-purpose flour, sifted

2 teaspoons baking powder

¾ teaspoon salt

8 tablespoons (1 stick) butter, at room temperature, plus more for the pan

1 cup sugar

2 tablespoons raw honey

4 large egg whites, plus 1 egg, at room temperature

Scrapings from 1 vanilla bean, or 1 teaspoon pure vanilla extract

½ cup whole milk, at room temperature

¼ cup water

Caramel Fleur de Sel Whipped Cream Frosting (recipe follows)

THIS CAKE MAKES ME think of garden parties on the lawn, with ladies in pastels under parasols sipping tea out of delicate teacups. The hostess (you) debuts this perfect confection, bursting with bright strawberries and whipped clouds of salted caramel cream. (Wipe drool off page here.) The perfect ladies go berserk.

Hopefully, your friends are more refined. Still, don't judge them when they refuse your offers of cutlery as they dig in. Oh, and get ready to brag your butt off, 'cause yeah, this cake is a winner, and yeah, you made it from scratch.

The plain cake layers can be stored in clean cake pans and covered with aluminum foil at room temperature or in the refrigerator. Just be sure to do the final assembly with frosting and strawberries right before you eat it.

1. In a food processor, puree 1 pint of the strawberries. Transfer to a medium saucepan and place over medium heat. Cook, stirring frequently so that the berries don't burn, until reduced by half, 10 to 12 minutes. Let stand until completely cool, or transfer the puree to a bowl and place in the freezer 15 minutes.

2. Preheat the oven to 350°F. Butter and flour two 8-inch round cake pans.

3. In a medium bowl, whisk together the flour, baking powder, and salt. Set aside.

4. Using an electric mixer with the paddle attachment or a hand mixer, beat the butter and sugar on medium-high speed until light

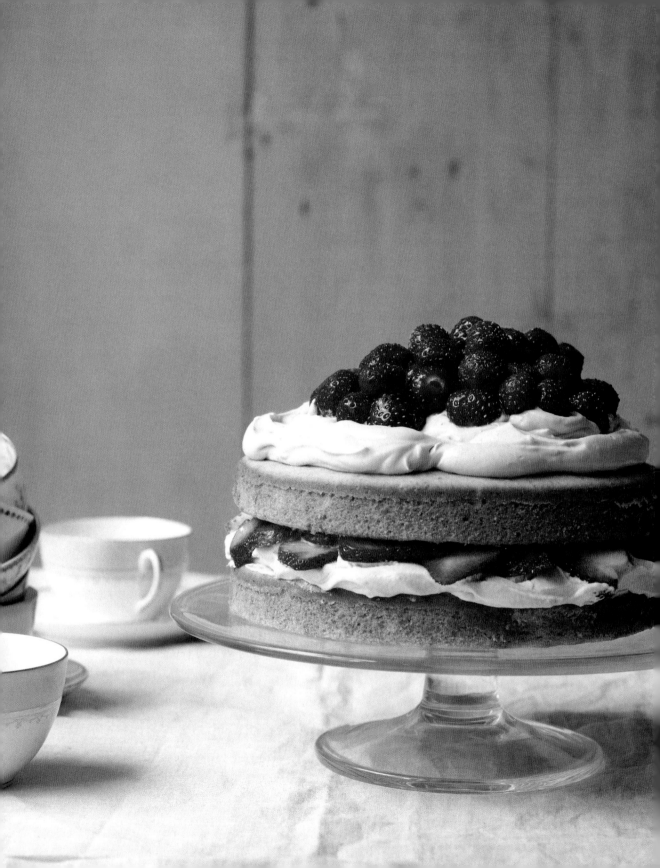

Carla Hall, my cohost on *The Chew*, showed me a great way to use leftover vanilla bean pods. Add ½ cup salt and 1 vanilla bean to your food processor, then pulse until the bean is evenly distributed throughout the salt to make vanilla salt. (You could, of course, do this with sugar, too!) It goes wonderfully sprinkled on everything from sweet cookies, ice creams, and crumbles (like this one), to seafood stews—even tangy salads and fresh fruit.

and fluffy, scraping down the sides of the bowl as needed. Add the cooled strawberry puree and the honey and beat until combined. One at a time, add the egg whites and egg, beating after each one. Beat in the vanilla.

5. On low speed, beat in half the flour mixture until combined, scraping down the sides of the bowl as needed. Beat in the milk and water until combined. Beat in the remaining flour mixture until just combined.

6. Evenly divide the batter between the 2 prepared cake pans. Bake, rotating the pans halfway through, until the cakes are golden and a wooden skewer inserted into the center comes out clean, about 25 minutes.

7. Transfer the pans to a cooling rack and let them cool for 10 to 15 minutes. Turn out the cakes right side up and set aside until completely cool.

8. Cut 10 to 15 of the most beautiful strawberries in half (these will go on top of the cake) and another 10 to 15 into thin lengthwise slices (these will go between the layers).

9. The less perfect-looking of the two layers will be the bottom layer. Center it on a pretty serving plate, then use a long, sharp knife to slice away the cake dome and create a flat surface. Dollop half of the frosting on the center and spread it to within a half inch of the edge. Arrange the sliced berries on top. Add the second cake layer to the top, right side up. Spread the remaining frosting on top of the cake. Heap the halved berries in the center of cake. Add a final sprinkle of salt, if desired. Enjoy immediately for maximum fluffy frosting clouds!

CARAMEL FLEUR DE SEL WHIPPED CREAM FROSTING

makes 3 cups

THIS WILL EITHER BE the hardest or the easiest icing you'll ever make, and it all comes down to whether or not you begin the process prepared—sort of like life! First, read through the entire recipe before you do anything so you know all the steps. Then, get all your tools out and ingredients measured ahead of time so that you're not scrambling to figure out just how much cream goes in as the caramel turns from luscious, golden amber to burnt. If you can manage this, you will be spooning soft clouds of whipped caramel cream into your mouth in no time!

½ cup sugar

2 tablespoons water

2 cups heavy cream

2 tablespoons (¼ stick) butter

1 teaspoon sea salt

1. In a heavy medium saucepan, combine the sugar and water. Place over medium-high heat and cook, stirring, until the sugar dissolves. Cook without stirring (you may swirl gently to avoid any dark spots) until the syrup turns deep amber, taking care not to burn it, 5 to 7 minutes. While whisking constantly, carefully pour ¾ cup of the cream down the side of the pan until smooth. Whisk in the butter and salt until melted. Let cool completely to room temperature.

2. Transfer the caramel to a bowl. Place it in the freezer until cooled and thickened but not solid, stirring occasionally, 20 to 25 minutes.

3. In an electric mixer with a whisk attachment, beat the remaining 1¼ cups heavy cream on medium-high speed until stiff. Gently fold the caramel into the whipped cream until combined.

CHOCOLATE FUDGE POPS

makes 6 frozen pops

One 13-ounce can original or "lite" coconut milk, shaken

5 tablespoons unsweetened cocoa powder

2 tablespoons raw honey

1 teaspoon pure vanilla extract

¼ teaspoon salt

THESE POPS ARE SO much better than the plastic-wrapped kind you pull out of your grocery-store freezer. With insane amounts of chocolate, real, wholesome ingredients, and total satisfaction for about 125 calories a pop, what more could you want?

Blend all the ingredients until smooth and pour the mixture into ice pop molds. Insert the base and freeze for at least 2 hours, or until set. Loosen by running the molds under warm water. Enjoy!

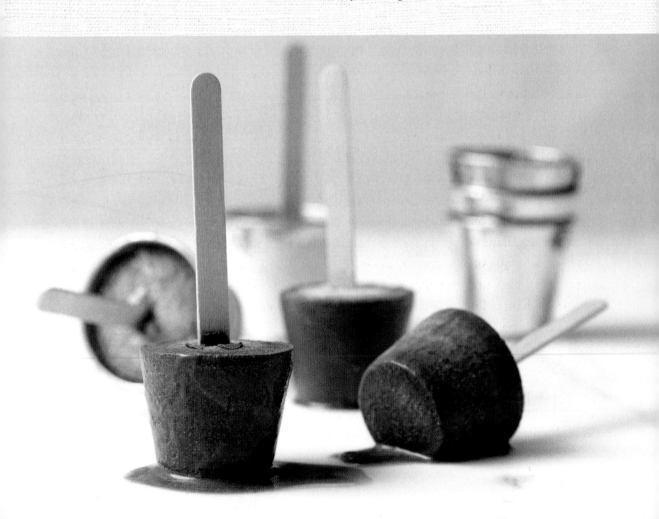

CONCLUSION

Well, you're here. Thirteen (my lucky number!) chapters later, and we've covered everything from what we consume to the passions that consume us, from the ways we stay fit to the ways we stay strong, from the lighting in the living room to the people who light up our lives.

At the end of the day, *Relish* is all about craving, savoring, grabbing, loving, wanting, taking, giving, delighting, igniting, and inciting. But it's also about prevention. Preventing what exactly? Regrets. If you live every day fully, there will be no need to look back and wish you'd done anything differently because each moment will have brought you closer to the happy you you are right now. If we want to live well, today, tomorrow, and in the future, we must pledge to eat happy so that our bodies are energized for the hard work ahead, to let go of our place-holder lives and stop postponing our commitment to living fully, to embrace self-sufficiency and be strong for ourselves so we can be strong for others.

So how do we do it? How do we continue to learn and grow but not miss the stage of life we're in right now? How do we avoid fast-forwarding through these years, the same years we're going to look back on one day and wish we'd paused to appreciate?

Here's my plan: I'm going to stay playful even when deadlines are approaching. I'm going to be forgiving of myself while maintaining top-notch standards. I'm going to work hard to manage what's in my control—and stop spinning my wheels in situations that I'll never be able to change. I'm going to decide to find fulfillment in myself as much as in the world around me. And I'm going to have fun trying to do it all (well, everything that interests me, anyway), one step at a time.

Relishing every minute of the journey comes down to knowing that creativity, curiosity, and joie de vivre are free and available right now. So cook with abandon and eat with delight. Love with passion and live with purpose. Buy the ticket and take the ride. The prize—your happiest, sweetest, most delicious life ever—is yours for the taking. *Relish* it.

ACKNOWLEDGMENTS

And now, for the most important part: a massive *thank-you* to all who helped make this book a glorious destination and an even more fun, fulfilling adventure along the way.

You may not even know you were an inspiration for this book, but if I've chatted your ear off about the glories of a particular dish; the fun of redesigning a space; the importance of making happy, healthy living easy and enjoyable; the bliss of loving relationships; mistakes I've made and the things I've learned to do better next time, then I thank you for lending your ear and your wisdom. That includes all of you, wonderful viewers of *The Chew* and readers of *The Dorm Room Diet*!

And for those who are truly saints among men—and women, of course—my heartfelt thanks go out to you:

John, for gamely taste testing every recipe time and time again; for lending your excitement, curiosity, and brilliance to everything we do together; and especially for showing me what it feels like to be the happiest little lady in the whole wide world. I love you.

Mommy and Grandmommy, for showing me that the kitchen could be my playground; that everything can be fixed—from broken batters to broken hearts; and for being the sources of all my good ideas and the touchstones in all my journeys.

Daddy (the man who taught me all things worth doing in life are worth doing well), Grandaddy (the king of Staten Island spaghetti sauce and stuffed artichokes), Baba Anne and Büyük Baba (who made their Istanbul home a neverending source of culinary inspiration), and my loving, supportive family of aunts, uncles, and cousins (for showing me exactly why a relished existence is worth living).

Sandra Bark, you were the voice in my head personified. Thank you for providing structure to my lifetime of musings and memories and for making the process of putting myself to page feel freeing and fun. I've loved every minute of it!

Ellen Silverman, you could not have made me a happier, prouder, hungrier girl each time you worked the magic of your lens. I am grateful for both your breathtaking images that bring this book alive and your friendship. Paige Hicks and Philippa Brathwaite, you brilliantly distilled all my wish lists into a singularly beautiful aesthetic that feels just like home. Susan Sugarman and Anna Helm Baxter, thank you for lending your loving hands to making every dish jump off the page with deliciousness. Samantha Napolitano, your digital genius was invaluable. Scott McFarlane, thank you for helping make my home picture perfect. Many thanks also to your teams: Penelope Gil, Maya Rossi, Eddie Barerra, Matt Clery, Rhoda Boone, Amy Lincoln, Brooke Deonarine, Yvette Dizon Hunter, and Tina DeGraff, and to ABC Carpet and Home, Canvas, Aero, Ochre, and Royal Copenhagen for making my heart flutter with so many gorgeous homewares.

Bucketloads of thanks must be showered upon: Cassie Jones, my brilliant editor and fearless guide through this project of a lifetime; Mary Schuck, Lorie Pagnozzi, and Kris Tobiassen, for enduring all my neurotic tweaks and developing a cover and book interior to make me swoon; Liate Stehlik, publisher extraordinaire, for seeing the potential of this project, giving me the opportunity to realize it, and jumping in headfirst with me; and the entire William Morrow team, without whom this book would still be just a pipe dream on my computer and not the even better reality in your hands: thank you, Kara Zauberman, Lynn Grady, Tavia Kowalchuk, Shelby Meizlik, Megan Swartz, Joyce Wong, and Nyamekye Waliyaya.

Massive thanks to my lovely literary agent, Erin Malone at William Morris Endeavor, for being as excited to read this book as I was to write it! And special thanks to Esther Margolis, the very first person to give forum to the things I thought were important to write about, and a mentor in all my literary pursuits.

To my spectacular cohosts—Carla, Clinton, Michael, and Mario—and my entire *Chew* family: thank you for making every day at "work" feel like playtime.

To my friends: Thank you for sharing a million meals, a million fits of laughter, a million adventures, a million fails, and a million success messages, all multiplied into infinite reasons to go on feeling like a million bucks every time we're together.

And finally, oodles of hugs and kisses for my siblings and partners in crime—Arabella, Zoe, and Oliver. You make every day worth relishing. Love you, Ozlings!

INDEX

Note: Page references in *italics* indicate photographs.